Women's and Men's Health

NEW CONTENT AUTHORS

Elizabeth Margaret Prusak, MD
Tewksbury, MA

Mark Itzkowitz, MD
Tewksbury, MA

SECTION EDITOR

Kaci L. Durbin, MD
OB Hospitalist and Director
Saint Anthony's Medical Center
St. Louis, MO

MEDICAL EDITOR

Qyana Kelly Griffith, MD
Los Angeles, CA

Table of Contents

WOMEN'S HEALTH

OBSTETRICS **11-1**
PRECONCEPTION CARE AND
  FAMILY PLANNING.................................. 11-1
    Overview... 11-1
    Genetic Risks....................................... 11-1
    Congenital Infections.......................... 11-1
    Environmental Toxins.......................... 11-1
    Tobacco, Alcohol, and Prescription /
      Nonprescription Drugs...................... 11-1
    Medical Conditions Affecting Pregnancy......... 11-2
    Exercise and Nutrition........................... 11-2
    Domestic Violence................................ 11-2
  VITAMIN AND NUTRITIONAL DEFICIENCIES
    AND PREGNANCY................................. 11-2
    Overview... 11-2
    Folic Acid... 11-2
    Iron... 11-3
    Calcium.. 11-3
    Zinc... 11-3
    Iodine.. 11-3
    Magnesium 11-3
    Vitamin A 11-3
    Vitamin B_{12} 11-3
    Vitamin B_6 11-3
  DRUGS AND MEDICATIONS IN PREGNANCY.... 11-3
  GASTROENTEROLOGY DISORDERS
    IN PREGNANCY................................... 11-5
    Endoscopic Workup 11-5
    GERD 11-5
    Crohn Disease Medications 11-5
    Constipation....................................... 11-5
    Pancreatitis.. 11-5
    Liver Disease 11-5
  PULMONARY DISORDERS IN PREGNANCY 11-5
    Asthma Treatment 11-5
    Tuberculosis Treatment 11-6
    Pulmonary Embolism and
      Deep Vein Thrombosis 11-6
  CARDIOLOGY DISORDERS IN PREGNANCY...... 11-6
    Normal Findings 11-6
    Cardiac Issues 11-6
  INFECTIOUS DISEASES IN PREGNANCY........... 11-7
    Bacterial Infections 11-7
    Parasitic Disease................................ 11-7
    Viral Infections................................... 11-7
    Fungal Infections 11-8
  NEPHROLOGY DISORDERS IN PREGNANCY 11-8
    Hypertension...................................... 11-8
    Systemic Lupus Erythematosus
      with Lupus Nephritis 11-10
    Chronic Renal Failure 11-10
    Renal Stones..................................... 11-10
  ENDOCRINOLOGY DISORDERS
    IN PREGNANCY................................... 11-10
    The Serum Osmostat 11-10
    Prolactin Levels................................. 11-10
    Pituitary Adenoma 11-10
    Thyroid Disease.................................. 11-10
    Polycystic Ovary Syndrome.................. 11-11
    Diabetes.. 11-11

  NEUROLOGY DISORDERS IN PREGNANCY.......11-11
    Migraine..11-11
    Pseudotumor Cerebri...........................11-11
    Seizures 11-11
    Carpal Tunnel 11-12
  RHEUMATOLOGY DISORDERS
    IN PREGNANCY 11-12
    Systemic Lupus Erythematosus.............. 11-12
    Avascular Necrosis of the Hip................ 11-12
  DERMATOLOGY DISORDERS
    IN PREGNANCY 11-12
  ALLERGY AND IMMUNOLOGY
    IN PREGNANCY 11-12

OFFICE GYNECOLOGY **11-12**
  NOTE 11-12
  ECTOPIC PREGNANCY 11-12
    Overview.. 11-12
    Presentation.......................................11-13
    Diagnosis...11-13
    Prognosis...11-13
    Treatment...11-13
  SEXUALLY TRANSMITTED INFECTIONS......... 11-13
  VAGINITIS 11-13
  PREMENSTRUAL SYNDROME...................... 11-13
  PREMENSTRUAL DYSPHORIC DISORDER........11-14
    Overview..11-14
    Diagnosis...11-14
    Pathophysiology..................................11-14
    Workup..11-14
    Clinical Course and Management 11-14
  CONTRACEPTIVE COUNSELING....................11-14
    Overview..11-14
    Methods of Contraception 11-14
    Emergency Contraception..................... 11-15
  ENDOMETRIOSIS..................................... 11-15
  OVARIAN CYSTS 11-15
  ABNORMAL UTERINE BLEEDING 11-15
    Overview.. 11-15
    Workup..11-16
    Diagnosis...11-16
    Treatment...11-16
  ANOVULATORY BLEEDING 11-16
    Overview..11-16
    Pathophysiology..................................11-17
    Etiologies...11-17
    Treatment...11-17
  POLYCYSTIC OVARY SYNDROME (PCOS) 11-17
    Overview..11-17
    Diagnosis...11-18
    Additional Testing...............................11-18
    Prognosis...11-18
    Treatment...11-18
  AMENORRHEA.. 11-18
    Overview..11-19
    Primary Amenorrhea 11-19
    Secondary Amenorrhea.........................11-19
  DYSMENORRHEA 11-19
  PERIMENOPAUSE AND MENOPAUSE..............11-19
    Overview..11-19
    Symptoms and Effects of Menopause........... 11-20
    Differential Diagnosis........................... 11-20
    Treatment... 11-20
  POSTMENOPAUSAL BLEEDING.................... 11-20
  ENDOMETRIAL CANCER 11-21

BREAST DISORDERS (NONCANCEROUS) 11-21
    Mastitis.. 11-21
    Cyclic Breast Pain 11-21

MEN'S HEALTH

BENIGN PROSTATIC HYPERPLASIA 11-21
    OVERVIEW... 11-21
    TREATMENT 11-22
ERECTILE DYSFUNCTION 11-22
    OVERVIEW... 11-22
    CLASSIC CAUSES OF ED 11-23
    DIAGNOSIS... 11-23
    TREATMENT OPTIONS.............................. 11-23
SCROTAL MASSES (NONCANCEROUS) 11-24
    OVERVIEW... 11-24
    TESTICULAR TORSION.............................. 11-24
    EPIDIDYMITIS... 11-25
    INGUINAL HERNIA 11-26
    HYDROCELE 11-27
    HEMATOCELE 11-27
    VARICOCELE.. 11-27

SEXUAL HEALTH CONCERNS
FOR WOMEN AND MEN

SEXUAL DYSFUNCTIONS.............................. 11-28
    OVERVIEW... 11-28
    DIAGNOSTIC FEATURES............................ 11-29
INFERTILITY.. 11-29
THE MEDSTUDY HUB: YOUR GUIDELINES
  AND REVIEW ARTICLES RESOURCE.............. 11-30

WOMEN'S HEALTH

OBSTETRICS

PRECONCEPTION CARE AND FAMILY PLANNING

PREVIEW | REVIEW

- What age is considered advanced maternal age in which the risk of abnormal chromosomes increases?
- Epileptic mothers have what percentage of risk of congenital abnormalities?

Overview

Patient care prior to conception improves pregnancy outcomes. Because 50% of pregnancies are unplanned, consider pregnancy as a possibility in your reproductive-aged female patients. Use other visits (e.g., work physicals, follow-up visits) as an opportunity to address preconception issues.

The following is a preconception visit checklist:

- Genetic risks
  ◦ Folic acid supplementation
  ◦ Carrier screening—ethnic background: sickle cell anemia, thalassemia, Tay-Sachs disease
  ◦ Carrier screening—family history: cystic fibrosis, spinal muscular atrophy, fragile X syndrome, or nonsyndromic hearing loss (*connexin-26* mutation)
- Congenital infections—screen for infectious diseases, immunize, and counsel.
- Environmental toxins, such as occupational and household chemical exposures
- Tobacco, alcohol, and prescription and nonprescription drug use
- Diseases and disorders
- Exercise and nutrition
- Domestic violence screen

Genetic Risks

Folic acid supplementation is discussed under Folic Acid on page 11-2.

Maternal age ≥ 35 years is considered advanced maternal age. As women age, the risk of fetal chromosomal abnormalities, medical complications during pregnancy, and infertility increases. Counsel all women about these risks and inform them about available testing for fetal aneuploidy, which includes noninvasive prenatal testing, amniocentesis, and chorionic villus sampling. Although risk increases as women get older, everyone should be offered these available tests regardless of age.

The American College of Obstetricians and Gynecologists recommends screening all pregnant women for hemoglobinopathies with CBC and RBC indices. Carrier screening is also recommended for the following hereditary conditions:

- Spinal muscular atrophy
- Cystic fibrosis
- Fragile X syndrome (only in patients with a family history of the disease)
- Congenital hearing loss (Screen for *connexin-26* mutation in patients with congenital hearing loss.)
- Spinal muscular atrophy and cystic fibrosis (for all women contemplating pregnancy)
- Tay Sachs disease (1:30 Ashkenazi Jews are carriers)

Congenital Infections

Preconception screening for HIV and syphilis are important. Highly active antiretroviral therapy (HAART) during pregnancy can decrease the risk of perinatal transmission to the fetus. Consider administering hepatitis B vaccine to women at risk (although it may be given during pregnancy).

Give the live vaccines for measles, mumps, and rubella ≥ 1 month prior to pregnancy. Give the varicella vaccine ≥ 3 months prior to pregnancy. Give influenza at any time, as it can be safely administered during pregnancy.

Educate pregnant women on toxoplasmosis and the need to avoid handling cat litter, garden soil, and raw meat. See more on toxoplasmosis under Parasitic Disease on page 11-7. Cytomegalovirus (CMV) and parvovirus B19 can be best prevented by good personal hygiene and hand washing, especially around young children. Advise patients to avoid contact with individuals with known infections. See more on CMV under TORCH on page 11-7.

Environmental Toxins

Advise women to avoid environmental toxins that can cause harm to the embryo or fetus:

- Metals such as lead and mercury
- Solvents (e.g., used in dry cleaning) such as trichloroethylene, chloroform, benzene, toluene
- Plastics in plastic manufacturing
- Pollutants and pesticides (e.g., garden sprays)
- Gases, including anesthesia and carbon monoxide
- Radiation exposure (e.g., medical use)

Tobacco, Alcohol, and Prescription / Nonprescription Drugs

Exposure to certain drugs can be harmful to the embryo or fetus. The FDA categorizes drugs to try to elucidate risks. See drug information publications for further information.

Avoid the following drugs in pregnancy:

- Misoprostol, oral contraceptives
- Benzodiazepines
- Warfarin (unless patient has mechanical heart valves)
- HMG-CoA reductase inhibitors

- Megadose vitamin A
- Nicotine, alcohol
- Thalidomide
- Nonprescription drugs such as cocaine, heroin, and marijuana

Smoking carries dose-dependent risks to the mother and developing fetus, including low birth weight, perinatal mortality, ADHD, and miscarriage.

Alcohol carries risks, such as intellectual disability and growth disorders.

Medical Conditions Affecting Pregnancy

Diabetes: See Diabetes on page 11-11.

Hypertension: See Hypertension on page 11-8.

Epilepsy: Note that infants of epileptic mothers have up to an 8% risk of congenital anomalies. If possible, use a single agent to control the mother's epilepsy. Many antiepileptic drugs are teratogenic; therefore, discuss medication teratogenicity with epileptic women of child-bearing age. Do not stop the patient's seizure medication without consulting the patient's neurologist.

Anxiety/Depression: Benzodiazepines may increase the risk of cleft lip, cleft palate, and withdrawal symptoms in the fetus. Discuss the risks and benefits of continuing antidepressant medications during pregnancy. Consult with the patient's psychiatrist regarding medication changes. Do not prescribe a woman of child-bearing age paroxetine. If she is already on paroxetine, consult with a psychiatrist for cross-titration of the medication to an alternate SSRI vs. discontinuing the drug—after a discussion of risks, benefits, and alternatives during pregnancy and lactation. Consult a psychiatrist if a woman is on mood stabilizers or antipsychotics.

Exercise and Nutrition

Recommend regular, moderate exercise. Hyperthermia is associated with an increased risk of congenital anomalies. Women who are pregnant or are trying to become pregnant should avoid extremes in exercise and extremes in temperature (e.g., hot tubs).

Counsel women who are overweight (BMI 25–30), obese (BMI > 30), or underweight (BMI < 18.5) on normal preconception weight.

Advise women to avoid the overuse of:

- Vitamin A (limit to 5,000 IU/day)
- Caffeine (limit to < 200 mg/day)

See Vitamin and Nutritional Deficiencies and Pregnancy for information on nutritional deficiencies.

Domestic Violence

Approximately 324,000 pregnant women are abused each year in the United States. Domestic violence is associated with pregnancy weight gain, infection, anemia, tobacco use, stillbirth, pelvic fractures, placental abruption, fetal injury, preterm delivery, and low birth weight. Violence can escalate during pregnancy—and consequently, homicide is a leading cause of maternal mortality.

Screen for domestic violence in a private setting without any other family members present. Inform patients that this is routine assessment and will be kept confidential.

VITAMIN AND NUTRITIONAL DEFICIENCIES AND PREGNANCY

PREVIEW | REVIEW

- Pregnancy requires a total of how many additional kcals?
- Neural tube defects can be reduced by taking which supplement?
- A patient with a history of a pregnancy with a neural tube defect should take how much folic acid daily?
- What is a common mineral deficiency in pregnant women who have not had prenatal care?
- How many additional milligrams of ferrous sulfate are needed in pregnancy?

Overview

Pregnancy only requires an additional 100–300 kcal/day. Although vitamin and nutritional deficiencies in pregnancy are rare in the United States, assess the risk of nutritional deficiencies in certain populations (e.g., patients with vegan diet, pica, milk intolerance, anemia).

Encourage a pregnant woman to eat a well-balanced diet and monitor her weight. Note that pregnancy has elevated vitamin and nutritional requirements for fetal development.

Folic Acid

The most important supplementation during pregnancy is folic acid. Ideally, women should start folic acid 400 mcg/day PO at least 1 month prior to conception and continue it for at least the first 3 months of pregnancy.

Neural tube defects can largely be prevented by a daily intake of folic acid 400 mcg through the preconception period. If a woman delivered a previous child with a neural tube defect, increase her daily intake to 4 mg/day. The dose should be consumed as a separate supplement. Additionally, patients on antiseizure drugs that affect folate levels should take 4 mg/day of folic acid.

Iron

Iron deficiency is commonly seen in pregnant women who have had no prenatal care. Pregnant women need an additional 27 mg/day of ferrous sulfate. Anemia of pregnancy is common, and the most encountered cause is iron deficiency anemia. The additional iron required is sufficiently provided in a daily prenatal vitamin.

Calcium

Ca^{2+} supplementation is not routinely required during pregnancy.

Zinc

There is no requirement for zinc supplementation in pregnancy because deficiency is rare. Observational data relating zinc deficiency to adverse perinatal outcomes has been conflicting. Some studies suggest zinc supplementation can prevent congenital malformations, such as cleft lip and palate, in cases of deficiency, but this has not been proven.

Iodine

Severe maternal iodine deficiency predisposes the offspring to cretinism, characterized by severe neurological defects. The use of iodized salt and bread is recommended during pregnancy, and no supplementation is necessary.

Magnesium

There is no requirement for Mg^{2+} supplementation, and deficiency is rare. However, deficiency can occur after gastric bypass surgery.

Vitamin A

Excess vitamin A is associated with birth defects. Supplemental vitamin A is not recommended.

Vitamin B$_{12}$

Vitamin B_{12} deficiency can occur in vegetarian or vegan women, as well as women who have had a gastric bypass. Measure B_{12} at the beginning of pregnancy and continue to measure monthly if there is a proven deficit. Supplementation may be needed if B_{12} levels are low. Because breast milk of a vegetarian or vegan contains little vitamin B_{12}, these women require supplementation during breastfeeding as well.

Vitamin B$_{6}$

Use vitamin B_6 combined with doxylamine to treat hyperemesis gravidarum. A typical dose is 10–25 mg orally, 3–4×/day.

DRUGS AND MEDICATIONS IN PREGNANCY

PREVIEW | REVIEW
- During which trimester is metronidazole contraindicated?
- Know Table 11-1 on page 11-4.
- Are ACE inhibitors safe in pregnancy?
- A pregnant woman has DVT. Which commonly used anticoagulant is not recommended?

Medications, prescriptions, and over-the-counter drugs should only be used when the benefit clearly outweighs the potential risk to mother or fetus. In 2015, the FDA replaced the former pregnancy risk letter categories (A, B, C, D, and X) on prescription drug labeling with new, more comprehensive labeling. Each drug now has listed narrative sections titled "pregnancy," "lactation," and "female and males of reproductive potential." Each section is further divided and discusses a risk summary, clinical considerations, and available data on the particular drug. Pregnancy exposure registry information is also included in the pregnancy narrative.

The following medications are considered safe in the treatment of common conditions in pregnancy:

- Pain/Fever—acetaminophen
- Pain/Fever—NSAIDs can be used up to 30 weeks of gestation. (Avoid after 30 weeks to prevent premature closure of ductus arteriosus and oligohydramnios.)
- Antibiotics—cephalosporins, penicillins, erythromycin, clindamycin, azithromycin. Avoid metronidazole and sulfonamide drugs in the 1st trimester, but they can be used during the 2nd and 3rd trimesters.
- Antivirals—acyclovir, famciclovir, valacyclovir
- Nausea/Vomiting—pyridoxine + doxylamine, diphenhydramine, meclizine; 2nd line therapies—prochlorperazine, metoclopramide, and ondansetron
- Gastroesophageal reflux disease (GERD) symptoms—H_2 blockers, proton pump inhibitors
- Insomnia—doxylamine, diphenhydramine
- Diarrhea—loperamide
- Constipation—docusate, bisacodyl, lactulose, magnesium hydroxide
- Anticoagulation—low-molecular-weight heparin (LMWH), unfractionated heparin
- Opioids—codeine, oxycodone, methadone (Note: They should be used for the shortest time possible to avoid neonatal abstinence syndrome.)

Know Table 11-1 on page 11-4.

Table 11-1: Frequently-Asked-About Drugs in Pregnancy

Avoid Use in Pregnancy if Possible	Effects on the Fetus	Safer Alternatives for Pregnancy (examples not all-inclusive)
ACE inhibitors, ARBs	IUGR, oligohydramnios, stillbirth	Clonidine, labetalol, calcium channel blockers, digoxin, propranolol, procainamide
Alkylating agents	Absence of digits	
Most aminoglycosides	Ototoxicity, nephrotoxicity	Gentamicin
Antiepileptic drugs	Neural tube defects, cardiac defects, cleft palate, skeletal abnormalities	Levetiracetam preferred antiepileptic agent
NSAIDs (e.g., ibuprofen, diclofenac, naproxen) after 30 weeks gestation	Premature closure of the ductus arteriosus and oligohydramnios	NSAIDs are safe prior to 30 weeks of gestation. After 30 weeks, use acetaminophen.
Diethylstilbestrol (DES)	Vaginal clear cell adenocarcinoma, congenital Müllerian anomalies	
Folate antagonists (e.g., methotrexate, antiepileptic drugs such as valproic acid)	Neural tube defects	Levetiracetam preferred antiepileptic agent
HMG-CoA reductase inhibitor	Possible delayed fetal development	
Lithium	Ebstein anomaly	
Misoprostol	Fetal death	
Paroxetine	Ventricular and atrial septal defects, neonatal withdrawal symptoms, serotonin syndrome	Fluoxetine, citalopram, or other SSRIs
Tetracycline	Inhibited bone growth, discolored teeth	
Thalidomide	Limb effects	
Warfarin	Bone deformities, fetal hemorrhage, abortion, ophthalmologic abnormalities	Unfractionated heparin, enoxaparin (a LMWH)
Thiazolidinediones (TZDs)	Possible IUGR, embryo-fetal toxicity (animal studies)	Metformin, insulins
Aspirin (full dose)	Premature fetal ductus arteriosus closure	Acetaminophen, low-dose aspirin
Benzodiazepines	Cleft lip and palate, neonatal withdrawal symptoms	
Bismuth subsalicylate	Premature closure of ductus arteriosus, IUGR	
Methimazole, ^{131}I	Fetal hypothyroidism	
Substances		
Alcohol	Fetal alcohol syndrome (most common preventable cause of birth defects and intellectual disability)	
Cocaine	Low birth weight (leading cause in developed countries), preterm birth, IUGR, placental abruption	
Smoking	Low birth weight, preterm birth, placental problems, SIDS, ADHD	
Other		
Iodine (lack or excess)	Congenital goiter or hypothyroidism (cretinism)	Propylthiouracil (PTU), levothyroxine
Maternal diabetes	Caudal regression syndrome, congenital heart defects, neural tube defects, macrosomia, polycythemia, hypoglycemia	
Methylmercury	Neurotoxicity	
Vitamin A excess	High risk of spontaneous abortions and birth defects (e.g., cleft palate, cardiac abnormalities)	
X-rays	Microcephaly, intellectual disability	

Adapted from: First Aid for the USMLE Step 1 2018

ACE = angiotensin-converting enzyme; ADHD = attention-deficit/hyperactivity disorder; ARB = angiotensin II receptor blocker; IUGR = intrauterine growth restriction; LMWH = low-molecular-weight heparin; SIDS = sudden infant death syndrome

GASTROENTEROLOGY DISORDERS IN PREGNANCY

Endoscopic Workup

Esophagogastroduodenoscopy (EGD) is the test of choice to work up many GI diseases during pregnancy to limit or preclude the use of radiation. However, only perform it if there is a strong indication, and when possible, delay it until the 2nd trimester.

Endoscopic ultrasonography (EUS) is normally used in evaluating pancreatic diseases. It can also be used to evaluate biliary duct disease. In nonpregnant individuals, endoscopic retrograde cholangiopancreatography (ERCP) is preferred, but this is best avoided in pregnancy.

GERD

Progesterone increases during pregnancy, leading to the relaxation of smooth muscle, including the lower esophageal sphincter (LES). Consequently, pregnant women are predisposed to reflux. LES pressure is also decreased by chocolate, smoking, and certain medications, especially those with anticholinergic properties. Ranitidine, famotidine, and lansoprazole are used for refractory GE reflux symptoms. Avoid bismuth subsalicylate due to the salicylate exposure.

Crohn Disease Medications

The following are medications used for Crohn disease that have no evidence of risk in pregnancy:

- Metronidazole (However, because of the lack of data, it is contraindicated in the 1st trimester.)
- Prednisone
- Sulfasalazine
- Mesalamine

Constipation

The altered progesterone and estrogen levels are the probable cause of constipation in pregnancy. Recommend dietary modifications, such as increased fluids and fiber, first. If constipation persists, over-the-counter medications are indicated. The following medications are also safe to use:

- Docusate
- Bisacodyl
- Lactulose
- Magnesium hydroxide

Pancreatitis

Pancreatitis is rare in pregnancy but is treated similarly to pancreatitis outside of pregnancy. Obtain an abdominal ultrasound on the patient to evaluate for cholelithiasis. Keep the patient NPO and hydrate with intravenous fluids.

Liver Disease

Pregnancy-associated liver disease can range from mild to life-threatening. During a normal pregnancy, albumin levels are lower due to hemodilution. Alkaline phosphatase is slightly elevated from the placental source. The remaining biochemical liver tests (aspartate aminotransferase [AST], alanine aminotransferase [ALT], bilirubin, and coagulation factors) are within normal range.

Signs and symptoms suggesting liver dysfunction include jaundice, pruritus, abdominal pain, nausea, and vomiting.

Initial workup includes LFTs, viral hepatitis panel, RUQ ultrasound, PT (prothrombin time)/INR, CBC, and BMP (basic metabolic panel). Liver biopsy is rarely needed.

Consider the following etiologies in working up a pregnant patient with hepatobiliary findings:

- **Hyperemesis gravidarum** occurs in the 1st trimester. It can cause volume depletion and mild increase in AST and ALT. It usually resolves with conservative symptomatic management.
- **Intrahepatic cholestasis of pregnancy** occurs in late pregnancy (3rd trimester), and pruritus is a common symptom. It is associated with prematurity and stillbirth. Treat with ursodeoxycholic acid and early delivery (36–37 weeks).
- **Acute fatty liver of pregnancy** occurs in late pregnancy. It is a very serious condition in which there is microvesicular fat deposition in the liver (i.e., Reye syndrome), with only a modest elevation of AST/ALT/bilirubin. Patients develop coagulopathy and can progress to liver failure. It is associated with encephalopathy, hypoglycemia, preeclampsia, pancreatitis, disseminated intravascular coagulopathy (DIC), and renal failure. Prompt delivery is the primary treatment.
- **HELLP syndrome** typically occurs at 28–36 weeks of gestation, but it can occur during the 2nd trimester or postpartum. For more on HELLP syndrome, see Hypertension on page 11-8.
- Hepatitis E (unlike hepatitis A) carries a very high risk for fulminant hepatitis in the 3rd trimester of pregnancy. It has a 20% fatality rate. Think of a pregnant woman traveling to Southeast Asia who contracts hepatitis E (fecal-oral transmission like hepatitis A).

PULMONARY DISORDERS IN PREGNANCY

Asthma Treatment

Treatment of asthma during pregnancy is not significantly different from asthma treatment for nonpregnant patients. It is important to minimize exacerbations and optimize control with the current medication regimen. Recommend smoking cessation because it decreases asthma symptoms, decreases hospitalizations and emergency department visits, and improves responses to treatment. Furthermore, smoking cessation is beneficial for the pregnancy because it decreases the risk of intrauterine growth restriction (IUGR), placental abruption, preterm birth, and stillbirth. Use a step-up approach for asthma control, including the use of inhaled corticosteroids and inhaled long-acting beta-agonists. Use IV or oral steroids, in addition to inhaled beta-agonists (albuterol) and anticholinergics, for acute exacerbations.

Budesonide is preferred in pregnancy, but all inhaled corticosteroids can be used.

Tuberculosis Treatment

Per the World Health Organization, treat a pregnant woman with tuberculosis (TB) with standard 1st line TB drugs, with the exception of streptomycin because it causes ototoxicity and nephrotoxicity. Pyridoxine supplementation is also recommended for all pregnant or breastfeeding women taking isoniazid.

Pulmonary Embolism and Deep Vein Thrombosis

The risk of pulmonary embolus (PE) and deep vein thrombosis (DVT), known collectively as venous thromboembolism (VTE), is increased up to 5-fold during pregnancy and postpartum. Risk factors for VTE in pregnancy include prior history of VTE, the presence of a thrombophilia, obesity, hemoglobinopathies, hypertension, and smoking.

If a DVT is suspected, the recommended diagnostic test is compression ultrasonography of the proximal veins. Patients with a PE should undergo a ventilation-perfusion scan or computed tomographic (CT) angiography. D-dimer is not recommended in pregnancy.

Treat a patient with a DVT or PE with anticoagulation. LMWH can be self-administered and requires little-to-no monitoring. Enoxaparin (an LMWH) is generally considered to be safe for both the mother and fetus in pregnancy. The 2012 American College of Chest Physicians guidelines recommend the use of LMWH during all phases of pregnancy for prevention and treatment of VTE in women with VTE or at elevated risk for VTE (e.g., antiphospholipid antibody syndrome).

Pregnancy is generally considered a contraindication for warfarin because of its teratogenic effects. (The exception is a patient with a mechanical heart valve, for whom warfarin is the only acceptable anticoagulant.) Unfractionated heparin is an option, but it poses challenges, such as parenteral dosing and the need for frequent monitoring.

CARDIOLOGY DISORDERS IN PREGNANCY

PREVIEW | REVIEW

- Is an S_3 gallop normal in pregnant women?
- Is electrical cardioversion possible during pregnancy?

- What do you have to rule out in a pregnant patient who presents with new-onset atrial fibrillation and pulmonary edema?
- How is peripartum cardiomyopathy treated?

Normal Findings

An S_3 and/or a systolic murmur are normal and commonly heard in pregnant women secondary to the increased cardiac output of pregnancy. The heart rate is typically elevated, with an average increase of 10–30 bpm. Jugular venous pressure typically increases. Additionally, most pregnant women experience some pedal edema.

Cardiac Issues

Absolute cardiac contraindications to pregnancy include pulmonary arterial hypertension (PAH) and Eisenmenger syndrome. Patients with secundum atrial septal defect (ASD), aortic stenosis, or dilated cardiomyopathy must be closely watched by an obstetrician who specializes in high-risk pregnancies. Patients with significant aortic stenosis or dilated cardiomyopathy are normally kept on bed rest. Secundum ASD patients are usually not at risk for cardiac decompensation, unless they develop atrial fibrillation. Cyanotic heart disease has very high risks.

Hypertension in pregnancy: See Hypertension on page 11-8. Cardiology, Book 4, and Pulmonary Medicine, Book 2, have additional information on pulmonary HTN.

Hypertensive cardiomyopathy (HCM) among asymptomatic women is not a contraindication for pregnancy. In women with HCM who are asymptomatic or whose symptoms are controlled with beta-blockers, the beta-blockers should be continued during pregnancy with increased surveillance for fetal bradycardia and intrauterine growth restriction. In women with HCM and resting or provocable LVOT obstruction (≥ 50 mmHg) and/or cardiac symptoms not controlled by medical therapy alone, pregnancy may carry an increased risk for heart failure, arrhythmia, and fetal loss; refer these patients to a high-risk obstetrician.

Peripartum cardiomyopathy of pregnancy is a condition in which, at the end of pregnancy, the patient experiences heart failure signs and symptoms and is found on echocardiogram to have a left ventricular ejection fraction < 45%. The etiology is unclear. Treatment is similar to other forms of heart failure. Beta-blocker and diuretic therapy is the mainstay of treatment. Nitrates + hydralazine and digoxin can be added as 2nd and 3rd line therapy. ACEIs (ACE inhibitors), ARBs, and spironolactone are not recommended during pregnancy. Patients with a persistently low ejection fraction (EF) of < 50% (or < 25% at the time of diagnosis) are advised against future pregnancies due to the risk of heart failure progression.

Atrial fibrillation: Like secundum ASD, the initial presentation of mitral stenosis in a pregnant patient can be new-onset atrial fibrillation and pulmonary edema. The increased blood volume in pregnancy can cause a precipitous exacerbation of mitral stenosis—so consider treating all pregnant mitral stenosis patients prophylactically with digoxin. Electrical cardioversion can be used in pregnancy.

In a pregnant patient presenting with new-onset atrial fibrillation and pulmonary edema, rule out both mitral stenosis and secundum ASD.

Aortic dissection: The 3rd trimester of pregnancy, systemic hypertension, cystic medial necrosis, bicuspid aortic valve, and coarctation of the aorta are all predisposing factors.

Valve surgery: Porcine valves (vs. mechanical valves) are often given to women of childbearing age to avoid the use of anticoagulants during pregnancy.

Controversy exists regarding the use of LMWH vs. warfarin for anticoagulation with mechanical prosthetic valves during pregnancy. Discuss the risks and benefits of warfarin (less risk of thrombosis for the mother; increased risk of defects for the infant, especially if given in 1st trimester; increased risk of fetal bleeding throughout pregnancy vs. LMWH (increased risk of thrombosis for the mother; decreased risk of defects for the infant). Most experts recommend warfarin in these patients.

Maternal **rubella infection** during pregnancy can cause patent ductus arteriosus (PDA), supravalvular aortic stenosis, branch pulmonic stenosis (peripheral PS), and other congenital cardiac defects. Rubella has been eradicated in the Americas.

INFECTIOUS DISEASES IN PREGNANCY

PREVIEW | REVIEW

- Should asymptomatic bacteriuria in a pregnant woman be treated?
- What is the maternal-to-fetal transmission rate of HIV without ART? With ART?

Bacterial Infections

UTIs are typically caused by *Streptococcus agalactiae* and *Escherichia coli*. Treat with penicillins, cephalosporins, or nitrofurantoin. Ciprofloxacin is not given to pregnant women due to concerns of joint problems developing in the fetus.

Listeria monocytogenes infections occur most in those with decreased cellular immunity syndromes such as AIDS, lymphoma, and leukemia, but they also are seen in neonates, the elderly, and pregnant women. The most common presentation is a woman in her 3rd trimester with a flu-like illness. It is diagnosed by blood culture.

Streptococcus agalactiae, a common urinary tract pathogen, is also a cause of postpartum endometritis and bacteremia; so, suspect this in any woman who develops a postpartum fever!

Gonorrhea is more likely to disseminate in pregnant women. The newborn is at risk for gonococcal conjunctivitis. Antibiotic ointment is applied to the infant's eyes at birth to prevent the conjunctivitis.

Approximately 5% of pregnant women have *Chlamydia trachomatis* in their genital tracts. Applying antibiotic ointment to the infant's eyes at birth does not prevent chlamydial conjunctivitis.

Treat asymptomatic bacteriuria in pregnant women, because 1/3 of cases progress to pyelonephritis without treatment.

Parasitic Disease

Toxoplasma gondii can cause congenital toxoplasmosis, which results in intellectual disability and chorioretinitis. The fetus is more likely to have a congenital infection if the disease is acquired later in pregnancy (15% in the 1st trimester; 70% in the 3rd trimester). Toxoplasmosis prior to pregnancy is generally not a concern during the pregnancy.

Viral Infections

TORCH

TORCH is an acronym for certain infections acquired *in utero* that are the most common causes of congenital problems. They include infections caused by:

- *T*oxoplasma (parasite; see topic above)
- *O*ther (i.e., syphilis, enteroviruses, varicella zoster, parvovirus B19)
- *R*ubella (no longer in the Americas)
- *C*MV (most common viral cause)
- *H*erpes simplex

Previously, the "other" designation only included syphilis. Lately enteroviruses, varicella zoster, and parvovirus B19 have been included.

Varicella zoster has a slight risk of causing congenital defects. The pregnant woman with chicken pox has a 10% chance of developing severe pneumonia.

Rubella, due to a successful vaccination program, has been declared eliminated in North and South America, but it continues to be a problem elsewhere. There are still a few cases seen in the Americas, but they are imported. Rubella can frequently cause miscarriages and congenital defects, such as cataracts, heart problems, and intellectual disability. The global incidence, however, is decreasing with the use of the rubella vaccine. Worldwide, rubella incidence declined from 670,894 cases in 2000 to 22,361 cases in 2016. Congenital rubella syndrome rates are highest in Africa and southeast Asia.

CMV is ubiquitous and the most common cause of congenital viral infection. 1–2% of all newborns have the infection *in utero*, but only a few have any abnormalities. These abnormalities, which range from mild neurologic problems to microcephaly, usually occur in mothers with a primary CMV infection.

HIV: Although not included in the TORCH acronym, there is a mother-to-fetus transmission risk of 30%. However, this is reduced to < 2% with 3-drug antiretroviral therapy (ART); therefore, ensure that all pregnant women with HIV receive ART. If viral load is ≥ 1,000 copies/mL, also give zidovudine at the time of delivery. Consider it for those with 50–1,000 copies/mL.

Zika Virus

Zika virus is a mosquito-borne (*Aedes* spp.) *Flavivirus* that causes symptoms in ~ 20% of infected patients. Zika virus is carried by the same mosquito that carries dengue and chikungunya viruses. Symptoms are milder but similar to those of dengue and chikungunya fevers, which include fever, muscle and joint pain, rash, and conjunctivitis.

In late 2015, an alarming rise in the number of infants born with microcephaly was seen in Brazil and linked to maternal Zika virus infection. This prompted the World Health Organization to declare a public health emergency of international concern. They issued an advisory that warns pregnant women and women considering pregnancy against travel to high-risk areas, including parts of Central and South America.

Sexual transmission of Zika virus has been reported. Recommend abstaining from sexual activity or using condoms during the pregnancy period. Women with Zika virus exposure may breastfeed.

There is no specific treatment or vaccine for Zika virus; treatment is symptomatic management.

For more on Zika virus, see Infectious Disease, Book 1.

Fungal Infections

The preferred treatment for fungal infections in pregnancy is topical antifungal creams.

High-dose (400–800 mg/day) fluconazole is contra-indicated in pregnancy because of associated fetal abnormalities of the cranium, face, bones, and heart. A single, low dose of fluconazole (150 mg) to treat yeast infection can be prescribed after the 1st trimester.

NEPHROLOGY DISORDERS IN PREGNANCY

PREVIEW | REVIEW

- List the 4 categories of hypertension in pregnancy.
- What are the defining features of preeclampsia?
- What are the diagnostic criteria for preeclampsia?
- What is HELLP syndrome?

Hypertension

Overview

In normal pregnancy, BP falls due to decreased systemic vascular resistance, so normal BP in pregnancy is always < 120/80 mmHg. HTN in pregnancy is defined as:

- mild if BP is 140–159/90–109 mmHg or
- severe if BP ≥ 160/110 mmHg.

Note: The JNC 8 (Eighth Joint National Committee) did not address HTN in pregnancy, so do not refer to the JNC 8 for a pregnant patient with HTN. There are 4 categories of HTN in pregnancy:

1) **Chronic HTN:** preexisting HTN or HTN diagnosed before the 20th week of gestation

2) **Preeclampsia:** New onset of HTN + proteinuria or other significant organ dysfunction after the 20th week of gestation in a woman with no history of HTN

3) **Gestational HTN:** Onset after the 20th week and no proteinuria in a woman with no history of HTN

4) **Chronic HTN with superimposed preeclampsia:** worsening HTN + new-onset proteinuria after the 20th week of gestation in a woman with history of chronic HTN

Diagnosis of Preeclampsia

Preeclampsia more commonly occurs in primigravidas, usually in the 3rd trimester, and resolves after delivery. However, it can present postpartum. In 2013, the American College of Obstetrics and Gynecology updated the diagnostic criteria for preeclampsia. Proteinuria is no longer required for the diagnosis if other signs or symptoms of significant organ dysfunction are present (see Table 11-2). Women with preeclampsia are considered to have severe features if any of the following are present:

- SBP ≥ 160 mmHg or DBP ≥ 110 mmHg
- Low platelets
- Elevated liver enzymes
- Acute kidney injury
- Pulmonary edema
- New-onset cerebral or visual symptoms (i.e., visual disturbances, severe headache, confusion, seizures)

HELLP syndrome is a severe form of preeclampsia with **h**emolytic anemia, **e**levated **l**iver enzymes, and **l**ow **p**latelets. **Eclampsia**, defined as generalized, tonic-clonic seizures in a woman with preeclampsia or gestational HTN, is also a manifestation of severe preeclampsia.

Risk Factors, Prevention, and Treatment of Preeclampsia

Risk factors for preeclampsia include diabetes mellitus, chronic hypertension, multiple gestations (e.g., twins, triplets), chronic kidney disease, and prior preeclampsia. In 2014, the USPSTF (U.S. Preventive Services Task Force) issued a recommendation that pregnant women at increased risk for preeclampsia take 81 mg ASA daily. Risk of preeclampsia is reduced by 24%! The risk of premature birth is decreased by 14% and IUGR by 20%.

Treat all severe hypertension occurring during pregnancy (regardless of category) to at least < 160 mmHg SBP and < 110 mmHg DBP. Beyond this, blood pressure treatment targets in pregnancy are controversial and not well addressed in any guidelines (remember, the JNC 8 does not discuss hypertension in pregnancy). Overzealous treatment of hypertension in pregnancy has the potential to cause reduced placental blood flow and low fetal birth weight. Treating to a DBP of 85 mmHg appears to be safe for the fetus and is probably a good target. Although chronic hypertension is a risk factor for preeclampsia, treatment of hypertension in pregnancy does not prevent preeclampsia (weird, but true).

Bed rest is no longer recommended for asymptomatic or mild preeclampsia—clinical trials show it does not improve outcomes. For women with symptoms or severe hypertension, give intravenous magnesium sulfate to prevent seizures (eclampsia). Monitor the renal function, CBC (look for hemolytic anemia or thrombocytopenia), and LFTs. Abnormalities in any of these indicate severe preeclampsia and warrant immediate delivery, which is the only definitive treatment for preeclampsia. Ultimately, care providers often need to balance what is best for maternal health (early delivery) with what is best for the baby (postponing delivery to avoid consequences of severe prematurity).

Preeclampsia and eclampsia can occur postpartum. A woman who presents with new-onset hypertension and cerebral or visual symptoms within 6 weeks of delivery has preeclampsia until proven otherwise. Monitor these women closely in an inpatient setting and treat with magnesium sulfate and antihypertensives.

Women who have had preeclampsia are at an increased risk for cardiovascular disease later in life. Regularly screen these women and treat them for modifiable cardiovascular risk factors, such as hypertension, obesity, and hyperlipidemia.

Chronic Hypertension in Pregnancy

Review medications of women with chronic HTN who are contemplating pregnancy or are already pregnant. Discontinue ACEIs/ARBs and (usually) diuretics. BP medications may often be discontinued in pregnant women with chronic HTN that is controlled, but frequently monitor BP and symptoms. (That's right! This is the one instance where antihypertensives are actually removed!) Reinstitute medications if SBP ≥ 160 mmHg or DBP ≥ 105 mmHg.

Antihypertensive Medications in Pregnancy

Oral antihypertensives that are safe to use in preeclampsia, gestational hypertension, and chronic hypertension in pregnancy include:

- Labetalol (other beta-blockers impair placental perfusion)
- Methyldopa
- Extended-release nifedipine
- Hydralazine

2nd line agents include diltiazem and verapamil, but watch for signs/symptoms of volume contraction, including oligohydramnios. Diuretics are generally not recommended in preeclampsia unless pulmonary edema is present. Know that the following antihypertensives are contraindicated: ACEIs/ARBs, direct renin inhibitors, and nitroprusside. ACEIs/ARBs and renin inhibitors are teratogenic; nitroprusside causes cyanide poisoning in the fetus.

Any pregnancy complicated by persistent, severe hypertension (SBP ≥ 160 mmHg or DBP ≥ 105 mmHg) may

Table 11-2: Diagnostic Criteria for Preeclampsia	
Blood pressure	SBP ≥ 140 mmHg or DBP ≥ 90 mmHg on 2 occasions at least 4 hours apart after 20 weeks of gestation in a woman with previously normal blood pressure When SBP ≥ 160 mmHg or DBP ≥ 110 mmHg, hypertension can be confirmed within minutes to facilitate timely antihypertensive therapy.
And	
Proteinuria	≥ 300 mg in a 24-hour urine collection, or Protein:creatinine ratio ≥ 0.3 mg/mg, or Urinary dipstick reading ≥ 1+ (only if quantitative methods are unavailable)
Or, in the absence of proteinuria, new-onset hypertension with new onset of any of the following:	
Thrombocytopenia	Platelets < 100,000µL (100 × 10⁹/L
Renal insufficiency	Creatinine > 1.1 mg/dL (97.2 µmol/L) or doubling of the serum creatinine
Impaired liver function	AST or ALT ≥ 2× normal
Pulmonary edema	Diagnosed by physical exam and chest radiograph
Cerebral or visual symptoms	Severe headache, blurry vision, scotomata, confusion, seizures

Adapted from: The American College of Obstetrics and Gynecologists Task Force on Hypertension in Pregnancy, 2013
ALT = alanine aminotransferase; AST = aspartate aminotransferase

require IV antihypertensives; labetalol and hydralazine are good options. Avoid rapid falls in maternal blood pressure to prevent fetal hypoperfusion.

Systemic Lupus Erythematosus with Lupus Nephritis

Systemic lupus erythematosus (SLE) with lupus nephritis: Pregnancy complicated by lupus is associated with a higher risk of maternal complications, including preterm labor, unplanned cesarean delivery, fetal growth restriction, preeclampsia, eclampsia, thrombotic events, and infections. Fetal complications include stillbirth, IUGR, and neonatal lupus syndromes. Fetuses of women with SSA (Ro) or SSA (La) antibodies are at risk for congenital heart block. Hydroxychloroquine is considered safe in pregnancy and should be continued.

Chronic Renal Failure

Chronic renal failure: Patients who are normotensive with a creatinine < 2 mg/dL (176.8 μmol/L) do not have an increased risk of abortion or malformation, and there is no increase in the rate of progression of the renal disease. All patients with chronic renal failure do have an increased risk of pregnancy-induced hypertension.

As renal failure progresses, a woman's fertility decreases. A dialysis patient rarely becomes pregnant. Stable renal transplant patients usually have a great pregnancy outcome!

Renal Stones

Increased Ca^{2+} absorption and excretion occur during pregnancy. Even so, the frequency of renal stones is the same as in the nonpregnant patient. The urinary tract of the pregnant patient is dilated, and if stones develop, most pass easily.

ENDOCRINOLOGY DISORDERS IN PREGNANCY

PREVIEW | REVIEW

- What is the treatment for postpartum thyroiditis?
- A pregnant woman has Graves disease. What can you do to treat her?
- Which medications commonly given to diabetic patients are contraindicated in pregnancy?
- When should pregnant women be screened for diabetes? What is the test of choice?
- What medication is used to treat gestational diabetes if diet and exercise fail to reach targets?

The Serum Osmostat

Pregnant women increase their circulating blood volume by almost 50%. This is a result of the osmotic set point resetting, causing the antidiuretic hormone to be released at a lower osmolality.

Prolactin Levels

Estrogen directly inhibits dopamine outflow, so elevated prolactin (PRL) levels can be seen in pregnant patients and in those taking estrogen.

Pituitary Adenoma

About 1/3 of pituitary macroadenomas, some of which cause increased PRL levels, enlarge during pregnancy. Ideally, a patient should be started on bromocriptine or cabergoline prior to conceiving. If a woman is diagnosed in pregnancy and the tumor is large enough to cause symptoms, start bromocriptine or cabergoline at that time. Bromocriptine is considered safe in pregnancy. Caution is advised for cabergoline because there is no human data available. Consider surgery if vision is threatened.

Note: Bromocriptine and cabergoline are FDA approved for hyperprolactinemia.

Thyroid Disease

Hyperthyroidism

Treatment with ^{131}I is contraindicated in pregnancy.

Hyperthyroidism in pregnancy is uncommon and often does not require treatment. However, there are a few circumstances when treatment is necessary to prevent fetal hyperthyroidism.

Gestational transient thyrotoxicosis does not require treatment. This is normal physiology of pregnancy in which human chorionic gonadotropin (hCG) stimulates thyroid stimulating hormone () receptors, resulting in a mild elevation in T_3/T_4 and suppression of TSH.

Subclinical hyperthyroidism (low TSH and normal free T_4) does not require treatment. Follow up thyroid labs every 4–6 weeks.

Symptomatic and/or overt hyperthyroidism requires treatment and is most commonly due to Graves disease or hCG-mediated hyperthyroidism. Treat with a beta-blocker and antithyroid medication (propylthiouracil or methimazole). Patients uncontrolled on medications require thyroidectomy. Monitor the fetus to prevent fetal thyrotoxicosis.

Postpartum thyroiditis is an autoimmune-mediated process caused by thyroid peroxidase antibody. It presents with a hyperthyroid phase followed by a hypothyroid phase. This entity usually resolves within 1 year and rarely requires treatment. Use propranolol for significant hyperthyroid symptoms. Use replacement thyroid medication for hypothyroid symptoms or when the TSH is > 10 mU/L in asymptomatic women. It is important to follow up with thyroid function tests (TSH, FT_4, and FT_3) every 4–6 weeks to ensure resolution and exclude Graves disease. 1/3 of patients are at risk for permanent hypothyroidism and require long-term replacement therapy.

During pregnancy, surgery may be indicated to treat Graves disease in patients with an associated cold nodule or relapse after radiation and in some young patients with a large goiter.

Hypothyroidism

Because their requirements increase, always treat pregnant hypothyroid patients and follow their TSH levels during pregnancy. Increase their dose to 50% more than the prepregnancy dose. Failure to treat maternal hypothyroidism during pregnancy can adversely affect the baby.

Polycystic Ovary Syndrome

See Treatment on page 11-18 for the treatment of polycystic ovary syndrome (PCOS).

Diabetes

Overview

Diabetes in pregnancy is classified as follows:

Preexisting (overt) diabetes: diabetes (Type 1 or Type 2) that existed prior to pregnancy. Note that preexisting diabetes is sometimes first recognized in the 1st trimester of pregnancy.

Gestational diabetes: transient diabetes due to the increased insulin resistance of pregnancy; typically diagnosed during the 2nd half of pregnancy.

Preexisting Diabetes

In women with preexisting diabetes who are planning for pregnancy, achieve strict glycemic control before conception. Maintain fasting plasma glucose (FPG) < 100 mg/dL (5.6 mmol/L) and HbA1c < 6% (< 6.5% in early pregnancy) per 2018 ADA guidelines. Preconception, blood glucose control reduces fetal malformation; during pregnancy, it reduces miscarriages, fetal anomalies/death, and newborn problems. Tight glycemic control decreases the risk of macrosomia (birth weight ≥ 9–10 lb) and shoulder dystocia in the newborn (which increases as birth weight increases).

During pregnancy, a diabetic patient requires ~ 50% more insulin due to insulin resistance from placental hormones. This increased requirement is gone immediately after delivery, so anticipate a reduction in insulin dosage of at least 33% postpartum and observe the patient carefully the day after delivery.

Insulin is the preferred agent for management of both Type 1 and Type 2 diabetes in pregnancy. In pregnancy, avoid the following medications commonly employed in diabetes management:

- Statins
- ACEIs and ARBs
- Most oral hypoglycemics

Gestational Diabetes

Like preexisting diabetes, gestational diabetes increases the risk of preeclampsia, macrosomia, and stillbirth. Gestational diabetes usually resolves after delivery, but it can recur in subsequent pregnancies. Women with gestational diabetes have an increased long-term risk for Type 2 diabetes and cardiovascular disease.

Screen all pregnant women for gestational diabetes between 24 and 28 weeks of gestation. The initial screening test is the 50-g, 1-hour glucose challenge. If this is abnormal, proceed to the 100-g, 3-hour glucose tolerance test to make the diagnosis. Screen pregnant women at high risk for pregestational diabetes at the 1st prenatal visit. Indications for early screening include being overweight or obese (BMI > 25) with one of the following risk factors: physical inactivity, 1st degree relative with diabetes, previous gestational diabetes, high-risk ethnicity, previous macrosomic infant, hypertension, hypercholesterolemia, PCOS, or cardiovascular disease.

Treat gestational diabetes first with nutritional counselling and exercise. Patients should monitor blood glucose, with target fasting blood glucose of < 95 mg/dL (5.3 mmol/L), 1-hour postprandial glucose < 140 mg/dL (7.8 mmol/L), and 2-hour postprandial glucose < 120 mg/dL (6.7 mmol/L). If these targets are not achieved with diet and exercise, insulin is the 1st choice agent. Glyburide and metformin are sometimes used in women who refuse or cannot comply with insulin therapy.

NEUROLOGY DISORDERS IN PREGNANCY

Migraine

Treat migraines in pregnancy first with acetaminophen, acetaminophen-codeine, or butalbital-acetaminophen-caffeine. Consider NSAIDs, such as naproxen, ibuprofen, and ketorolac, prior to 30 weeks of gestation. Use triptans for moderate-to-severe symptoms.

Pseudotumor Cerebri

Pseudotumor cerebri usually occurs in premenopausal obese women (90%) and may occur during pregnancy. See more on pseudotumor cerebri in Neurology, Book 4.

Seizures

Among pregnant women on seizure medications, the risk of birth defects is 4–6%. However, uncontrolled seizures can cause placental abruption, early labor, and premature delivery. When the risk of teratogenicity is compared to the problems that seizures cause during pregnancy, the risk of uncontrolled seizures is greater.

Maintain a pregnant woman on monotherapy and at the lowest dose of medication possible because the risk of malformation increases as each drug is added. Consult a neurologist to assist with any medication changes.

There is no "safe" antiepileptic drug (AED), but valproate is more likely to cause neural tube defects than other commonly used antiepileptics; avoid when possible.

The teratogenic risk of AEDs is decreased by folic acid. All women of childbearing age on antiepileptic drugs should take 4 mg/day of folic acid.

Inadequate evidence exists to determine if newborns of women taking AEDs have an increased risk of hemorrhagic complications. The American Academy of Neurology concluded in its 2009 Practice Parameter Update that there is not enough evidence to recommend for or against the use of prophylactic vitamin K to prevent bleeding in the neonate.

Carpal Tunnel

Pregnancy can cause an acute presentation of carpal tunnel syndrome (CTS), which typically improves after delivery. Treat conservatively with wrist splints.

RHEUMATOLOGY DISORDERS IN PREGNANCY

Systemic Lupus Erythematosus

SSA (Ro) and SSB (La) antibodies are associated with neonatal lupus and congenital heart block. General internists need to know about this risk when counseling women with lupus about pregnancy.

Patients with SLE have a higher incidence of failed pregnancies. Risk of pregnancy complications (flare or fetal problems) is much greater if the disease is active (especially renal manifestations) or if the mother has anti-dsDNA or antiphospholipid antibody syndrome (APS). Treat pregnant women with APS and a history of recurrent miscarriages with heparins (low-molecular-weight or unfractionated) plus low-dose aspirin—to decrease the risk of miscarriage. Heart block starting in the 3rd trimester can be seen in fetuses of mothers with SLE who have SSA (Ro) and/or SSB (La) antibodies.

If an SLE patient wishes to become pregnant and has had a recent lupus flare, continue the glucocorticoids and or hydroxychloroquine. Measure baseline complements, anti-dsDNA, SSA/SSB, and a 24-hour urine protein before or very early in the pregnancy. Manage flares during pregnancy with glucocorticoids. Refer pregnant women with SLE to a high-risk obstetrician (and pediatric cardiologist if appropriate).

Avascular Necrosis of the Hip

Causes of avascular necrosis of the hip include pregnancy, steroid use, sickle cell disease, HIV/AIDS, alcoholism, trauma, Gaucher disease, and hypercoagulable states.

DERMATOLOGY DISORDERS IN PREGNANCY

Acne is more pronounced in pregnancy due to increases in progesterone. Treatment is focused on safer topical agents (i.e., erythromycin, clindamycin, azelaic acid) and avoidance of other agents known to be harmful (i.e., isotretinoin, tazarotene, tetracycline, minocycline). Topical benzoyl peroxide is also generally not used.

Pruritic urticarial papules and plaques of pregnancy (PUPPP) is a common erythematous, pruritic papular rash that spreads outward to form plaques. PUPPP presents within the striae of the abdomen then spreads to the body, sparing the face, soles, and palms. It typically presents at around 35 weeks of gestation but can develop later in pregnancy or up to 2–3 weeks after delivery.

ALLERGY AND IMMUNOLOGY IN PREGNANCY

Persistent nasal congestion can accompany pregnancy (rhinitis of pregnancy). It is generally treated with non-pharmacological measures, including:

- Keep pets out of the room.
- Encase pillows/mattress in covers that protect against dust mites.
- Avoid outdoor activities when pollen counts are high.
- Change clothes after spending time outdoors.
- Shower to remove pollen from the hair and skin.

Intranasal steroids have not been shown to be effective.

OFFICE GYNECOLOGY

PREVIEW | REVIEW

- What are the risk factors for an ectopic pregnancy?
- How is an ectopic pregnancy diagnosed?

NOTE

Some office gynecology topics are also discussed in other sections of Internal Medicine Core. Especially review infections during pregnancy in Infectious Disease, Book 1. Pap smear, ovarian cancer, and breast cancer are covered in Oncology, Book 3. Amenorrhea is discussed in Endocrinology, Book 4. Osteoporosis is discussed in General Internal Medicine, Book 5.

ECTOPIC PREGNANCY

Overview

An ectopic pregnancy is the result of the implantation of a fertilized ovum in a site other than the uterus (ampulla of the fallopian tube 95% of the time). It occurs in 1–2% of pregnancies, and it accounts for 9% of all pregnancy-related deaths. Risk factors include prior history of ectopic pregnancy, history of infertility, prior tubal surgery, salpingitis, history of multiple sexual partners, ruptured appendix, advanced maternal age, smoking, and *in utero* diethylstilbestrol exposure. Women using an intrauterine device (IUD) or tubal sterilization for contraception are at an increased risk of an ectopic pregnancy if they become pregnant.

Presentation

Patients typically present with sudden lower abdominal/pelvic pain or 1st trimester bleeding. Bimanual cervical exam may reveal adnexal tenderness or an adnexal mass. A ruptured ectopic pregnancy may present with diffuse abdominal pain, rebound tenderness, vital sign instability, and shock. The risk of rupture is about 30% in the first 48 hours; it then falls to about 5–10%.

Diagnosis

Ultrasound is indicated in all women with a suspected ectopic pregnancy to look for an intrauterine pregnancy, an adnexal mass, or free pelvic fluid. An elevated β-hCG in the absence of an intrauterine pregnancy is highly suspicious of an ectopic pregnancy.

Differential diagnosis:

- Spontaneous abortion
- Molar pregnancy
- Adnexal mass (e.g., ovarian torsion, tuboovarian abscess, cyst rupture)
- Pelvic inflammatory disease (PID)
- Appendicitis
- Pyelonephritis
- Urinary tract infection (UTI)
- Nephrolithiasis
- Diverticulitis
- Ulcerative colitis

No physical exam findings are specific to ectopic pregnancy because the findings may mimic those listed in the differential above. No single serum β-hCG level is diagnostic of an ectopic pregnancy; therefore, it is necessary to perform serial serum β-hCG levels to differentiate between normal and abnormal pregnancies and to monitor resolution of ectopic pregnancy once therapy has been initiated (β-hCG will decrease). Confirmed diagnosis can be made by visualization of ectopic pregnancy on ultrasound or by laparoscopy/laparotomy.

Prognosis

Spontaneous resolution occurs in 88% of ectopic pregnancies with hCG levels < 200 mU/mL and in 59% of ectopic pregnancies with hCG levels < 2,000 mU/mL. In the U.S., mortality is 0.5/100,000 live births. The recurrence rate is about 10% in women with 1 previous ectopic pregnancy, and it rises to over 25% in women with 2 previous ectopic pregnancies.

Treatment

Treatment may vary depending on the presentation. Watchful waiting is an option if the patient is asymptomatic, there is evidence of spontaneous resolution, and the patient accepts the risk of rupture. Surgery or methotrexate therapy may be appropriate 1st line therapy for an unruptured ectopic pregnancy.

Give methotrexate to stable patients with a fetal crown-rump length < 4 cm and no fetal embryonic cardiac activity. CBC and comprehensive metabolic panel (CMP) are necessary prior to administering methotrexate. The following are absolute contraindications:

- Intrauterine pregnancy or breastfeeding patient
- Immunodeficiency
- Moderate-to-severe anemia, leukopenia, or thrombocytopenia
- Active pulmonary disease
- Active peptic ulcer disease
- Hepatic or renal dysfunction
- Ruptured ectopic and/or unstable patient
- Patient inability to participate in follow-up
- Sensitivity to methotrexate

Patients who receive methotrexate need serial hCG levels on post-treatment days 4 and 7. If the decrease in hCG is < 15%, give additional methotrexate.

Surgery is indicated for a ruptured ectopic pregnancy, as indicated by a patient who is hemodynamically unstable or has an acute abdomen. Surgery may also be performed in stable and unruptured patients who are not candidates for or who decline methotrexate. Consult a gynecologist for all patients with suspected ectopic pregnancies.

SEXUALLY TRANSMITTED INFECTIONS

See Infectious Disease, Book 1, for information on sexually transmitted infections (STIs).

VAGINITIS

See Infectious Disease, Book 1, for information on vaginitis.

PREMENSTRUAL SYNDROME

Premenstrual syndrome (PMS) is a group of symptoms that most often start during the late luteal phase and are gone within 1–2 days of the onset of menses. The biochemistry of this dysfunction has not been established.

No single treatment has been proven effective, but the cause may be multifactorial, so there are many avenues of treatment to explore with each patient. You can achieve ovulatory suppression with oral contraceptives or the progestin-only pill. Other options include medroxyprogesterone and levonorgestrel implants.

Dietary changes, such as avoiding caffeine, salt, sugar, alcohol, and/or chocolate, can help some patients reduce or eliminate symptoms.

PREMENSTRUAL DYSPHORIC DISORDER

PREVIEW | REVIEW

- What are the diagnostic criteria for PMDD?
- What organic syndromes can cause symptoms similar to PMDD?

Overview

Premenstrual dysphoric disorder (PMDD) is a cluster of affective, behavioral, and somatic symptoms recurring monthly during the luteal phase of the menstrual cycle. The prevalence of PMDD is between 1.8% and 8% of menstruating women. The heritability percentage of PMDD is unknown; however, heritability of premenstrual symptoms is between 30% and 80%.

Diagnosis

PMDD is diagnosed by the DSM-5 as follows:

At least 5 symptoms (listed below) must be present in the final week before menses, improve within a few days of menses, become minimal after menses, and be observed daily for 2 cycles:

- ≥ 1 of the following mood symptoms:
  ◦ Marked affective lability: mood swings, sudden tearfulness, increased sensitivity to rejection
  ◦ Marked irritability, anger, increased conflicts
  ◦ Marked depressed mood, hopelessness, self-deprecating thoughts
  ◦ Marked anxiety or tension
- Plus ≥ 1 of the following symptoms:
  ◦ Decreased interest
  ◦ Difficulty concentrating
  ◦ Lethargy, easily fatigued
  ◦ Change in appetite, cravings
  ◦ Hypersomnia or insomnia
  ◦ Overwhelmed feeling or loss of control
  ◦ Breast tenderness/swelling, joint/muscle pain
  ◦ Symptoms that interfere with daily functioning and are not due to substances, another mental disorder, or a medical disorder

Risk factors include anxiety or depressive disorders (especially peripartum depression), increased age, stress, lack of exercise, history of interpersonal trauma, seasonal changes, and family history of PMDD.

Pathophysiology

The exact cause of PMDD is unknown. It is postulated that fluctuations in estrogen and progesterone lead to serotonin deficiency.

Workup

Exclude organic syndromes with manifestations similar to those of PMDD, including thyroid disorder (TSH), anemia (CBC), and perimenopause/menopause (FSH).

Clinical Course and Management

Onset of PMDD can occur at any point after menarche. Anecdotally, many individuals report worsening symptoms as they approach menopause. Symptoms cease after menopause, although hormone replacement can trigger the reexpression of symptoms. Treat with oral contraceptives and/or SSRIs. Combined oral contraceptives, with a 24/4 regimen and containing drospirenone or levonorgestrel as the progestogenic component, have been shown to relieve both psychological and physical symptoms of PMDD. SSRIs, while also considered a 1st line treatment, are effective for psychological symptoms only. Treat severe PMDD, unresponsive to other therapies, with GnRH agonists.

CONTRACEPTIVE COUNSELING

PREVIEW | REVIEW

- The copper IUD, Paragard, is effective for up to how many years?
- How frequently is the medroxyprogesterone injection given?
- What is the most common of the least effective contraceptive methods?

Overview

The 2 main goals of discussing contraception are to formulate a reproductive life plan and to reduce unintended pregnancies. Discussing a reproductive life plan helps dictate which contraception type is most beneficial for the patient at that time in her life. Unintended pregnancies can result in significant depression, financial burden, poor prenatal care, and abortions.

Although there is no perfect contraception aside from abstinence, the most effective method is a personal decision for each patient. The best method for a woman will depend upon her individual needs, such as religious beliefs, tolerance of side effects, effects on menstruation, cost, and the ability to use a contraception properly (e.g., take an oral pill daily). Additionally, the need or contraindication of hormones plays a large role in selecting the method.

Methods of Contraception

Contraceptive methods are divided into 3 categories:

1) Most effective
   - Permanent sterilization
   - Long-acting, reversible contraceptives, including IUDs and implants
   - Lowest pregnancy rate

2) Effective
- OCP (oral contraceptive pill), vaginal ring, or patch
- MPA (medroxyprogesterone acetate) injection
- Diaphragms
- Low pregnancy rate but dependent upon patient use

3) Least effective
- Condoms, spermicides, rhythm method, and pull-out method
- Associated with a high risk of unintended pregnancies

Most effective: There are 2 types of IUDs. Both have an unintended pregnancy rate of < 1% per year. Nonhormonal IUDs (called Paragard) contain copper, disrupt cervical mucus, and are a sperm inhibitor. They are effective for up to 10 years. Hormonal IUDs contain progesterone, lessen menses, thin the lining of the uterus, and inhibit sperm entry. They are effective for 3–5 years, depending on the type.

The etonogestrel implant, with a 0.5% failure rate, is effective for up to 3 years and is inserted in the office in the nondominant arm. It contains progestin hormone, can affect menses, and inhibits ovulation.

Effective: The most common effective method is the OCP, which has a 9% unintended pregnancy rate. OCPs are composed of estrogen and progesterone and are a hormonal ovulation inhibitor. They reduce the menstrual flow and make menses more predictable. OCPs need to be taken daily to be effective, and there is typically a placebo week indicated by a lighter color at the end of the pill pack.

The vaginal ring is inserted monthly; it stays in the vagina for 3 weeks and comes out for 1 week.

The patch is changed weekly (on 3 weeks and off 1 week). Efficacy is similar to OCPs for both the ring and the patch.

MPA is an injection given once every 3 months in the office. It contains progesterone, lessens menses, and is associated with long-term, mild weight gain. The pregnancy rate is ~ 6% per year.

Diaphragms, used less commonly today, have a failure rate of about 12%.

Least effective: The most common of the least effective methods, the condom, has a failure rate of 18%. Condoms are hormone-free, available for purchase over the counter, and made of latex or nonlatex materials. Of note, lambskin condoms do not protect against sexually transmitted infections. Female condoms, withdrawal methods, and spermicides have failure rates > 20%.

Emergency Contraception

Use emergency contraception to prevent pregnancy after unprotected intercourse. The FDA has approved ulipristal acetate (30 mg oral) and levonorgestrel (1.5 mg oral), called the "morning after pill," for this indication. Ulipristal can be used up to 120 hours after unprotected sex, while levonorgestrel can be used up to 72 hours after unprotected sex. Additionally, specific combined progestin-estrogen pills and the copper IUD can be used as emergency contraception. If oral contraceptives or a copper IUD are desired for emergency contraception, refer to a gynecologist experienced in this area. No serious adverse events have been reported with emergency contraception. Typical side effects include nausea, headache, and irregular bleeding.

ENDOMETRIOSIS

Endometriosis is characterized by endometrial glands and stroma occurring outside the uterine cavity. It is a benign, inflammatory, estrogen-dependent condition. Women present with pelvic pain, infertility, or an ovarian mass. Definitive diagnosis can only be made surgically with peritoneal biopsy. Treat with NSAIDs and OCPs. A progesterone IUD, medroxyprogesterone, GnRH agonist, or aromatase inhibitors are other options for treatment in patients who have failed or are not candidates for NSAIDs and OCPs. Surgical resection may be needed for refractory cases, fertility-related endometriosis, and obstructive symptoms.

OVARIAN CYSTS

Ovarian cysts are fluid-filled sacs within or on the surface of ovaries. Most ovarian cysts are asymptomatic and disappear over time. However, some can cause pain or fullness, especially those that have ruptured. Treat symptomatic cysts conservatively with pain medication, including NSAIDs. Large, symptomatic, or persistent cysts or those suspicious for malignancy may need to be surgically removed; refer these patients to gynecology. Ruptured cysts that result in hemodynamic instability require hospitalization for expectant management.

ABNORMAL UTERINE BLEEDING

PREVIEW | REVIEW

- What test is indicated in all women with abnormal uterine bleeding?
- What are the indications for an endometrial biopsy in women with abnormal uterine bleeding?

Overview

Abnormal uterine bleeding (AUB) refers to either heavy menstrual bleeding or intermenstrual bleeding. (The use of the terms dysfunctional uterine bleeding, menorrhagia, and metrorrhagia are no longer recommended.) Rule out pregnancy prior to any other workup. Address hormonal contraceptive use, which is also a common cause of abnormal bleeding.

The differential diagnosis of AUB in nonpregnant women who are not taking oral contraceptives is broad. Structural causes include endometrial polyps, adenomyosis, uterine fibroids, endometrial hyperplasia, or endometrial malignancy. Nonstructural causes include coagulopathies, ovulatory dysfunction, or infections. See Table 11-3 for differential diagnosis by age.

Table 11-3: Abnormal Uterine Bleeding—Age-Based Differential Diagnosis	
Patient Age	Common Diagnoses
13–18	Physiologic anovulation (immature hypothalamic-pituitary-ovarian axis) Hormonal contraceptive use Pregnancy Pelvic infections Coagulopathies
19–39	Pregnancy Structural lesions (usually polyps or fibroids) Anovulatory bleeding (usually PCOS) Hormonal contraceptive use Endometrial hyperplasia
40 to menopause	Physiologic anovulatory bleeding (secondary to declining ovarian function) Endometrial hyperplasia or carcinoma Endometrial atrophy Uterine fibroids

Workup

When taking a medical history, ask about bleeding patterns, pain associated with bleeding, family history of bleeding, or other bleeding problems (including gum bleeding, nosebleeds, or easy bruising). Ask about potential medications that might cause AUB, including anticoagulants, NSAIDs, or hormonal contraceptives.

Note physical signs of excessive weight, acne, hirsutism, or any acanthosis nigricans that may suggest PCOS. Additionally, look for signs of a bleeding disorder, including petechiae or ecchymoses. Perform a pelvic examination, including both speculum examination and bimanual examination, to assess for cervical lesions, vaginal lesions, or uterine enlargement or irregularity. Chlamydia and gonorrhea cervicitis swabs may be obtained as well.

Obtain a pregnancy test, CBC, and thyroid-stimulating hormone (TSH) level in all women. Order a transvaginal ultrasound to evaluate the uterus. The exception is adolescents 13–18 years of age; unless there are signs of a bleeding disorder, a pregnancy test is usually sufficient.

Perform an endometrial biopsy on all women > 45 years of age. Perform an endometrial biopsy on a woman < 45 years of age if she is obese, has a history of unopposed estrogen exposure, or has previously failed medical management for AUB.

Diagnosis

Diagnose structural lesions by ultrasound. A thickened endometrium can be indicative of an endometrial polyp, endometrial hyperplasia, or malignancy; however, this finding is nonspecific. Adenomyosis and fibroids can also be seen on ultrasound.

Diagnose coagulation disorders with laboratory testing. Among patients with suspected bleeding disorders based on history, order a CBC and coagulation studies. The most common bleeding disorder, von Willebrand disease, is diagnosed by decreased von Willebrand factor antigen or decreased ristocetin cofactor activity.

Diagnose anovulatory bleeding clinically. Anovulatory cycles are those that vary in length from one cycle to another. Patients with anovulation also do not have premenstrual symptoms, such as breast discomfort or premenstrual cramping and bloating. Further workup of anovulatory bleeding is discussed under Anovulatory Bleeding.

Diagnose infections, such as chlamydia or gonorrhea, with a cervical swab using culture, antigen, or nucleic acid detection methods.

Treatment

Treatment depends on the etiology of the bleeding. Treat patients with suspected anovulatory bleeding and an otherwise normal workup with combined oral contraceptives or progestins (including cyclic oral progesterone or the levonorgestrel IUD). Treat any infections with appropriate antibiotics (see Infectious Disease, Book 1, for treatment of STIs).

Refer patients with suspected bleeding disorders to a hematologist. Refer patients with structural lesions, including uterine fibroids or polyps, to a gynecologist.

ANOVULATORY BLEEDING

PREVIEW | REVIEW

- What hormone is lacking in patients with anovulatory bleeding?
- What blood work should be ordered to rule out an androgen-secreting tumor?
- What is the typical treatment for an adolescent (13–18 years of age) with anovulatory bleeding?

Overview

Anovulatory bleeding is a type of abnormal uterine bleeding resulting from a lack of regular ovulation. Patients who are anovulatory have cycles that vary in length by > 10 days from one cycle to the next. Ovulatory dysfunction can result in 2 types of bleeding patterns:

1) Oligomenorrhea—cycles > 35 days and < 6 months apart

2) Amenorrhea—no menstruation for 6–12 months after the establishment of a cyclical pattern (See more on this topic under Amenorrhea on page 11-18.)

Pathophysiology

During normal ovulatory cycles, follicular development occurs, followed by ovulation. Once ovulation occurs, the corpus luteum develops and then undergoes luteolysis. Estrogen rises during the first 1/2 of the cycle, and then progesterone rises after ovulation.

In patients with anovulation, estrogen continues to rise as no ovulation or corpus luteum development occurs. No progesterone is secreted by the ovary. Consequently, unopposed estrogen production leads to uncontrolled endometrial proliferation without progesterone-induced withdrawal bleeding. The endometrium is vascular and without stromal support, leading to abnormal bleeding patterns.

Etiologies

Like AUB in general, the differential diagnosis for anovulatory bleeding is broad. The most common causes are physiologic anovulatory bleeding, commonly seen after menarche, and polycystic ovarian syndrome (See Polycystic Ovary Syndrome (PCOS)). Differential diagnosis and recommended diagnostic workup is listed in Table 11-4.

Treatment

Treat bothersome physiologic anovulation in adolescents with combined oral contraceptives or other progestin contraceptives. Adolescents 13–18 years of age with a negative pregnancy test and signs of anovulatory bleeding can be started on hormonal treatment without any other workup.

Treatment of PCOS is discussed in detail under the next topic. Hypothyroidism is treated with levothyroxine. Treat patients with hyperprolactinemia secondary to a pituitary adenoma with bromocriptine. Counsel patients with hypothalamic amenorrhea on nutrition. These women should increase their caloric intake. Give patients with primary ovarian insufficiency oral contraceptives.

Refer patients with congenital adrenal hyperplasia, 3- beta-hydroxysteroid dehydrogenase deficiency, androgen-secreting tumors, Cushing syndrome, or acromegaly to an endocrinologist specializing in these disorders.

POLYCYSTIC OVARY SYNDROME (PCOS)

PREVIEW | REVIEW

- The Rotterdam criteria for PCOS requires how many signs of PCOS?
- What are 3 clinical features of hyperandrogenism?

Overview

Polycystic ovary syndrome (PCOS) is one of the most common endocrine disorders of women of reproductive-age in the U.S., with a prevalence of 4–12%. It is characterized by menstrual dysregulation (e.g., oligomenorrhea, amenorrhea), high levels of masculinizing hormones (resulting in hirsutism and acne), decreased fertility, and metabolic syndrome. The onset is at about 16 years of age; however, syndrome recognition may be delayed as the symptoms can be interpreted as normal

Table 11-4: Differential Diagnosis of Anovulatory Bleeding		
Suspected Diagnosis	**Additional Signs and Symptoms**	**Diagnostic Testing**
Physiologic anovulatory bleeding	None except irregular menses; patient will be within 3 years of menarche	None
PCOS	Hirsutism, polycystic-appearing ovaries on ultrasound	Testosterone, pelvic ultrasound
Hypothyroidism	Fatigue, weight changes, thyroid nodule, or goiter	TSH
Hyperprolactinemia	Lactation, headaches, visual disturbances	Prolactin, MRI of brain (if prolactin elevated)
Late-onset congenital adrenal hyperplasia	Hirsutism	Early-morning 17-hydroxyprogesterone
Hypothalamic amenorrhea	Disordered eating, over-exercising, low body weight	LH, FSH, estradiol
Primary ovarian insufficiency	Hot flashes	FSH, estradiol
Androgen-secreting tumors	Virilization, deep voice, clitoromegaly	Testosterone, DHEA-S, urine level 17-ketosteroids Imaging of the ovaries and adrenals
Cushing syndrome	Buffalo hump, striae, hypertension	Cortisol and dexamethasone suppression testing
Acromegaly	Changes in hat and hand size, protruding jaw, impaired vision	Insulin-like growth factor

DHEA-S = dehydroepiandrosterone sulfate; FSH = follicle stimulating hormone; LH = luteinizing hormone; PCOS = polycystic ovary syndrome; TSH = thyroid stimulating hormone

maturation during the few years after menarche. The etiology of PCOS is unknown, but it may be due to peripheral insulin resistance leading to hyperinsulinemia with consequent stimulation of excess ovarian androgen production. Family history may be notable for diabetes, obesity, menstrual disorders, infertility, adrenal enzyme deficiencies, or hirsutism.

Diagnosis

The diagnosis of PCOS is based on 3 criteria. Of the signs listed below, the NIH criteria confirms a diagnosis of PCOS if the first 2 signs are present, and the Rotterdam criteria requires 2 of the 3 signs. The PCOS Society criteria is fulfilled if hyperandrogenism and 1 of the other signs is found. The criteria are:

1) Hyperandrogenism
2) Oligomenorrhea (70–75% of cases)
3) Polycystic ovaries

Hyperandrogenism presents with:

- Acne
- Androgenic alopecia (i.e., male-pattern baldness)
- Male pattern hirsutism
- Elevated levels of testosterone or dehydroepiandrosterone sulfate (DHEA-S)

Other signs and symptoms of PCOS may include:

- Infertility (30–70% of cases)
- Obesity and metabolic syndrome (40% of cases)
- Diabetes
- Obstructive sleep apnea

Polycystic ovaries are present when:

- at least 1 ovary has ≥ 12 follicles, or 25 follicles using more modern ultrasound techniques, or
- 1 ovary has a volume of 10 mL.

Note that 65 % of patients with normal ovulatory patterns may have ovaries fulfilling these criteria.

See Figure 11-1 for ultrasound images of PCOS.

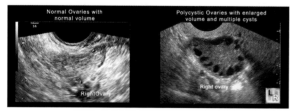

Figure 11-1: Ovaries of PCOS

As adolescent females commonly have oligomenorrhea after menarche, many experts suggest that all 3 criteria (hyperandrogenism, oligomenorrhea, and polycystic ovaries) be present to diagnose an adolescent with PCOS.

In addition to hyperandrogenism, physical findings include increased abdominal adiposity (monitor BMI); cutaneous findings include skin tags and acanthosis nigricans (brown to black, velvety hyperpigmentation of the skin found on the neck, on axillae, under breasts, or on the vulva).

Additional Testing

In addition to the aforementioned tests of testosterone or DHEA-S levels and pelvic ultrasound, perform the following testing on patients with PCOS:

- TSH, prolactin, 17-hydroxyprogesterone levels (to exclude other common causes of anovulatory bleeding if not done yet)
- 2-hour oral glucose tolerance test (screening for diabetes and impaired glucose tolerance)
- Fasting lipid and lipoprotein levels

Prognosis

Up to 40% of women with PCOS have insulin resistance, placing them at an increased risk of Type 2 diabetes and cardiovascular and cerebrovascular diseases. Screen women for Type 2 diabetes, hypertension, dyslipidemia, as well as obstructive sleep apnea (given likelihood of obesity). Women with PCOS are also at an increased risk for endometrial hyperplasia and carcinoma due to chronic anovulation (resulting in continuous endometrial stimulation).

Treatment

Recommend lifestyle modifications, such as improved diet and increased physical activity, for all women with PCOS. A reduction in body weight is associated with improved pregnancy rates, improved glucose levels, and decreased hirsutism. If a patient does not desire pregnancy, treat PCOS with hormonal contraception or progesterone medication to prevent endometrial hyperplasia, mitigate irregular menses, decrease hirsutism, and improve acne.

Use metformin to treat insulin resistance and obesity. Treat excessive hair with spironolactone. Recommend depilatory methods if the patient desires. Treat acne with topical creams. If a patient desires pregnancy, do not prescribe spironolactone.

If a patient wants to become pregnant, refer her to a subspecialist. Infertility secondary to anovulation is typically treated with ovulation induction agents, including letrozole, an aromatase inhibitor, and clomiphene citrate, an estrogen receptor modulator.

AMENORRHEA

PREVIEW | REVIEW

- What is the definition of primary amenorrhea?
- What is the radiologic test of choice when performing an evaluation for amenorrhea?
- What radiology study should be ordered in patients with unexplained elevated PRL level?

Overview

Amenorrhea is the absence of menses and can be intermittent or permanent depending on the etiology.

Primary Amenorrhea

Primary amenorrhea is the absence of menses by 15 years of age. It is the result of a genetic cause or an anatomical problem, the most common of which are Turner syndrome, Müllerian agenesis, constitutional benign delay, anorexia, vaginal septum, and PCOS.

To determine etiology, think of the organs affecting the menstrual cycle:

- Ovary (e.g., Turner syndrome gonadal dysgenesis)
- Uterus (e.g., Müllerian agenesis)
- Hypothalamus (e.g., anorexia)
- Pituitary (e.g., hypopituitarism)
- Vagina (e.g., transverse vaginal septum)

An abnormality at any one of these locations can cause primary amenorrhea. Take a thorough history by asking questions to determine recent stress, weight loss, family history of delayed or absent puberty, drug use, and completed stages of puberty.

Next, determine if a uterus is present or not via a physical exam or ultrasound. Perform a vaginal examination to evaluate for pubic hair growth and vaginal patency. Look for the presence of breast development and any evidence of hirsutism. Initial laboratory evaluation includes hCG, FSH, TSH, and PRL. This is primarily a pediatric condition and requires evaluation and management by a gynecology specialist.

Secondary Amenorrhea

Secondary amenorrhea is the absence of menses for:

- ≥ 3 months in a woman who previously had regular menstrual cycles or
- ≥ 6 months in a woman who has had irregular menses.

As with primary amenorrhea, identify the involved organs to help determine the cause. The most common causes of secondary amenorrhea are pregnancy, PCOS, and functional hypothalamic amenorrhea. Primary amenorrhea typically occurs because of an anatomical or a genetic abnormality; however, the conditions that cause secondary amenorrhea can also present as primary amenorrhea. Diagnostic tests include β-hCG, TSH, FSH, and PRL.

Assess estrogen status with a progesterone challenge test; give a dose of progesterone for up to 10 days; stop at 10 days or when bleeding occurs (whichever comes first). If withdrawal bleeding occurs, it signifies the presence of endogenous estrogen exposure. Order a brain MRI for patients with unexplained elevated PRL levels to evaluate for a pituitary or hypothalamic lesion. Other causes of elevated PRL can include antipsychotic drug use.

Manage a patient with secondary amenorrhea by correcting the underlying pathology to prevent long-term complications, such as osteoporosis, and to help the woman achieve fertility if desired.

DYSMENORRHEA

PREVIEW | REVIEW

- What hormone is released from the uterine lining that causes painful menstruation?

Dysmenorrhea, or painful menstruation, is divided into primary and secondary categories. Primary dysmenorrhea is the presence of recurrent, crampy pain during menstruation in the absence of an identifiable cause. Secondary dysmenorrhea has similar clinical features, but the symptoms are specific to a cause.

Risk factors for developing dysmenorrhea include smoking, BMI < 19 or > 30, history of sexual assault, and < 30 years of age. Dysmenorrhea is thought to result from painful uterine contractions initiated by prostaglandins.

Dysmenorrhea is a clinical diagnosis and does not have any laboratory or radiology features. To make the diagnosis, a good history and physical exam are necessary, focusing on the symptoms and complaints of the patient. It is important to exclude identifiable causes by evaluating the severity of the disease; e.g., days missed from school or work, amount of medication (e.g., NSAIDs) taken, and grading of the pain. Consider miscarriage, ectopic pregnancy, ruptured ovarian cyst, fibroids, and endometriosis as possible identifiable causes.

Nonhormonal and hormonal treatment options for dysmenorrhea include NSAIDs, OCPs, IUDs, and progesterone injectables.

PERIMENOPAUSE AND MENOPAUSE

PREVIEW | REVIEW

- What is the definition of menopause?
- What is the median age of menopause?
- Menopause prior to what age is considered primary ovarian insufficiency?
- What hormonal treatment is given to patients who suffer from vaginal atrophy?
- What are the risks of hormone replacement therapy?

Overview

Menopause is defined as the permanent cessation of menses; it occurs secondary to the loss of ovarian activity. Patients are postmenopausal after 1 full year of amenorrhea, making menopause a retrospective diagnosis. The median age is 51 years. The transition to menopause is called perimenopause and occurs naturally any time after

40 years of age. Primary ovarian insufficiency, menopause prior to 40 years of age, is abnormal, and occurs in approximately 1% of women.

During perimenopause, FSH levels are higher than LH, and both rise to even higher values than those seen during normal menstruation. The FSH rise precedes the LH rise. Persistently high FSH levels combined with 12 months of amenorrhea indicate menopause.

Symptoms and Effects of Menopause

Symptoms of perimenopause are hot flashes, mood swings, vaginal dryness, irregular periods, and lack of sexual desire. Perimenopause lasts for about 4 years before the final menstrual period occurs. Many women go through this time naturally and do no need medical treatment.

Hot flashes (a.k.a. night sweats) are the most common symptom reported during perimenopause. The mechanism of action is unknown. Hot flashes are described as a flush of heat that lasts up to 4 minutes starting in the chest and rising up to the face. Hot flashes can persist past menopause, which is normal. They occur mainly at night and can cause sleep disturbances.

Vaginal dryness and libido: Naturally, the vagina becomes dry with the lack of estrogen as a woman goes into menopause. This can manifest as painful sex and even pain with daily walking activities. Secondary to painful sex and the changing appearance of the vagina, many women then experience a decrease in sexual desire. On exam, the vagina will appear pale and raw. The introital opening narrows and the vagina becomes narrower.

With decreasing estrogen, a woman is susceptible to an increased risk of **cardiovascular disease** and **osteoporosis**. Furthermore, LDL increases during the menopause transition, and **bone loss** is significant.

Differential Diagnosis

The differential diagnosis for menopause includes hyperthyroidism, pregnancy, malignancy, or pheochromocytoma.

Treatment

Many patients attain menopause naturally, with no treatment needed. However, for those who do require treatment, hormone replacement therapy (HRT) is the mainstay for severe symptoms of the menopausal transition. Patients with a uterus need estrogen combined with progesterone either in the form of a transdermal patch/gel/spray or a daily pill. Transdermal estrogen formations are preferred over oral pills because they bypass the gastrointestinal conversion of estradiol to estrone, resulting in lower triglyceride levels and clotting factors. Case control studies show a lower risk of venous thromboembolism with transdermal preparations. Additionally, vaginal rings have been used for hormone replacement and, similarly, achieve a lower risk of blood clots.

Regardless of the type of estrogen used, progesterone must be given so that the uterine wall is not hyperstimulated from unopposed estrogen. If a patient has had a hysterectomy, prescribe estrogen alone.

Give vaginal estrogen to patients who suffer from painful sex and atrophy. Typically, these patients do not require progesterone supplementation.

HRT is contraindicated in patients with the following risk factors:

• History of breast cancer
• Coronary heart disease
• Previous venous thromboembolism
• Previous stroke or transient ischemic attack
• Active liver disease
• Unexplained vaginal bleeding
• History of endometrial cancer

Prescribe HRT at the lowest dose and for the shortest period of time to relieve symptoms. Counsel patients on the risks and individualize treatment based on patient desires and symptoms. The risks of HRT are:

• Venous thromboembolism
• Stroke
• Breast cancer
• Endometrial cancer (unopposed estrogen)
• Coronary heart disease (in women > 60 years of age)

Give hormonal alternatives to patients who are not candidates for or who do not want estrogen. Alternatives to hormones for the treatment of vasomotor symptoms include paroxetine, clonidine, and gabapentin; only paroxetine is FDA approved. Alternative methods, such as herbals, vitamins, black cohosh, or vitamin E, have not been proven to help ease symptoms of the menopausal transition.

POSTMENOPAUSAL BLEEDING

Perform an endometrial assessment (transvaginal ultrasound or endometrial biopsy) if a woman has postmenopausal bleeding:

• In the absence of HRT therapy
• After she has been on combined HRT continuously for 1 year without bleeding
• At an unexpected time during cyclic replacement

Postmenopausal bleeding is cancer until proven otherwise. If a transvaginal ultrasound reveals an endometrial thickness of ≤ 4 mm, it has a 99% negative predictive value for endometrial cancer, and endometrial biopsy is not indicated. If the thickness is > 4 mm, perform an endometrial biopsy because endometrial cancer cannot be excluded.

ENDOMETRIAL CANCER

Endometrial cancer is the most common gynecological cancer in the United States. The average age of diagnosis is 61 years. Unopposed estrogen exposure is the main risk factor. Surgery is usually curative for low-risk patients. Adjuvant chemotherapy is offered to high-risk patients. See Oncology, Book 3, for more on endometrial cancer.

BREAST DISORDERS (NONCANCEROUS)

PREVIEW | REVIEW

- What is the most common infectious organism that causes mastitis?
- When during breastfeeding is mastitis most likely to occur?
- What antibiotic is used to treat mastitis?
- Cyclic breast pain typically happens how many weeks prior to menses?
- What location on the breast is cyclic pain most common?
- Does cyclic breast pain occur more commonly in larger or smaller breasted women?
- What are some physical signs of breast cancer?
- What is the only FDA-approved drug to treat cyclic breast pain?

Mastitis

Mastitis, breast inflammation typically due to infection, frequently occurs in lactating women. Puerperal, or lactational, mastitis is caused by prolonged engorgement, oversupply of milk, infrequent feedings, or a blocked milk duct. Organisms grow in the static milk and result in infection. The most common infectious organism that causes mastitis is *Staphylococcus aureus*. If infection does not resolve, an abscess results. Although possible, it is rare that mastitis occurs in nonlactating women secondary to TB, foreign bodies, sarcoidosis, histoplasmosis, or idiopathic causes.

Pain, swelling, and redness are the typical clinical symptoms of puerperal mastitis. It is most common during the first 3 months of breastfeeding.

Diagnosis is made clinically; labs are not needed.

Therapy includes NSAIDs, cold compresses, continuance of breastfeeding, and antibiotics. Treat *S. aureus* with dicloxacillin 500 mg 4×/day. If the patient has an allergy to beta-lactam antibiotics, use clindamycin. If improvement does not occur after 48 hours with antibiotic use, do an ultrasound to rule out an abscess. Differential diagnosis includes inflammatory breast cancer and breast abscess.

There is no proven prevention of puerperal mastitis; however, consistent breastfeeding, assuring that the infant is well attached during breastfeeding, and breastfeeding for 4–6 months is recommended.

Cyclic Breast Pain

Breast pain, most commonly cyclical, is a common complaint seen in the office. Cyclic breast pain is related to the menstrual cycle and presents the week prior to menses. The location is usually in the upper outer quadrant of the breast, and the pain is bilateral. Women with larger breasts are more likely to have cyclic breast pain than women with smaller breasts. Most cyclic breast pain resolves within 3–4 months and returns intermittently throughout a woman's lifetime. Although cyclic breast pain is not typically associated with breast cancer, it is important to evaluate whether the pain is pathological or physiological.

Include the following information in the history and physical:

- Location of the pain
- Whether or not the pain is bilateral
- Relation of the pain to any activity
- Recent trauma to the breast
- Whether or not the pain is phasic

The goal of the physical exam is to exclude any signs of a possible malignancy, such as nipple retraction, a solid mass, or bloody nipple discharge. Also examine the axillary lymph nodes for enlargement or tenderness. If a mass or signs of malignancy are observed, order a mammogram and breast ultrasound.

Most women who present with cyclic and diffuse breast pain only need a physical exam and reassurance.

Those who experience severe pain that interferes with their lifestyle may benefit from hot compresses and support bras. Danazol is the only FDA-approved drug to treat cyclic breast pain; acetaminophen and NSAIDs are also effective. Tamoxifen is rarely used due to its side effects of hot flashes, vaginal dryness, and an increased risk of blood clots. Reduction of caffeine and vitamin E have not been proven to help.

MEN'S HEALTH

BENIGN PROSTATIC HYPERPLASIA

PREVIEW | REVIEW

- How does prostatic hyperplasia affect PSA levels?
- What is the initial treatment for BPH? Which medications are commonly used for treatment?

OVERVIEW

Benign prostatic hyperplasia (BPH; also incorrectly called benign prostatic hypertrophy) is an enlarged prostate gland. The prevalence of BPH increases from about 10% at 30 years of age to > 80% at 85 years of age. About 15% of these patients have impaired urination. We still do not understand what causes BPH and have yet to identify any specific risk factors—except age. BPH does not increase the chance of prostate cancer.

Symptoms of BPH are secondary to urinary retention and include frequency, hesitancy, urgency, nocturia, and difficulty starting and stopping the stream, as well as reduced stream. Other diseases can also cause these symptoms (e.g., bladder cancer, cystitis) and should be considered before making a diagnosis of BPH. Know that serum prostate-specific antigen (PSA) levels increase as the prostate increases in size, so PSA screening for prostate cancer is less specific in men with BPH (more false positives).

Do the 2 definitive tests:

1) Digital rectal exam to palpate the prostate: A smooth, rubbery, and symmetrical gland is normal, while a hard, irregular, and asymmetrical gland is suggestive of malignancy.

2) Urinalysis to assess for hematuria (with a culture if infection is suspected)

The American Urologic Association (AUA) does not recommend serum PSA or serum creatinine in the workup of BPH whereas the European Urologic Association does. Experts in the U.S. go either way.

TREATMENT

Treat BPH only if it significantly affects the patient adversely and/or if it causes outlet obstruction that leads to hydronephrosis or acute kidney injury.

Start treatment of symptomatic patients with behavioral therapy. Make sure patients know to reduce the intake of caffeine and alcohol (diuretics), stay away from fluids before bed, and attempt to urinate twice to completely empty the bladder.

Medical therapy:

- 1st line: alpha-blocker (i.e., terazosin, doxazosin, tamsulosin, alfuzosin, silodosin)
- Add a 5-alpha-reductase inhibitor (finasteride or dutasteride) if needed.

The most common side effects of these medications are postural hypotension and lightheadedness. Be careful about combining sildenafil or vardenafil with these drugs because the combination worsens hypotension.

The 5-alpha-reductase inhibitors, which inhibit conversion of testosterone to dihydrotestosterone, take at least 6 months to decrease prostate size and relieve symptoms. These drugs work better for large prostates and have a more durable effect. The major side effect is impairment of sexual function (decreased libido and delayed ejaculation). Finasteride, a type of 5-alpha-reductase inhibitor, can decrease microvessel density in the prostate, especially the suburethral prostate because it reduces episodes of recurrent hematuria in patients with BPH. 5-alpha-reductase inhibitors decrease serum PSA, even in cancer patients.

Transurethral resection of the prostate (TURP) is the treatment of last resort and is used when drugs fail to work.

ERECTILE DYSFUNCTION

PREVIEW | REVIEW

- What percentage of males by age group experience ED?
- What is the most common cause of neurogenic ED?
- Which medications most commonly cause ED?
- If an exam presents a young male with ED who is on no medications, what is the most likely etiology?
- What is the mechanism of action for sildenafil?

OVERVIEW

The most common type of male sexual dysfunction is **erectile dysfunction (ED)**, which is defined as the inability to achieve or maintain an erection sufficient for satisfactory sexual intercourse. It is not uncommon for men to experience brief episodes of ED, often secondary to stress, anxiety, or alcohol. However, true ED caused by a physiologic problem typically causes a gradual decrease in function over time. There is a strong age-related increase in problems with erection in men > 50 years of age: 2% of men < 40 years of age complain of frequent problems with erections, while 40–50% of men > 60 years of age may have significant problems with erections.

The smooth muscle in the flaccid penis is in a state of tonus or contraction due to alpha stimulation by norepinephrine. Cyclic guanosine monophosphate (cGMP) and cyclic adenosine monophosphate (cAMP) are made by the norepinephrine and vasoactive intestinal peptide (VIP) pathways. This cGMP causes the relaxation of the smooth muscle in the penis, which increases the inflow through the helicine artery into the erectile tissue. The swelling of this tissue causes compression of the outflow venules, resulting in a sustained erection.

Men with ED have problems with this pathway. Atherosclerosis can lead to a decrease in blood flow through the helicine artery, preventing venous compression and, therefore, an erection. Nerve damage from a stroke, spinal cord injury, or diabetes can also prevent relaxation of the smooth muscle of the penis, leading to ED.

Many men with ED can have low self-esteem and depression and may fear or avoid future sexual encounters, resulting in decreased sexual satisfaction and reduced sexual desire in the individual's partner. Risk factors for acquired erectile disorder include age, smoking tobacco, lack of physical exercise, diabetes, and decreased desire. Associated factors include neurotic and submissive personality traits, depression, and PTSD.

Erectile failure on first sexual attempt has been found to be related to having sex with a previously unknown partner, concomitant use of drugs or alcohol, not wanting to have sex, or peer pressure. There is minimal evidence regarding the persistence of erectile failure after the first attempt.

The natural history of lifelong erectile disorder is unknown. Most episodes of ED remit spontaneously without professional intervention, but some men may continue to have episodic problems. In contrast, acquired erectile disorder is often associated with an organic cause (e.g., vascular disease), and persists.

CLASSIC CAUSES OF ED

ED can be caused by organic or psychological problems, or a side effect of medications (25% of cases). Most causes of ED are at least partially organic.

Causes of ED:

- **Organic**: The organic causes are neurogenic, vascular, hormonal, and normal aging. Onset is usually slow, and they present with loss of nocturnal and morning erections.
  - **Neurogenic**: The most common neurogenic cause of ED is diabetes mellitus. Other causes are surgical procedures (especially prostate), MS (multiple sclerosis), ALS (amyotrophic lateral sclerosis), Parkinson's, and other causes of peripheral neuropathy. Cyclists who spend > 3 hours/week on an upright bicycle can experience ED due to pressure that the seat places on the pudendal nerves (reducing blood flow to the cavernosal artery).
  - **Vascular**: The most common vascular cause is peripheral arterial disease. Those with diabetes can also have vascular damage, compromising blood flow. Other causes are surgical procedures, inflammatory conditions, or pelvic fracture. In elderly men, ED is caused by vascular compromise in 50% (indicated by a low penile brachial pressure index [PBPI]). ED due to vascular compromise indicates increased risk of present and future major vascular disease.
  - **Hormonal**: often accompanied by a loss of libido. Symptoms can include a gradual onset of frontal headaches or visual disturbances (space-occupying tumor); hot flashes and a decreased need for shaving (decreased androgens); fatigue + weight gain + dry skin + constipation (hypothyroidism).
  - **Normal aging**: Sexual potency does decrease with age.
- **Psychological**: typically, acute onset. This is the most common cause of ED in younger patients. They continue to have nocturnal and morning erections, but libido is lost. ED is directly correlated with depression. Unfortunately, SSRIs used for the treatment of depression are also associated with a very high incidence of sexual dysfunction (generally delayed ejaculation).

- **Medications:** especially antidepressants (e.g., SSRIs), clonidine, spironolactone, beta-blockers, and thiazide diuretics. Tricyclics (TCAs), MAOIs, benzodiazepines, antipsychotics, antihistamines, antihypertensives, diuretics, NSAIDs, and finasteride can also cause ED.
- **Drugs of abuse:** nicotine (85% more common in smokers), alcohol, cocaine, opiates

DIAGNOSIS

Perform a thorough physical examination (rule out hernia). Blood tests include:

- Serum chemistry
- CBC
- LFTs
- Lipid profile
- Hemoglobin A1c
- Urine toxicology
- Testosterone
- TSH
- LH
- FSH
- PRL
- PSA
- U/A

Diagnostic tests include:

- Duplex ultrasound
- Penile nerve function
- Nocturnal penile tumescence (NPT)
- Penile biothesiometry
- Dynamic infusion cavernosometry and cavernosography (DICC)
- Corpus cavernosometry
- Magnetic resonance angiography (MRA)

TREATMENT OPTIONS

1st line treatment for ED:

- **Sildenafil citrate** (Revatio, Viagra) inhibits phosphodiesterase Type 5 (PDE5), an enzyme that inactivates cGMP. It works very well for many causes of ED, including psychogenic. Side effects are due to its vasodilatory properties—headaches, flushing, dyspepsia, bluish hue in the vision. Reports of sudden onset sensorineural hearing loss have also been documented.
- **Vardenafil** (Levitra, Staxyn) is similar to sildenafil in mechanism, effectiveness, and side effects.
- **Tadalafil** (Adcirca, Cialis) has the same mechanism of action as sildenafil and vardenafil but with a longer half-life. Erectile function may be improved for up to 36 hours. This drug is approved for daily use. One specific side effect is back pain. Tadalafil is FDA approved as a treatment for BPH symptoms when used on a daily basis, although the mechanism remains unclear.
- **Avanafil** is similar to sildenafil in mechanism, effectiveness, and side effects.
- **PDE5 inhibitors** are more likely to cause hypotension when taken with nonselective alpha-blockers (prazosin, doxazosin, and terazosin). Uroselective

alpha-blockers (tamsulosin and alfuzosin) are less likely to cause hypotension. There is a risk of hearing loss with all the PDE5 inhibitors. Contraindications are any concurrent nitrates. Relative contraindications are heart failure, hypotension, unstable angina, hypertensive cardiomyopathy (HCM), and severe aortic stenosis.

- **Yohimbine** is a naturally occurring alpha-blocker. It has minimal effect, but, because it is inexpensive and has minimal side effects, it is often tried on patients with a mostly psychogenic etiology. It is better than a placebo but much less effective than sildenafil.
- **Vacuum devices** work well but are clumsy to use. They are indicated only when oral therapy is contraindicated or the patient prefers them to oral therapy.

2nd line treatment for ED:

- **Alprostadil** (prostaglandin E_1) injected into the corpora cavernosa of the penis works well. It is especially useful in patients with ED due to neurologic dysfunction.

3rd line treatment for ED:

- **Penile implants**: There are various types—hydraulic, semirigid, and flexible rods. This option is normally used only for those who have failed all other therapy. The surgery can cause complications, and there is a risk of postsurgical infection. Scarring can cause erections to curve. Tissue erosion can occur. If there are no complications, penile implants are effective and patient satisfaction rates are high.
- **CBT** (individual and couples therapy) can also be beneficial.

SCROTAL MASSES (NONCANCEROUS)

PREVIEW | REVIEW

- How does ultrasound help in the diagnosis of testicular torsion?
- If surgery is done within 6 hours of symptom onset of testicular torsion, what is the success rate in salvaging the testicle?
- What are common ultrasound findings in epididymitis?
- What are common causes of acute epididymitis in younger men?
- How is acute epididymitis treated empirically?
- How does a hydrocele develop?
- On which side do most varicoceles develop?

OVERVIEW

Scrotal masses vary in origin from benign causes to surgical emergencies. We'll discuss scrotal masses of nonmalignant origin. (See Oncology, Book 3, for testicular cancer.) The anatomy of the scrotum is described in Figure 11-2. See Table 11-5 for a summary of scrotal masses. Figure 11-3 on page 11-26 summarizes the evaluation of a scrotal mass.

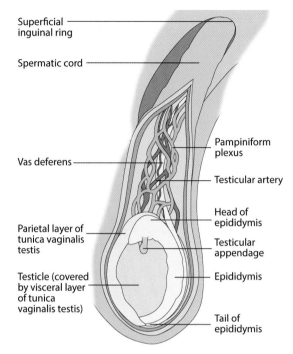

Figure 11-2: Anatomy of the scrotum

History and examination are very useful in evaluating scrotal masses. An initial assessment of pain is important. Painful masses suggest more emergent problems, such as testicular torsion or epididymitis.

TESTICULAR TORSION

Testicular torsion occurs when there is twisting of the spermatic cord within the tunica vaginalis and subsequent occlusion of the arterial blood supply to the testicle. It most commonly occurs in adolescent boys but can occur in older men as well. Torsion can lead to testicular loss (due to ischemia), within about 6 hours if not corrected surgically.

Presenting symptoms are scrotal pain, nausea, and vomiting. The most accurate sign of testicular torsion is an absent ipsilateral cremasteric reflex—a reflex observed in males when stroking the inner part of the thigh results in contraction of the cremaster muscle that pulls up the testis ipsilaterally. Other signs on examination include fever, swelling of the scrotum, and a testicle that is positioned horizontally or riding higher than normal.

Patients with a suggestion of testicular torsion warrant emergent urologic evaluation and surgical exploration. Doppler ultrasound may assist the diagnosis by demonstrating absent testicular blood flow. Time is of the essence; there is a 90% salvage rate if surgery is done

Table 11-5: Summary of Scrotal Masses			
Cause	**Presentation**	**Diagnosis**	**Treatment**
Testicular torsion	Pain and swelling Possible absent cremasteric reflex Horizontal or high position of the testicle Nausea/Vomiting Fever	Clinical, with Doppler ultrasound	Orchiopexy within 6 hours, manual detorsion if surgery unavailable Bilateral orchiopexy is recommended because the contralateral testis is at risk for torsion.
Epididymitis/Epididymo-orchitis	Acute unilateral pain and swelling	Clinical, with Doppler ultrasound	Ceftriaxone and doxycycline; consider adding fluoroquinolone
Testicular appendage torsion	Acute unilateral pain Blue dot sign	Ultrasound	Pain control
Hematocele	History of trauma Pain and swelling	Ultrasound or surgical exploration	Pain control; surgery if needed
Testicular cancer	Firm, unilateral nodule	Ultrasound, tumor markers	Surgery
Inguinal hernias	Pain with bending, lifting, coughing, or straining Pain and scrotal bulge with Valsalva maneuvers	Physical examination, ultrasound	Surgery
Hydrocele	Painless scrotal swelling (Unless very large; these present with painful scrotal swelling and lower back pain.)	Transillumination, ultrasound	Watchful waiting, hydrocelectomy and aspiration, pain control
Varicocele	Dilation of tortuous spermatic veins, which look like a "bag of worms"	Ultrasound	Observation, surgery, or embolization

within 6 hours, which drops to 50% if surgery is not performed within 12 hours of symptoms.

If surgery is not an option, attempt manual detorsion. With torsion, the testicles usually twist medially so you typically must twist laterally to achieve detorsion. For example, when detorsing the patient's left testicle, stand in front of the patient. Using the right forefinger and thumb, rotate the testicle clockwise 180° at a time. Repeat as needed. It may take up to 4 tries because the torsion can have rotations up to 720°. Successful detorsion is made evident by immediate pain relief. Detorsing the patient's right testicle requires counter-clockwise rotation. Follow up with ultrasound to ensure good vascular flow. Surgery is still required to ensure full detorsion and for bilateral testicular fixation. Keep in mind that intermittent torsion of the testicle may occur and also requires urologic evaluation.

Torsion of the testicular appendage may occur. Examination reveals the "blue dot sign," a bluish hue from the ischemic appendage. Finally, the torsion of the appendix epididymis may occur as well.

EPIDIDYMITIS

Epididymitis occurs when there is pain and inflammation of the epididymis. Orchitis is an inflammation of the testes, and it can be related to epididymitis infection that has spread to the testicles. If both the epididymis and testicles are affected, it is called epididymoorchitis.

Presenting symptoms are similar to testicular torsion. Patients present with acute onset, unilateral scrotal pain and erythema. Physical examination reveals localized tenderness and swelling of the affected testicle. If severe, patients can present with fever, scrotal wall erythema, and a reactive hydrocele.

Ultrasound can help differentiate epididymitis from testicular torsion. Epididymal swelling and hyperemia suggest epididymitis. Color Doppler ultrasound shows absent blood flow with testicular torsion (see previous topic), and increased vascularity of the epididymis with epididymitis.

Urology consultation is often helpful, especially if the diagnosis is uncertain.

Acute epididymitis lasts < 6 weeks and frequently coexists with urethritis (which may be asymptomatic). Chronic epididymitis lasts > 6 weeks.

In younger men, acute epididymitis commonly results from sexually transmitted infections caused by *Chlamydia trachomatis* or *Neisseria gonorrhoeae*. Men who engage in anal intercourse (as the insertive partner) may develop acute epididymitis caused by enteric organisms such as *E. coli* and *Pseudomonas* species. As men age, urinary outflow obstructive disease (e.g., benign prostatic hyperplasia) with bacteriuria may result in acute epididymitis. Other etiologies of epididymitis include immunosuppression, surgery, and systemic illness

TB may lead to chronic epididymitis with granuloma formation, which can be bilateral. Consider TB as the cause in men with a history of TB exposure.

Gram stain of urethral secretions can demonstrate leukocytes in epididymitis, and if *N. gonorrhoeae* is the cause, intracellular gram-negative diplococci may be present. Perform further testing with culture, nucleic acid hybridization, and amplification testing of urine and/or urethral swabs to isolate chlamydial and gonorrheal infection.

Epididymitis is generally self-limiting and heals without complications with analgesics and rest in prepubertal boys. Treat epididymitis empirically with ceftriaxone and doxycycline, and if enteric organisms are causative, consider adding fluoroquinolone. Tailor treatment depending on culture results. In addition to antibiotics, supportive

therapy includes reduction in physical activity, scrotal support and elevation, NSAIDs/analgesics, sitz baths, and ice packs.

Refer sexual partners for evaluation. Epididymitis in the setting of HIV expands the differential diagnosis to include CMV, *Salmonella*, *Toxoplasma gondii*, *Ureaplasma urealyticum*, *Corynebacterium* species, *Mycoplasma* species, and *Acinetobacter lwoffii* (formerly *Mima polymorpha*).

INGUINAL HERNIA

Inguinal hernia is an extremely common disorder that occurs when fat or intestine displace through the inguinal canal (indirect) or when there is a weak area or tear in the abdominal wall (direct). Primary symptoms are pain with bending, lifting, coughing, or straining. Inguinal hernias may lead to scrotal masses that are visible and may

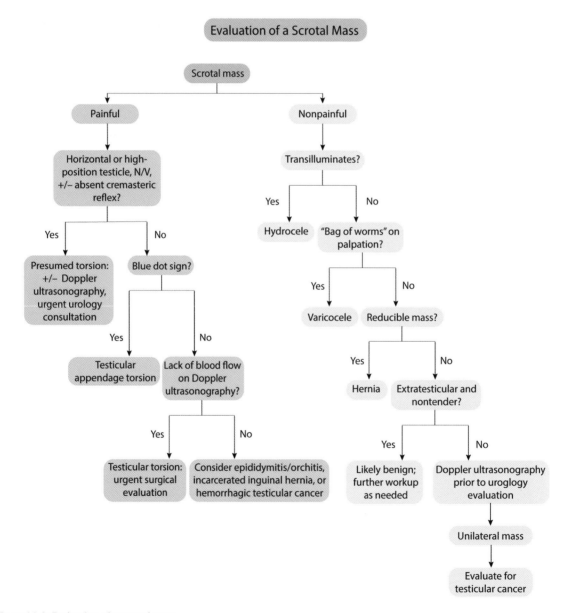

Figure 11-3: Evaluation of a scrotal mass

increase in size with Valsalva maneuver. If not obvious, a hernia may be palpated by placing a finger through the scrotal sac to the inguinal canal and having the patient cough. Generally, treat symptomatic hernias surgically.

HYDROCELE

Hydrocele results from accumulation of serous fluid between the layers of the tunica vaginalis surrounding the testicle (Figure 11-4). Patients typically present with painless swelling of the groin or scrotum on one or both sides. (Larger hydroceles may cause scrotal or lower back pain).

Hydrocele may result from infection, trauma, and neoplasm. Inguinal hernias may also be contributory.

Diagnose a hydrocele clinically, using transillumination. Hydroceles transilluminate well, unlike hematoceles, hernias, or solid masses.

Classic presentation is a tense, painless, fluid-filled swelling in the scrotum/groin that easily transilluminates. Use ultrasonography if palpation and transillumination are inconclusive.

Surgical exploration is warranted if any of the following signs or symptoms exist:

- Inability to clearly delineate or palpate the testicular structure
- Tenderness, fever, or any gastrointestinal symptoms
- Shadows on transillumination

Treatment includes watchful waiting, hydrocelectomy, aspiration (if necessary), and pain control if the hydrocele is large. Hydroceles may recur.

HEMATOCELE

Hematocele is a collection of blood outside of the testicle but within the tunica vaginalis. It can appear similar to a hydrocele; however, it does not transilluminate, differentiating the two conditions. Furthermore, a hematocele is typically caused by trauma or surgery. It results in pain and swelling of the testicle. Larger hematoceles can cause distortion of the testis and may resemble malignancy. Ultrasound and MRI are useful in diagnosis. Treatment includes surgery and pain control.

VARICOCELE

A varicocele is an abnormal dilation of the spermatic veins due to an anatomical abnormality. Malfunctioning vein valves result in retrograde flow of blood into the scrotum, leading to tortuous spermatic veins. See Figure 11-5 on page 11-28 for the difference between normal and tortuous spermatic veins.

A patient with a varicocele will present with complaints of dull, aching pain in the scrotum, typically on the left side. Diagnose varicoceles clinically. The scrotum will

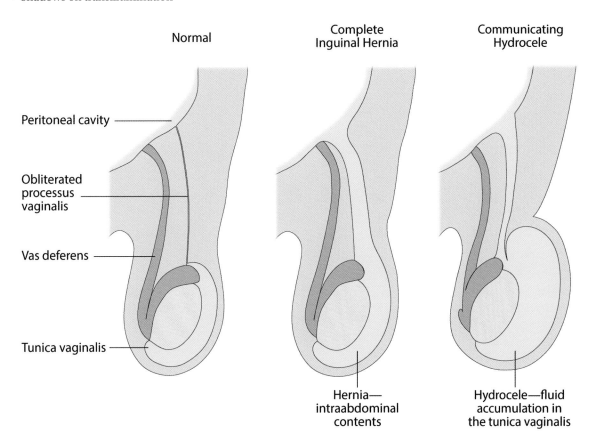

| Normal | Complete Inguinal Hernia | Communicating Hydrocele |

Peritoneal cavity

Obliterated processus vaginalis

Vas deferens

Tunica vaginalis

Hernia— intraabdominal contents

Hydrocele—fluid accumulation in the tunica vaginalis

Figure 11-4: Inguinal hernia vs. communicating hydrocele

feel like "a bag of worms" on palpation. Diagnosis can be confirmed with ultrasound.

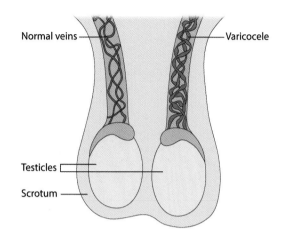

Figure 11-5: Left varicocele

Varicoceles are also a common, often reversible, cause of male infertility. Treatment options include observation, surgery, and embolization, depending on the suspected impact of the varicocele upon male fertility, the patient's age, and overall health.

SEXUAL HEALTH CONCERNS FOR WOMEN AND MEN

SEXUAL DYSFUNCTIONS

PREVIEW | REVIEW

- Which class of commonly used antidepressants can lead to sexual dysfunction in men and women?
- What mechanism of contraception can lead to sexual dysfunction in women?
- Know the prevalence of sexual dysfunctions by age and type.

OVERVIEW

Sexual dysfunctions are a heterogeneous group of disorders characterized by a clinically significant disturbance in a person's ability to respond sexually or to experience sexual pleasure. An individual can have several sexual dysfunctions at the same time. It is important to diagnose and treat properly.

Table 11-6: Female Sexual Dysfunctions			
	Female Sexual Interest / Arousal Disorder	Female Orgasmic Disorder	Genito-Pelvic Pain / Penetration Disorder	Substance- / Medication-Induced Sexual Dysfunction
Definition	Persistent or recurrent deficiency of sexual desire, aversion to sexual activity, or inability to complete sexual activity with adequate lubrication	Persistent or recurrent delay or absence of orgasm	Persistent or recurrent pain during intercourse and/or fear or anxiety regarding pain during intercourse	Persistent or recurrent disturbance in sexual function secondary to an exogenous substance, a medication, or withdrawal from that substance or medication
Prevalence	10–19%	3–6%	8–22%	Unknown
Etiology	Stress Anxiety or depression Relationship issues Medication use (i.e., SSRIs, OCPs)	Stress Anxiety or depression Relationship issues Medication use (i.e., SSRIs, OCPs)	Physical conditions (numerous—e.g., endometriosis, vulvodynia, pelvic adhesions) Vaginismus Sexual abuse history	Alcohol or other sedatives Opioids Anxiolytics Stimulants
Diagnosis	Based on history	Based on history	Based on history, physical examination, and/or pelvic ultrasound	Urine or blood toxicology screen
Treatment	Stop SSRIs or OCPs Sex or couples therapy Individual therapy Flibanserin (only FDA-approved treatment for premenopausal women with female sexual interest/ arousal disorder) Testosterone (used off-label) Bupropion (used off-label)	Stop SSRIs or OCPs Sex or couples therapy Individual therapy	Varies depending on etiology (broad)	Discontinue substance in question

OCPs = oral contraceptive pills; SSRIs = selective serotonin reuptake inhibitors

DIAGNOSTIC FEATURES

Sexual dysfunctions cause significant distress for at least 6 months and are not better explained by nonsexual mental disorder, severe relationship distress, substances, or another medical condition. They are either lifelong (since the start of sexual activity) or acquired (start after period of normal sexual activity). Sexual dysfunction is either generalized (not limited to certain situations) or situational (only occurs with certain types of stimulation, situations, or partners).

Sexual dysfunctions for women and men include those listed in Table 11-6 and Table 11-7, respectively.

INFERTILITY

PREVIEW | REVIEW

- When should an infertility workup be considered?
- How can you tell if a woman is ovulatory?
- What lifestyle modifications have been shown to improve pregnancy rates among patients with infertility?

Infertility has many potential causes, and for many couples, both male and female factors are present. Causes of female infertility include both endocrine disorders (e.g., prolactinoma, primary amenorrhea, PCOS, congenital adrenal hyperplasia [CAH]) and gynecologic causes (e.g., endometriosis, tubal obstruction and other fallopian tube abnormalities, pelvic adhesions). Male infertility

	Male Hypoactive Sexual Desire Disorder	**Erectile Disorder**	**Premature Ejaculation**	**Delayed Ejaculation**	**Substance- / Medication-Induced Sexual Dysfunction**
Definition	Persistently or recurrently deficient/absent sexual/erotic thoughts or fantasies and desire for sexual activity	Difficulty obtaining or maintaining adequate erection during sexual activity	Persistent or recurrent pattern of ejaculation occurring during partnered sexual activity within 1 minute following vaginal penetration	Marked delay, infrequency, or absence of ejaculation	Persistent or recurrent disturbance in sexual function secondary to an exogenous substance, a medication, or withdrawal from that substance or medication
Prevalence	6% age 18–24, 41% age 66–74	10–25%	20–30%	1%	Unknown
Etiology	Stress Anxiety or depression Relationship issues Medication use (i.e., SSRIs) Low testosterone	Vascular disease Neurogenic etiologies (e.g., diabetes, stroke) Low testosterone	Stress Anxiety or depression Prior sexual abuse Prostatitis	Neurologic disorders Stress Anxiety or depression Prostate surgery Medication use (i.e., SSRIs, alpha-blockers)	Alcohol or other sedatives Opioids Anxiolytics Stimulants
Diagnosis	Based on history Testosterone level	Based on history CBC, CMP, A1c hepatic panel for cardiovascular, atherosclerotic, renal, and liver disease	Based on history Urinalysis	History Neurologic examination	Urine or blood toxicology screen
Treatment	Stop SSRI Sex or couples therapy Individual therapy Testosterone replacement	Treat medical issues Sex or couples therapy Individual therapy Phosphodiesterase inhibitors Alprostadil Penile prosthesis/ vacuum pump devices	SSRIs Local anesthetics Individual therapy	Stop SSRIs Stop alpha-blockers if possible Individual therapy	Discontinue substance in question

SSRIs = selective serotonin reuptake inhibitors

can also be caused by endocrine disorders (e.g., prolactinoma, CAH, other causes of secondary hypogonadism), but the majority are due to primary (testicular) defects in sperm production.

An infertility workup for a couple can start when a couple fails to conceive after 1 year of frequent, unprotected intercourse (6 months if the woman is > 35 years of age because time is running out!). Evaluate the woman and man simultaneously when possible. Initial workup includes:

• Semen analysis (for sperm count, motility, and morphology)
• Assessment of ovulation: Women with regular menstrual cycles are likely to be ovulatory, and ovulation can be confirmed with a serum progesterone level on day 21 of the menstrual cycle. Women with irregular cycles should have a progesterone drawn 7 days before their presumed menses, and then drawn weekly until menstruation occurs.
• Hysterosalpingogram to assess the patency of fallopian tubes and integrity of the uterus
• Assessment of ovarian reserve with biochemical testing, such as FSH and estradiol on day 3 of the menstrual cycle, and/or anti-Müllerian hormone levels.

Counsel all patients, both men and women, with infertility on the following lifestyle modifications:

• Stop smoking.
• Limit or stop alcohol consumption.
• Reduce BMI to between 18.5 and 29.9, or ideally between 18.5 and 24.9

All patients with infertility should be referred to an obstetrician-gynecologist or reproductive endocrinology specialist. If abnormalities are detected on the above testing, refer the patient(s) directly to a reproductive endocrinologist. Treatment of infertility depends on the cause but can include medications to induce ovulation, metformin (for PCOS), surgical procedures to fix fallopian tube obstruction, and assisted reproductive technologies (e.g., *in vitro* fertilization).

THE MEDSTUDY HUB: YOUR GUIDELINES AND REVIEW ARTICLES RESOURCE

For both review articles and current internal medicine practice guidelines, visit the MedStudy Hub at

medstudy.com/hub

The Hub contains the only online consolidated list of all current guidelines focused on internal medicine. Guidelines on the Hub are easy to find, continually updated, and linked to the published source. MedStudy maintains the Hub as a service to the medical community and makes it available to anyone and everyone at no cost to users.

MedStudy

Neurology

SECTION EDITOR

Nicholas J. Silvestri, MD
Associate Professor of Clinical Neurology
University at Buffalo Jacobs School of
  Medicine and Biomedical Sciences
Buffalo, NY

REVIEWER

J. Chad Hoyle, MD
Associate Professor of Neurology
Residency Director, Department of Neurology
Director of Medical Education (Neurology,
  Psychiatry, and IM Clerkship Ring)
The Ohio State University
Columbus, OH

MEDICAL EDITOR

Theresa A. Buck, MD
Department of Veterans Affairs
Pulmonary/Critical Care
Bay Pines, FL

Table of Contents

CENTRAL NERVOUS SYSTEM:
Brain — Cortex

COMA...12-1
  OVERVIEW 12-1
  APPROACH TO COMA................................12-1
    Neurologic Exam Findings...........................12-1
    Workup...12-2
    Evaluation of Findings.................................12-2

COMA MIMICS 12-3
  LOCKED-IN SYNDROME.............................12-3
  VEGETATIVE STATE 12-3
  AKINETIC MUTISM......................................12-4
  CATATONIA 12-4
  BRAIN DEATH 12-4

SEIZURES 12-4
  OVERVIEW 12-5
  SEIZURE CLASSIFICATION 12-5
  SEIZURE EXAMPLES 12-6
  PSYCHOGENIC NONEPILEPTIC SEIZURES 12-6
  SEIZURE AURA 12-6
  SEIZURE MANAGEMENT 12-7
    History...12-7
    Scans and Lab...12-7
    Acute Treatment of Seizures 12-7
    Chronic Treatment of Seizures....................12-7
    Drug Interactions with AEDs.......................12-8
    Treatment of Seizures During Pregnancy.........12-9

DEMENTIA 12-9
  DEFINITION..12-10
  WORKUP 12-10
    Diagnosis of Dementia 12-10
    Mild Cognitive Impairment 12-10
    Reversible Causes 12-10
  SPECIFIC CAUSES OF DEMENTIA 12-11
    Normal Pressure Hydrocephalus.................12-11
    Alzheimer Disease.......................................12-11
    Vascular Dementia 12-12
    Frontotemporal Dementia...........................12-12
    Creutzfeldt-Jakob Disease...........................12-12
    Parkinson Disease Dementia.......................12-13
    Progressive Supranuclear Palsy 12-14
    Huntington Disease......................................12-14
    AIDS...12-14
    Depression..12-14

DELIRIUM..12-14

CNS: Brain — Subcortex

DEMYELINATING DISEASES.........................12-15
  MULTIPLE SCLEROSIS 12-15
    Overview...12-15
    Clinical Manifestations of MS......................12-15
    Diagnosis of MS 12-16
    Treatment of MS...12-16
  PROGRESSIVE MULTIFOCAL
    LEUKOENCEPHALOPATHY......................12-17
  OSMOTIC DEMYELINATION SYNDROME.......12-17

MOVEMENT DISORDERS.............................12-17
  PARKINSONISM.......................................12-17

PARKINSON DISEASE 12-18
  Overview...12-18
  Diagnosis..12-18
  Treatment..12-18
PROGRESSIVE SUPRANUCLEAR PALSY..........12-19
TREMORS..12-19
  Overview...12-19
  Exaggerated Physiologic Tremor 12-20
  Essential Tremor......................................12-20
TARDIVE DYSKINESIA 12-20
OTHER MOVEMENT DISORDERS 12-20
  Neuroleptic Malignant Syndrome...............12-20
  Hemifacial Spasm....................................12-20
  Tourette Syndrome...................................12-20
  Focal Dystonias.......................................12-21

CNS: Brain — Ventricles / CSF

INFECTIONS 12-21
  BACTERIAL CNS INFECTIONS.....................12-21
    Acute Meningitis 12-21
    Brain Abscess 12-21
  VIRAL CNS INFECTIONS 12-21
    CSF in Viral Encephalitis 12-21
    Herpes Simplex Encephalitis 12-21
    Mosquito-Borne Arboviruses......................12-22
    Diagnosis of Viral Encephalitis....................12-22
    Viral Myelitis 12-22
    Slow Viruses and Prions.............................12-22
    HIV 12-22
    Progressive Multifocal
      Leukoencephalopathy..............................12-23
    AIDS Myelopathy..12-23
  PARASITIC CNS INFECTIONS......................12-23
    Toxoplasmosis...12-23
    Neurocysticercosis......................................12-23
  FUNGAL CNS INFECTION 12-23

HEADACHE AND FACIAL PAIN.......................12-24
  OVERVIEW 12-24
  MIGRAINE...12-24
    Presentation...12-24
    Diagnosis of Migraine 12-25
    Acute Treatment of Migraine 12-25
    Prophylactic Treatment of Migraine............12-26
  CLUSTER HEADACHE..................................12-26
  TENSION HEADACHE 12-26
  BENIGN SEXUAL HEADACHE 12-27
  CONCUSSION 12-27
  POSTTRAUMATIC HEADACHE.....................12-27
  GIANT CELL ARTERITIS..............................12-27
  TRIGEMINAL NEURALGIA..........................12-28
  IDIOPATHIC INTRACRANIAL HYPERTENSION
    / PSEUDOTUMOR CEREBRI......................12-28

CNS: Brain — Cortex,
Subcortex, and Brainstem

STROKE AND TIA...12-28
  OVERVIEW 12-29
  TIA..12-29
  COMPLICATIONS OF TIA 12-29
  CLASSIFICATION OF STROKES 12-30
  PRIMARY PREVENTION OF STROKE
    AND TIA..12-30

IMAGING OF STROKES.............................. 12-30
ISCHEMIC STROKES 12-31
   Thrombotic vs. Embolic Strokes.................. 12-31
   Anterior Circulation............................. 12-31
   Posterior Circulation............................ 12-32
   Lacunar Infarcts 12-33
   Evaluation of Ischemic Stroke.................... 12-33
   Acute Treatment of Ischemic Stroke............. 12-34
   Chronic Treatment of Ischemic Stroke 12-35
   Cerebral Venous Thrombosis 12-35
CEREBRAL HEMORRHAGE........................ 12-36
   Overview...................................... 12-36
   Intracerebral Hemorrhage....................... 12-36
   Subarachnoid Hemorrhage...................... 12-37
   Cocaine Use 12-38
   Subdural Hematoma............................ 12-38
   Epidural Hematoma............................ 12-38
TRANSIENT GLOBAL AMNESIA —
   STROKE AND TIA MIMIC 12-38

CNS: Spinal Cord

MYELOPATHIES...................................... 12-39
   OVERVIEW 12-39
   METABOLIC MYELOPATHY —
   SUBACUTE COMBINED DEGENERATION
   OF SPINAL CORD................................ 12-39
   INFECTIOUS MYELOPATHIES 12-39
   AIDS... 12-39
   Epidural Abscess................................ 12-40
   Tuberculosis 12-40
   Syphilis 12-40
   INFLAMMATORY MYELOPATHY —
   TRANSVERSE MYELITIS........................... 12-40
COMPRESSION-INDUCED MYELOPATHIES 12-41
   Cervical Spondylosis with Myelopathy 12-41
   Thoracic Myelopathy 12-41
   Lumbosacral Myelopathy 12-41
MISCELLANEOUS MYELOPATHIES................ 12-42
   Ischemic Myelopathy 12-42
   Syringomyelia 12-42
   Anterior Horn Cell Disorders.................... 12-42

PERIPHERAL NERVOUS SYSTEM

RADICULOPATHIES................................... 12-42

NEUROPATHIES...................................... 12-43
   OVERVIEW 12-43
   MONONEUROPATHIES 12-43
   Focal / Compressive 12-43
   Mononeuritis Multiplex.......................... 12-44
   Bell's and Other Facial Nerve Palsies............ 12-45
   Diabetic Mononeuropathies 12-45
   POLYNEUROPATHIES.............................. 12-45
   Demyelinating vs. Axonal Polyneuropathies... 12-45
   Autoimmune, Inflammatory Polyneuropathies
   — Guillain-Barré Syndrome 12-45
   Chronic Inflammatory
   Demyelinating Polyneuropathy................. 12-46
   Charcot-Marie-Tooth Disease.................... 12-46
   Diabetic Peripheral Neuropathy................. 12-47
   Alcoholic Peripheral Neuropathy................. 12-47
   Other Causes of Axonal Neuropathies.......... 12-47
   Time of Onset.................................. 12-47

NEUROMUSCULAR JUNCTION

DISEASES OF THE NEUROMUSCULAR
   JUNCTION.................................. 12-47
   MYASTHENIA GRAVIS................................. 12-47
   LAMBERT-EATON MYASTHENIC
   SYNDROME.. 12-48

MUSCLE

MYOPATHIES.. 12-49
   NOTE 12-49
   INFLAMMATORY MYOPATHIES.................. 12-49
   ENDOCRINE MYOPATHIES....................... 12-49
   METABOLIC MYOPATHIES 12-49
   MUSCULAR DYSTROPHIES 12-49
   AIDS-RELATED MYOPATHY....................... 12-50

MISCELLANEOUS DISORDERS

CNS TUMORS... 12-50
   BRAIN TUMORS 12-50
   SPINAL CORD TUMORS......................... 12-50

CNS METASTASES...................................... 12-51

METABOLIC AND TOXIC DISORDERS.............. 12-51
   WERNICKE'S / KORSAKOFF'S 12-51
   LITHIUM TOXICITY............................... 12-52
   ANTICHOLINERGIC TOXICITY..................... 12-52

NARCOLEPSY... 12-52

VISUAL DISORDERS..................................... 12-52
   ACUTE-ONSET UNILATERAL BLINDNESS....... 12-52
   DIPLOPIA 12-53
   VISUAL FIELD DEFECTS........................... 12-53
   Scotomas...................................... 12-53
   Hemianopia and Quadrantanopia................ 12-53

NYSTAGMUS... 12-54

DIZZINESS / VERTIGO................................... 12-54
   SIGNS AND SYMPTOMS 12-54
   CAUSES OF VERTIGO............................. 12-55
   Benign Paroxysmal Positional Vertigo........... 12-55
   Vestibular Neuritis 12-55
   Aminoglycoside Toxicity 12-55
   Ménière Disease................................ 12-55
   Vertebrobasilar TIAs or Stroke................... 12-55

TINNITUS 12-56

NEUROMA... 12-56

COMPLEX REGIONAL PAIN SYNDROME.......... 12-56

THE MEDSTUDY HUB: YOUR GUIDELINES
   AND REVIEW ARTICLES RESOURCE.............. 12-56

CENTRAL NERVOUS SYSTEM: BRAIN — CORTEX

COMA

PREVIEW | REVIEW

- Which pupil finding can be seen with uncal herniation?
- What is the significance of doll's eyes?

OVERVIEW

Lethargy, confusion, stupor, obtundation, and coma are terms that apply to different degrees of the level of alteration of consciousness. The reticular activating system (RAS) and at least one of the cerebral cortices must be working effectively to sustain normal consciousness.

The RAS resides principally within the brainstem, so injury to the brainstem, such as from a hemorrhage, basilar artery ischemic stroke, or structural herniation affecting the pons or midbrain, can cause coma. The RAS also sends projections to the thalamus and hypothalamus (with the thalamus also being a relay center of information for the cortex). Thus, bilateral dysfunction of these structures may also cause coma.

Finally, diffuse processes affecting both cerebral hemispheres are common causes of coma. Therefore, severe metabolic derangements, toxic exposures, infection, anoxic brain injury, extensive traumatic brain injury, extensive bilateral cortical lesions, and nonconvulsive status epilepticus (NCSE) all may present with coma.

APPROACH TO COMA

Neurologic Exam Findings

Overview

A thorough history and neurologic exam are necessary to establish the diagnosis and to ascertain the etiology of coma. This includes a review of underlying medical and mental health illnesses, medications, ingestions, and intoxications. Use the Glasgow Coma Scale to assess responsiveness of patients with cerebral trauma. However, using this scale to evaluate other etiologies of acute coma provides little insight into the localization of the anatomical dysfunction. A full comatose exam includes the following:

- Assessment of level of consciousness to see if there is any response to verbal or painful stimuli
- Cranial nerve exam (especially pupillary reaction, oculocephalic maneuver or cold caloric testing, corneal reflex, and gag reflex)
- Evaluation of motor responses, reflexes, and observation of respiration (including specific respiratory patterns or whether the patient is breathing over the ventilator)

Vital signs, including temperature, pulse, respiratory rate, and blood pressure, can provide clues to the diagnosis, as can evaluation for nuchal rigidity and motor tone. Focal exam findings imply a structural cause of coma, while a nonfocal exam is more suggestive of a toxic-metabolic etiology.

Motor Responses

Motor responses related to cortical function include grimacing, localization of pain stimulus, and withdrawal to pain. Lack of reactivity to pain in one extremity or asymmetrical response implies a focal weakness or sensory loss. Posturing responses such as decerebrate and decorticate are subcortical responses that can help to localize the site of injury:

- **Decerebrate posturing** is a type of rigidity that occurs when the tonic labyrinthine reflex, which resists gravitational force, acts without modulation of the higher brain, causing extension of all extremities.
  ◦ This posturing can be seen during either uncal or cerebellar tonsillar herniation. Uncal transtentorial; see Evaluation of Findings on page 12-2)
  ◦ Decerebrate posturing implies brainstem dysfunction or severe neurologic dysfunction and is a worse sign than decorticate posturing.
- **Decorticate posturing** is a type of rigidity characterized by flexion of upper limbs with extension of lower limbs. It is caused by lesions at a more rostral level of injury to both corticospinal and rubrospinal tracts resulting from damage to brain areas that can include the cerebral white matter, internal capsule, and thalamus. These are upper motor neuron lesions. Causes include anoxic or traumatic brain injury, stroke, intracranial hemorrhage, brain tumors, and encephalopathy.

With uncal herniation, patients can progress from decorticate to decerebrate posturing.

Respirations

Cheyne-Stokes respiration is a pattern of breathing in which the patient has periods of hyperventilation alternating with apnea. This pattern occurs in bilateral cerebral disease, impending herniation, and brainstem lesions; it can also be due to cardiac and metabolic causes.

Apneustic breathing is characterized by a series of slow, deep inspirations, each one held for 30 seconds or longer, after which the air is expelled by elastic recoil of the lungs, followed by an apneic pause. The rate of apneustic breathing is commonly around 1.5 breaths per minute. It is due to a lesion of the lower pons.

Ataxic breathing is very irregular and typically indicates a lesion of the medulla.

Central neurogenic hyperventilation: Lesions of the lower midbrain/upper pontine tegmentum cause

NEUROLOGY

central neurogenic hyperventilation, which produces an increase in the rate and depth of respiration, resulting in advanced respiratory alkalosis.

Note that many of these patterns may not be seen in comatose patients because they often will be intubated to protect the airway. Assessment of whether a patient is breathing over the ventilator provides useful information.

Pupils

Remember that any significant asymmetry between the sizes of the pupils must be considered pathologic (Table 12-1). Carefully assess light reactivity and perform funduscopic examination to exclude papilledema (a sign of increased intracranial pressure [ICP]).

Oculovestibular Testing

Oculocephalic (doll's eyes) and ice-water caloric testing (eyes look toward the cold) test the same vestibular-brainstem-ocular muscle pathway. The complete absence of eye movement in response to oculovestibular testing indicates either severe disruption of brainstem at the level of the pons or a profound overdose of sedative, anesthetic, or anticonvulsant drugs.

Doll's eyes:

- Definition: When the head is turned, the eyes keep "looking" in the initial direction (eyes do not follow the movement of the head). Doll's eyes (i.e., a positive oculocephalic reflex) in a comatose person indicates that the brainstem is working normally. Absent doll's eyes, similar to no eye movement with cold caloric testing, implies dysfunction of the brainstem at the level of the pons and is a poor prognostic indicator. Generally, doll's eyes are preserved in early metabolic coma. One exception is metabolic coma due to barbiturates.
- Test for doll's eyes, which requires moving the head, only after C-spine injury is ruled out.

Reduction or absence of spontaneous blinking and loss of corneal reflexes are signs of deepening coma or brainstem dysfunction along the blink reflex arc involving afferent input from cranial nerve 5 and bilateral efferent input from cranial nerve 7.

Workup

Quickly obtain a CT or MRI of the brain to narrow the differential, especially when the cause is unclear.

In your workup, include CBC, electrolytes, BUN, creatinine, glucose, LFTs, ammonia level, ABGs, urinalysis, and a toxicology screen for illicit drugs.

Other tests, such as an EEG, are helpful in identifying NCSE, especially when there is a prior history of seizures. In one series of comatose patients in whom the cause was unknown, 8% were found by EEG to be in NCSE.

Finally, you may need to do a cerebrospinal fluid examination (including the usual bacterial and viral tests) if you suspect meningitis or encephalitis.

Evaluation of Findings

Supratentorial coma is due to an injury of the hemisphere(s).

There are 2 mechanisms:

1) Uncal (lateral) herniation: An expanding asymmetric mass lesion (i.e., tumor, stroke, hemorrhage) forces the uncus through the middle opening in the tentorium. This puts pressure on the brainstem and, therefore, the RAS. Because of the course of the 3rd cranial nerve, the herniating uncus compresses this nerve, causing an enlarged pupil ipsilateral to the supratentorial lesion.

2) Central herniation: Injury to the thalamus (such as hemorrhage) results in diminished consciousness very early in its course. Later, the pupils are in

	Size	Description	Cause	Examples
	⬤ ●	One dilated, nonreactive, or sluggish pupil	Parasympathetic nerve problem	Oculomotor nerve compression from uncal herniation, aneurysm of the posterior communicating artery
	· ●	One pinpoint pupil (miosis)	Sympathetic nerve problem (Horner's)	Lateral medullary syndrome, hypothalamus injury, Pancoast tumor, carotid dissection
	● ●	Two midpoint, nonreactive pupils	Parasympathetic and sympathetic nerve problem	Midbrain disruption (can affect one or both pupils), anoxia, hypothermia, anticholinergics, severe barbiturate overdose
	⬤ ⬤	Two dilated, nonreactive pupils		Anoxia, hypothermia, anticholinergics, severe barbiturate overdose
	· ·	Two pinpoint, reactive pupils		Opiates, pontine destruction

Table 12-1: Pupil Size in Coma

midposition and become fixed. As the herniation continues, the course begins to merge with that of uncal herniation. In other words, central and uncal herniation syndromes can be differentiated early on, but later their courses merge.

Note, however, that on CT scan of the brain, horizontal shift of the pineal body can help correlate with consciousness level:

Pineal shift on CT	Consciousness level
0–3 mm	Alert
3–4 mm	Drowsy
6–8 mm	Stupor
8–13 mm	Coma

Infratentorial coma is due to an injury that causes destruction or compression of the brainstem. Signs of infratentorial herniation include bilateral reactive pinpoint pupils (due to pontine involvement) and respiratory abnormalities, including Cheyne-Stokes breathing, apneusis (deep gasping), and ataxic breathing. There are 3 possible causes:

1) Basilar artery occlusion with pontine infarction

2) Cerebellar infarction or hemorrhage

3) Posterior fossa neoplasms

Expansion of the contents of the posterior fossa forces the contents of this compartment in 1 of 2 directions: up (upward herniation) or down (downward herniation). Upward herniation pushes the posterior fossa contents up under the tentorium, compressing the brainstem. Downward herniation forces the cerebellar tonsils down through the foramen magnum, compressing the medulla.

Metabolic coma has many causes including ischemia, hypoglycemia, hypothyroid (myxedema coma), thiamine deficiency (Wernicke encephalopathy), organ disease (e.g., lung [hypoxia and hypercapnia], liver [hepatic encephalopathy], kidney [uremia]), severe electrolyte derangements (such as Na^+ and Ca^{2+}), and drugs. Early in metabolic encephalopathy, patients have changes in respiratory pattern and mentation. The pupils are typically reactive until the terminal stages. Exceptions include anticholinergic toxicity and severe barbiturate intoxication, which cause fixed, dilated pupils. In addition, both hypothermia and anoxia/ischemia can cause fixed pupils of varying size. Anoxic-fixed pupillary dilatation lasting longer than a few minutes implies severe and, usually, irreversible brain damage.

COMA MIMICS

PREVIEW | REVIEW

- What is the presentation of locked-in syndrome?

- What is the definition of a persistent vegetative state?

- What are the etiologies of akinetic mutism and catatonia?

- How is brain death diagnosed? Is an EEG required?

- What is an apnea test?

LOCKED-IN SYNDROME

Locked-in syndrome is rare and most often caused by a lesion of the ventral pons as a result of basilar artery occlusion. The lesion commonly spares the somatosensory pathways and the ascending RAS responsible for arousal and wakefulness, as well as midbrain structures that allow the eyelids to be raised. Thus, the lesion interrupts the corticobulbar and corticospinal pathways, leaving the patient unable to speak. Those with locked-in syndrome are awake and aware of the surrounding environment but only have the ability to control eye movements. Typically, they can communicate only by using eye blinks and vertical eye movements. (The efferent abducens nerve fibers controlling horizontal eye movements are usually destroyed.) Because the cerebral cortex is spared, an EEG is normal. Some patients can recover some function, so include multidisciplinary and physical and speech therapy, pulmonary rehab, and help with swallowing in patient treatment. Locked-in syndrome highlights the need to carefully assess the level of consciousness in presumed comatose patients to avoid misdiagnosis.

VEGETATIVE STATE

Vegetative state results from severe bilateral cerebral dysfunction, often following a period of coma. Vegetative state is often caused by anoxic brain damage (e.g., after cardiac arrest) and can be the final stage of progressive cortical degenerative diseases, such as Alzheimer's and Creutzfeldt-Jakob's.

These patients typically have normal sleep-wake cycles but no discernible cognitive function. Respiratory rate can increase in response to manual stimulation, and they can have automatisms, such as swallowing, bruxism, grimacing, grunting, and moaning. There is loss of sphincter control. EEG abnormalities include low-amplitude delta-frequency background activity, burst suppression, widespread alpha and theta activity, an alpha coma pattern, and sleep spindles. Stimulating the patient causes minimal, if any, change in background EEG activity.

Neuropathology shows cortical laminar necrosis, which is often extensive, with a relative or complete sparing of brainstem structures (including the RAS).

Comatose patients who enter into vegetative states may recover or progress to death—normally within 2 weeks. A vegetative state that persists > 3 months is called a persistent vegetative state. Patients in a persistent vegetative state following traumatic brain injury (TBI) are more likely to recover than patients with anoxic injury. Up to 39% of TBI patients who are vegetative > 3 months recover consciousness by 1 year, whereas only 6% of nontraumatic patients do. After 6 months of vegetative state, 19% of TBI patients recover consciousness but only 1% recover in nontraumatic patients. Generally, within 5 years, demise occurs from pneumonia, urosepsis, or sudden death.

AKINETIC MUTISM

Patients with akinetic mutism are profoundly apathetic, although they register most of what is happening around them. They may speak normally and relate events from the recent and distant past. This state is caused by bilateral lesions generally of the anterior parts of the frontal lobes, leaving the motor and sensory pathways intact.

CATATONIA

Catatonia is a state of stupor and neurogenic motor immobility that can be caused by psychiatric states, such as schizophrenia, depression, PTSD, and drug abuse, as well as a wide range of underlying medical conditions. Patients with catatonia are unresponsive, although they preserve oculocephalic responses (doll's eyes). Some patients display a waxy flexibility of passive limb movement and hold limb postures that appear uncomfortable for long periods of time. Unusual motor mannerisms or repetitive motions, seen in a number of these patients, can give the impression of seizures. There are no signs of structural brain disease. EEG is typically normal, although it shows diffuse slowing with malignant catatonia. Treat with a trial of benzodiazepines or, in severe cases, consider electroconvulsive therapy.

BRAIN DEATH

The central features of brain death are an irreversible absence of all cerebral and brainstem functions, including spontaneous respiration. This regularly results from catastrophic brain damage (e.g., trauma, cardiac arrest, cerebral hemorrhage), but you need to exclude reversible causes, such as drug overdose.

Signs indicating the absence of cerebral function are the presence of deep coma along with the lack of spontaneous movement and motor and vocal responses to all visual, auditory, and cutaneous stimulation, as well as lack of brainstem reflexes and spontaneous respiration.

Diagnostic criteria for brain death:

- Knowledge of the preceding catastrophic event (clinical or imaging) responsible for the current status
- All possible metabolic confounders (e.g., electrolyte abnormalities) excluded
- Toxins excluded
- Core temperature > 97.0° F (36.1° C)

- Systolic blood pressure (SBP) > 100 mmHg (pressors allowed)
- Absence of brainstem function on exam, as indicated by the following:
  - Loss of spontaneous eye movements
  - Midposition of the eyes
  - Lack of oculocephalic (doll's eyes) and oculovestibular (caloric) responses
  - Presence of dilated or midpoint fixed pupils (4–9 mm)
  - Paralysis of bulbar musculature (no facial movement or gag, cough, corneal, or sucking reflexes)
  - Absence of motor and autonomic responses to noxious stimuli
  - Absence of spontaneous respiratory movements

If all the above criteria are fulfilled, carry out an apnea test.

Apnea test: Preoxygenate the patient with 100% O_2; pCO_2 should be normal. Then, disconnect the ventilator for 10 minutes and observe for respiration. A positive test occurs when there is no respiration, even with a $pCO_2 > 60$ mmHg or > 20 mmHg from baseline.

Diagnosis of brain death is made only by fulfilling the above clinical criteria.

Tests that can support a diagnosis of brain death (but are not mandatory except in children) include:

- Evaluation of brain blood flow
  - Angiography
  - Transcranial Doppler
  - MRA/CT angiography
  - SPECT (single-photon emission computed tomography)
- EEG

SEIZURES

PREVIEW | REVIEW

- Name some environmental triggers for seizures in susceptible people.
- What are some differences between generalized and focal seizures?
- What is the treatment of status epilepticus?
- Which test should you order if you suspect recurrent PNES?
- Which drug is used to treat absence seizures?
- Which AEDs decrease the effectiveness of oral contraceptives?
- Which AED serum concentration is reduced by estrogens?
- Which AED reduces the serum concentration of progestins?

OVERVIEW

Convulsion is an intense paroxysm of involuntary, repetitive muscular contractions, and it does not always have to be present during seizures. **Seizure** is preferable as a generic term because it includes all paroxysmal electrical discharges originating in the cerebral cortex that cause loss of consciousness, alteration of perception or impairment of psychic function, convulsive movements, disturbance of sensation, or some combination thereof. **Epilepsy** is a history of ≥ 2 unprovoked seizures occurring at least 24 hours apart. The condition of prolonged or repetitive convulsive seizures is termed **status epilepticus** and can be life-threatening.

It is crucial to determine whether the seizures are primary (idiopathic) or secondary.

In susceptible individuals, triggers for seizures include intense emotions, strobe lighting, loud music, stress, menstruation, and lack of sleep.

Metabolic or toxic causes of seizures do not constitute epilepsy. This type of seizure can be provoked by severe or rapid metabolic derangements (Na^+, Ca^{2+}, low Mg^{2+}, hypoglycemia); drugs, such as cocaine and amphetamines; and alcohol withdrawal (within 7–48 hours after last drink).

SEIZURE CLASSIFICATION

The 2017 International League Against Epilepsy (ILAE) changed the way seizures were classified and created a new framework with different levels for categorization, the International Classification of Epileptic Seizure. The levels are meant to provide consistency across diagnoses, research, and treatments. Review Figure 12-1 as you go over the following.

Seizure type indicates where the current seizure began in the brain: focal onset, generalized onset, or unknown onset—with no history of or with a new-onset seizure, this is often the only information you have. Onset locations:

- Focal onset seizure is subclassified by the patient's level of awareness (impaired or not), and whether or not there are motor symptoms at the onset.
- Generalized onset seizure is subclassified as motor or nonmotor (i.e., absence).
- Unknown onset

Epilepsy type is the 2nd level of diagnosis. It assumes that the patient has a diagnosis of epilepsy using standard criteria and testing (e.g., EEG). The patient has recurrent seizures that have been diagnosed as:

- Focal
- Generalized
- Combined generalized and focal
- Unknown

Epilepsy syndrome is the 3rd level of diagnosis. These syndromes are reliable concurrences of the above findings (e.g., seizure types and EEG patterns) with other factors such as age of onset and remission, diurnal variation, triggers, best treatment, and prognosis. Examples of syndromes with idiopathic generalized epilepsies (IGEs) are childhood absence epilepsy, juvenile absence epilepsy, juvenile myoclonic epilepsy, and generalized tonic-clonic seizures. There are several self-limited focal seizure syndromes that begin in childhood.

Etiology is considered from the very first seizure. These etiologies may be combined. For instance, a genetic

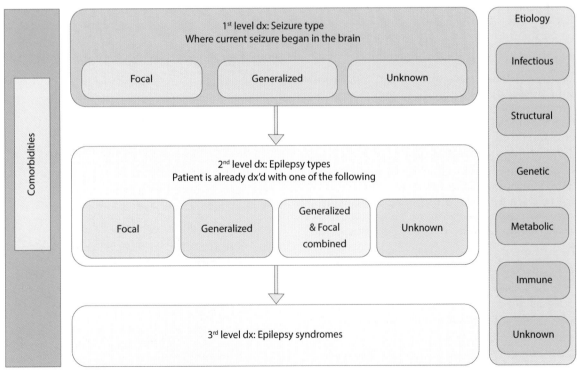

Figure 12-1: ILAE framework for seizure classification

abnormality may cause a metabolic or structural abnormality. The 6 etiologic groups are:

1) Infectious (most common cause worldwide; e.g., neurocysticercosis, HIV, cerebral toxoplasmosis, cerebral malaria, and congenital infections, such as Zika virus and CMV).

2) Structural (may be genetic or acquired; e.g., due to tumor, stroke, trauma, infection)

3) Genetic (based on family history, population research, or gene research)

4) Metabolic (most are genetic but may be acquired; e.g., cerebral folate deficiency, alcohol withdrawal)

5) Immune (e.g., antibody)

6) Unknown (cause is simply not yet known)

Comorbidities are associated with many epilepsies. There are often psychological, behavioral, and learning problems. Severe epilepsies can have motor deficits and movement disorders. Any comorbidity can cause psychosocial concern.

SEIZURE EXAMPLES

The following has 2 examples of generalized seizure (motor and nonmotor) and 2 of focal seizure (without and with impaired level of awareness):

1) **Generalized tonic-clonic** (previously grand mal) seizures involve both hemispheres, with resulting bilateral motor involvement. Consciousness is impaired with a pronounced postictal period. These seizures can be generalized from the start, or they can be focal seizures with secondary generalization.

2) **Absence** (previously petit mal) seizures are a type of generalized seizure. These are nonconvulsive, generalized seizures with no aura and no postictal symptoms. The attacks occur without warning and consist of a sudden interruption of consciousness during which the patient stares and briefly stops talking or ceases to respond. They can be induced by hyperventilating. Absence seizures have a characteristic 3-per-second spike and wave pattern on EEG. 2/3 of affected children outgrow absence seizures.

3) **Focal** seizures originate in a small area of the cortex. Consciousness is preserved. The symptoms of a focal seizure depend on the region of cortex from which the event is generated. For instance, a focal seizure arising in the occipital lobe (visual cortex) can be manifested by complex visual hallucinations; e.g., spinning colorful spheres. A focal seizure affecting the motor cortex can cause focal motor convulsions. These can spread to involve more of one side of the body ("Jacksonian march") as the seizure progresses. Postictally, patients may temporarily have weakness of the affected limb.

4) **Focal seizures with diminished consciousness** have many causes. A common type is the temporal lobe seizure in which the preceding aura may be a hallucination or perceptual illusion. There is a period of altered behavior and consciousness for which the patient is later found to be amnesic. The motor components of the temporal lobe seizure take the form of automatisms (e.g., lip-smacking, chewing or swallowing movements, salivation, fumbling of the hands, shuffling of the feet).

Status epilepticus is the term reserved for prolonged seizure activity. Prolonged seizures lead to neuronal cell death and long-term consequences. It is considered a medical emergency. A cause can be determined about 2/3 of the time. Usual causes in adults include stroke, alcohol or other drugs, stopping or changing seizure medications, hypoxia, CNS infection, metabolic causes, tumor, and trauma.

Status epilepticus is defined as a seizure lasting > 30 minutes or a series of ≥ 2 seizures without regaining consciousness in between. In practice, most seizures last only 1–2 minutes, so when a seizure lasts ≥ 5 minutes, become aggressive with abortive treatment to avoid prolonged status epilepticus.

PSYCHOGENIC NONEPILEPTIC SEIZURES

Psychogenic nonepileptic seizures (PNES; a.k.a. pseudoseizures) are not due to abnormal brain activity but are psychogenic. Features that suggest PNES include: forced eye closure during event, pelvic thrusting, crying, awareness during a spell of bilateral convulsing, side-to-side head movements, or absence of a postictal state.

Order video EEG monitoring if PNES is suspected or when the events do not respond to treatment and the diagnosis is not clear. Prolactin levels are elevated about 10 minutes after a generalized motor seizure, but they are not elevated with PNES. Note, however, that 20% of patients with PNES also have epilepsy.

SEIZURE AURA

An aura is a perceptual disturbance that may precede a focal seizure. Auras do not occur with primary generalized seizures. Note that auras do occur with migraine, but all discussion here is in reference only to seizures.

Auras have various manifestations affecting the senses. They can be somatosensory perceptions, such as pain, numbness or tingling, or related to other senses. They can be mostly motor, ranging from tremors or shaking to gross motor movement. They can also be:

• Visual with lights, patterns, or seeing objects
• Auditory with voices, noises, tones, and other sounds
• Olfactory, typically with a burnt rubber smell
• Gustatory with the perception of strange tastes

Know: Auras, in the context of seizures, are used as a warning manifestation of seizure and allow the patient to take precautions. These auras are thought to be produced by early seizure activity.

A focal seizure can evolve into a focal seizure with diminished consciousness, and either of these can evolve secondarily into a generalized seizure. In any of these situations, the preceding seizure is also called an aura by some.

SEIZURE MANAGEMENT

History

When obtaining the history, check for alcohol or drug use, recent medication changes, head injury, sleep deprivation, diabetes, and thyroid or parathyroid surgery.

Scans and Lab

Include glucose, Na^+, Ca^{2+}, MG^{2+}, LFTs, toxicology, drug levels (i.e., lithium, phenytoin), and BUN in lab tests to evaluate for provoking causes of a seizure. Order either an MRI with gadolinium or a CT with contrast (if MRI is contraindicated) after a first unprovoked seizure to exclude a structural abnormality; MRI is the best neuroimaging test. An EEG showing epileptiform abnormalities suggests the diagnosis of epilepsy, but a normal EEG does not exclude the diagnosis of a seizure disorder. Catching a seizure while a patient is hooked up to an EEG definitively distinguishes between seizure and nonepileptic causes of spells. However, typically, an EEG is obtained interictally, and one routine EEG only has a 50% sensitivity for detecting an abnormality between seizures.

Whether or not to start anticonvulsive therapy after an initial seizure depends on the following:

- Start antiepileptic drug therapy after 1 unprovoked seizure with the following, as the risk of recurrence is high:
  ◦ An abnormal EEG
  ◦ History of a prior neurologic injury
  ◦ Focal abnormality on exam
  ◦ Nocturnal seizure
  ◦ An abnormality on MRI
- Unless a patient has a 2nd unprovoked seizure, hold off on starting antiepileptic drug therapy with:
  ◦ Normal EEG
  ◦ Normal MRI
  ◦ Normal exam
  ◦ Absence of risk factors

Remember to consider CNS infection in a patient with seizure, headache, and fever or with meningeal signs. Obtain imaging prior to lumbar puncture (LP).

In approximately 70% of all patients with epilepsy, medications can control the seizures completely or almost completely; in an additional 20–25%, the attacks are significantly reduced in number and severity, but some may remain refractory. Epilepsy surgery and other options are available for treatment in refractory cases.

Acute Treatment of Seizures

Acute treatment of seizures: Intravenous benzodiazepines (e.g., diazepam, lorazepam, midazolam) are the drugs of choice. Phenytoin is also effective, but it takes longer to infuse. Treat alcohol withdrawal seizures acutely with IV benzodiazepines.

Typical treatment of status epilepticus in adults: Give thiamine and then 50 mL of D50 if the blood glucose level is low. Also give benzodiazepine (lorazepam preferred × 2 doses) followed by a loading dose of phenytoin or equivalent fosphenytoin for all status epilepticus patients. Fosphenytoin lacks the injection site necrosis and cardiac rhythm complications of intravenous phenytoin infusion but is much more expensive and can result in lower initial brain phenytoin levels (because of the time required for conversion from fosphenytoin to phenytoin). Nevertheless, the infusion rate is 3× faster than for phenytoin; therefore, fosphenytoin is frequently used in the emergency department. Also consider IV levetiracetam or IV valproic acid for status epilepticus, particularly in patients with known generalized epilepsy; though in general, fosphenytoin is 1st line treatment.

If the patient is still seizing after the initial treatment options noted above, give a 3rd dose of lorazepam, maximize the phenytoin dose, and then proceed to a barbiturate (phenobarbital or pentobarbital) or propofol. Endotracheal intubation and ICU-level care are generally needed if seizures are not controlled by the first 2 doses of lorazepam and a dose of phenytoin.

Chronic Treatment of Seizures

Antiepileptic drugs (AEDs) are the mainstay of treatment, with monotherapy the preferred goal (Table 12-2 on page 12-8). AEDs in epilepsy are generally started after ≥ 2 unprovoked seizures but are typically used after 1 focal unprovoked seizure if EEG is abnormal or if there is a head injury history. The risk of seizure recurrence after 2 seizures is ~ 60%, and after 1 seizure the risk is ~ 35%.

The choice of AED depends primarily on the seizure type, with additional considerations including cost, side-effect and metabolism profile, and patient preference for a dosage schedule.

Focal seizures: Almost all available AEDs are effective in the treatment of focal seizures. The notable exception is ethosuximide, which is used to treat only absence seizures. Further, with few exceptions, the AEDs are equally effective. The main differences are that older AEDs are generally cheaper, whereas newer AEDs are typically better tolerated and have fewer side effects.

Generalized tonic-clonic seizures: The list of effective agents includes:

- Topiramate
- Lamotrigine
- Valproic Acid
- Levetiracetam

- Felbamate
- Rufinamide
- Zonisamide

Generalized absence seizures: The list of effective agents includes:

- Lamotrigine
- Ethosuximide
- Valproic acid

When can you stop the medication? This must be individualized. Risk factors include a seizure within the last 2 years, epileptiform spikes on the EEG, abnormal MRI, and a late age of onset of the seizures. Patients who are seizure-free for 2–4 years and have their AEDs gradually withdrawn have ~ 40% risk of recurrent seizures within 2 years.

Options for intractable epilepsy include resective surgery (best for temporal lobe epilepsy), vagus nerve stimulation (does not work as well as surgery), and the ketogenic diet (works well in children).

Driving restrictions vary from state to state and continue to evolve. The Epilepsy Foundation has updated information for your state: www.epilepsy.com/driving-laws.

Drug Interactions with AEDs

AEDs and OCPs

Certain AEDs reduce the efficacy of oral contraceptive pills (OCPs):

- Phenytoin
- Phenobarbital

Table 12-2: Notable Advantages and Disadvantages of Antiepileptic Drugs		
Drug	**Used to Treat**	**Notable Advantages / Disadvantages**
Carbamazepine	Focal[1] Generalized tonic-clonic (alternative)	Good: Toxicity is uncommon. Bad: hyponatremia, leukopenia, thrombocytopenia, aplastic anemia, hepatotoxicity, teratogenic, liver inducer; reduces the efficacy of OCPs; risk of SJS in Asians with HLA-B* 1502
Clonazepam	Absence (short-term adjunctive use only)	Bad: loses efficacy
Ethosuximide	Absence[1] only	Bad: can cause bone marrow suppression (rare)
Gabapentin	Focal (adjunctive use)	Good: the only one with no significant drug interactions; renal clearance, so useful in those with liver disease Bad: ataxia, amnesia, limited efficacy
Lamotrigine	Focal (adjunctive use) Generalized	Good: wide spectrum, good efficacy, well tolerated in elderly patients Bad: can cause severe rash and SJS with rapid titration; reduces efficacy of OCPs
Levetiracetam	Focal and generalized (monotherapy)	Good: well tolerated in elderly patients; safe in Asian patients with HLA-B*1502 at increased risk for SJS; renally excreted, so no interaction with levels of other AEDs; IV form available Bad: depression, fatigue, irritability, and personality change
Oxcarbazepine	Focal	Good: generally well tolerated, metabolized in liver Bad: SJS, aplastic anemia, angioedema, hyponatremia; reduces the efficacy of OCPs
Phenobarbital	Focal (last choice)	Bad: sedation in adults, hyperactivity in children, among other cognitive changes; teratogenic; reduces the efficacy of OCPs; liver inducer: decreases levels of carbamazepine, felbamate, lamotrigine, tiagabine, and valproic acid
Phenytoin	Generalized	Good: wide spectrum, good efficacy Bad: gingival hypertrophy, decreases bone density, rash and SJS (especially in Asian descent with HLA-B* 1502), interferes with efficacy of OCPs, liver inducer, and increases risk of fetal malformations. Toxic levels can induce seizure.
Topiramate	Focal (monotherapy or adjunctive) Generalized (monotherapy or adjunctive)	Good: weight loss, headache prophylaxis if present Bad: kidney stones and increased glaucoma, weight loss, paresthesias, cognitive dysfunction; teratogenic; reduces efficacy of OCPs
Valproic acid	Generalized tonic-clonic[1] Absence (alternative) Focal (alternative, esp. if it generalizes)	Good: wide spectrum, good efficacy, IV form available Bad: GI side effects (fewer with extended release formulation); can rarely cause bone marrow suppression and hepatotoxicity/liver failure; teratogenic (neural tube defects), tremor, weight gain, hair loss; inhibits the metabolism of some seizure medications, such as carbamazepine, phenobarbital, phenytoin, and lamotrigine

[1]Primary drug
Note: Any of the above AEDs can cause ataxia, dizziness, and somnolence.
Also of note: Overall, use of antiepileptic medications confer a small increased risk of suicidal thoughts.
OCP = oral contraceptive pill; SJS = Stevens-Johnson syndrome; AED = antiepileptic drug

- Carbamazepine
- Lamotrigine
- Oxcarbazepine
- Topiramate

Advise women taking these AEDs to use a method of birth control other than oral contraceptives.

Note: Oral contraceptives that contain estrogen can decrease the drug concentration of the AED lamotrigine, and, thus, doses may need to be increased empirically. Conversely, lamotrigine can decrease serum concentrations of progestins (minipill). Thus, women on progestin-only contraceptives are at risk of getting pregnant; counsel them to switch to alternate methods of contraception.

AED Interactions

Phenytoin, phenobarbital, carbamazepine, and primidone are the earlier generation "enzyme-inducing" AEDs that stimulate a variety of cytochrome P450 enzymes. Because many other drugs are metabolized by these enzymes, patients on enzyme-inducing AEDs often need their dosage of other medications increased.

These can affect the metabolism of each other, requiring a change of dose. One counterintuitive example: Even though phenytoin increases the metabolism of primidone, the active metabolite of primidone is phenobarbital—so you may need to decrease the primidone dosage.

Valproic acid is different from other older-generation AEDs in that it inhibits some of these same enzymes! Especially watch for an increase in levels of phenobarbital, carbamazepine, phenytoin, and lamotrigine.

Newer AEDs do not have the same broad inducement of enzymes. Still, some have more specific effects; e.g., as mentioned above, some can increase the metabolism of OCPs.

Treatment of Seizures During Pregnancy

Know!

The background risk for birth defects is 2–3%. The goal of treatment during pregnancy is to control the seizures—uncontrolled seizures can cause placental abruption, early labor, and premature delivery. When the risk of teratogenicity is compared to the problems that seizures cause during pregnancy, the risks of uncontrolled seizures are greater!

Maintain a pregnant woman on monotherapy at the lowest dose of medication possible; risk of malformations increase as each drug is added.

Many AEDs are teratogenic. The most significant teratogens include phenytoin, phenobarbital, carbamazepine, topiramate, and valproic acid.

Valproic acid is more likely to cause neural tube defects than other commonly used AEDs and is associated with lower IQs of children exposed to this drug *in utero*—therefore, avoid if pregnancy is planned. The teratogenic risk of AEDs is decreased by folic acid, and thus, advise all women of childbearing age on antiepileptic drugs who can become pregnant to take 1 mg of folate daily—4 mg of folic acid daily in patients taking valproic acid or carbamazepine.

Note: Physicians generally give prophylactic vitamin K during the last month of pregnancy in patients on AEDs, based on reports indicating increased bleeding in patients on AEDs. However, the 2009 American Academy of Neurology (AAN) guidelines state there is not enough evidence to recommend for or against use of prophylactic vitamin K.

DEMENTIA

PREVIEW | REVIEW

- What is the definition of dementia?
- Which 6 domains may be impaired in patients with dementia?
- What is the definition of mild cognitive impairment?
- What is the clinical triad in normal pressure hydrocephalus?
- Compare and contrast the features of normal pressure hydrocephalus, AD, and vascular dementia.
- How is Alzheimer disease (AD) diagnosed?
- Which class of drugs is the 1st line treatment for AD?
- Which drug is used with a cholinesterase inhibitor for the treatment of advanced AD?
- What is a potential complication from the use of atypical antipsychotics in elderly patients with dementia?
- How does the clinical presentation of frontotemporal dementia differ from that of AD?
- Is CJD insidious or rapid?
- How do you diagnose CJD?
- What is the problem with using antipsychotic drugs to treat patients?
- Which feature is prominent in progressive supranuclear palsy with Parkinson disease dementia?
- What are the clinical features of Huntington disease?
- Name some features that distinguish depression from dementia.

DEFINITION

Dementia is defined as a chronic cognitive decline with or without behavioral impairment that:

- Is progressive
- Interferes with normal daily functioning
- Is not due to delirium or an underlying psychiatric disorder

Note how this definition contrasts with encephalopathy, which causes altered states of consciousness—from delirium to stupor.

WORKUP

Diagnosis of Dementia

Basic principles:

1) Perform a thorough H&P that includes obtaining history from the patient and an additional informant (because history from a potentially demented patient is not always reliable).

2) Perform an objective cognitive assessment using a validated tool (e.g., the Montreal Cognitive Assessment, the Mini-Mental State Exam).

3) Evaluate for depression that can mimic cognitive decline and for other secondary (reversible) medical causes of cognitive decline as outlined under Reversible Causes.

4) Consider detailed neuropsychological testing to fully map out affected domains of cognition to help solidify the correct diagnosis.

Dementia is diagnosed when abnormalities exist in ≥ 1 of the following 6 domains and are also progressive and interfere with daily functioning and independence:

1) **Learning and memory**—acquiring and/or remembering new information. Do they ask repetitive questions, lose items, or get lost?

2) **Executive function**—reasoning. Do they understand appropriate danger? Can they perform their activities of daily living (ADLs), such as grocery shopping?

3) **Perception and motor function**—assessing visuospatial orientation. Do they recognize faces and objects? Can they dress themselves? Do they get lost in their house?

4) **Language**—comprehension and speaking appropriate language. Do they have problems recalling common words without hesitations?

5) **Social cognition**—behaving normally and appropriately. Is there undue agitation, apathy, loss of empathy, or compulsive behavior?

6) **Complex attention**—ability to perform complex steps. Can they balance a checkbook or pay a grocery bill with cash?

Psychosis is a common feature of advanced dementia.

Mild Cognitive Impairment

When ≥ 1 of the domains is in decline, but the impairment does not significantly impact daily functioning, the diagnosis is mild cognitive impairment (MCI). If MCI is diagnosed, obtain an assessment of functional status.

MCI can be either amnestic or nonamnestic. Amnestic MCI is more common. Not all patients with MCI deteriorate into dementia. MCI progresses to dementia at a rate of about 5–10% per year. Such progression is more likely in patients with a family history of Alzheimer disease. Patients with amnestic MCI have memory impairment that does not significantly impact daily living, and general cognition is intact. Those with amnesic MCI are more likely to deteriorate to Alzheimer disease.

Patients with nonamnestic MCI have impairment in ≥ 1 of the other domains (executive function, perception, language, social, or complex attention), but daily living is not impacted.

Reversible Causes

In evaluating dementia, consider the following treatable causes of impaired cognition:

- Medications
- Vitamin B$_{12}$ deficiency (may have associated polyneuropathy/myelopathy)
- Hypothyroidism
- Chronic subdural hematomas (consider especially in alcoholics, in patients on anticoagulants, and in elderly patients with a history of falls)
- Normal pressure hydrocephalus
- Tumors, especially involving the frontal lobes
- Infection and inflammation (consider with clinical clues or a subacute, rather than indolent, decline)
  - AIDS
  - Neurosyphilis
  - Neurosarcoidosis
  - Chronic meningitis
  - Lupus cerebritis
  - Vasculitis
- Autoimmune encephalopathy (such as Hashimoto encephalopathy or paraneoplastic/autoimmune encephalitis)
- Heavy metal poisoning (arsenic, mercury, and lead)

In practice, an initial medical evaluation of cognitive disturbance entails imaging of the brain (MRI preferred, if possible), as well as thyroid and B$_{12}$ testing. Additional lab testing, such as for syphilis or HIV, is based on risk factors. Consider a much more expanded work up based on other clinical clues or a more rapid, subacute decline in cognition (see above again for the broad differential of reversible causes of cognitive decline).

Diagnosing a specific subtype of dementia is based on a range of clinical clues and presentations (see next).

SPECIFIC CAUSES OF DEMENTIA

Normal Pressure Hydrocephalus

Hydrocephalus is enlargement of the CSF spaces. There are various types:

- Normal pressure hydrocephalus (NPH) has enlarged ventricular size with normal opening pressures on LP.
- Noncommunicating (obstructive) hydrocephalus has enlarged ventricles due to a physical blockage in the small passages between ventricles—often in the aqueduct of Sylvius between the 3rd and 4th ventricles. This is usually a congenital issue (i.e., aqueductal stenosis), but it can be acquired in adults (e.g., hemorrhage, tumor, infection). ICP is elevated.
- Communicating hydrocephalus has enlarged ventricles due to decreased CSF resorptive capabilities. ICP is elevated.
- Hydrocephalus *ex vacuo* is a compensatory enlargement of the ventricles due to atrophy of the brain substance as a result of stroke, injury, or diffuse white matter changes (e.g., from diabetes or hypertension; see Vascular Dementia on page 12-12). ICP is normal.

NPH causes the classic triad of:

1) Gradually worsening dementia
2) Gait apraxia (a wide "magnetic" gait, like walking on a boat)
3) Bladder issues (detrusor overactivity with urinary urgency/frequency and incontinence)

Patients can present with frequent falls due to gait instability. Often, the mental issues and gait problems precede the bladder control issues. NPH rarely causes headaches.

NPH can occur as a result of prior head trauma, acute or ongoing chronic meningitis, or subarachnoid hemorrhage.

NPH has no associated cerebral atrophy. The opening pressure on LP is normal, and there is no papilledema. With early diagnosis, further neurologic deterioration can be improved, but not always sustained, with the placement of a ventricular shunt. An MRI or CT shows enlarged ventricles with normal size sulci. The course of dementia, while slowed with shunt placement (see below), is similar to Alzheimer's.

Note that hydrocephalus *ex vacuo* from diffuse white matter changes can present with the same clinical triad as NPH.

Diagnosis: Suggestive review of symptoms and physical exam findings. There is no papilledema, and opening pressure on LP is normal. Observing the clinical response to a high-volume LP (such as pre- and postgait assessments) remains the most utilized clinical diagnosis.

Treatment for NPH is ventriculoperitoneal or ventriculoatrial shunt. Certain indicators help identify patients who are most likely to respond to shunting:

- NPH secondary to subarachnoid hemorrhage, acute or ongoing chronic meningitis, or head trauma
- < 6 months of symptoms
- Gait abnormality > cognitive abnormality

Dementia for > 2 years or significant white matter disease or atrophy on imaging are indicators of poor shunt responsiveness.

Alzheimer Disease

Diagnosis of Alzheimer Disease

Alzheimer disease (AD) is the most common cause of dementia after 60 years of age. 1st degree relatives have a 4× normal risk of developing it.

AD is diagnosed when the illness is found to be insidious, progressive, and marked by impairments in ≥ 2 domains (memory, executive functioning, perception, language, behavior, and complex attention), such that there is significant impairment in normal daily functioning. As with MCI (see Mild Cognitive Impairment on page 12-10), the amnestic presentation of AD is the most typical. Patients with Alzheimer's have normal LP parameters.

Initial signs of AD usually reflect hippocampal dysfunction, with poor immediate recall and short-term memory. Impairment of naming can also be an early sign. As the disease progresses, impairments emerge in perception, social, complex, and executive domains, reflecting dysfunction in the parietal and frontal lobes. Changes in environment (such as vacations or hospital stays) can be disorienting, and the patient may become lost on walks or while driving.

Do not use any of the following for a definitive diagnosis of AD:

- MRI scans that show disproportionate atrophy
- PET scans demonstrating amyloid deposition or decreased tracer uptake
- CSF tau and amyloid measurements

These biomarkers are not specific enough, and abnormalities sometimes are seen in patients with normal cognition or MCI only.

Additionally, do not diagnose AD as a cause of dementia if the patient:

- has a history of significant cerebrovascular disease,
- has clinical features of frontotemporal dementia (see Frontotemporal Dementia on page 12-12) or dementia with Lewy bodies (DLB; more under Parkinson Disease Dementia on page 12-13),
- has evidence of another psychiatric or neurologic illness, or
- takes a medication that can cause cognitive impairment.

You must rule these out as causes of the dementia symptoms. In an elderly patient presenting with dementia without a movement disorder, the main diagnoses to consider are AD, vascular dementia, and mixed dementia (with both neurodegenerative and vascular components).

Treatment of AD

The 1st line treatment for Alzheimer's is cholinesterase inhibitors (CIs):

- Donepezil (Aricept)
- Rivastigmine (Exelon)
- Galantamine (Razadyne)

Additive drug treatment includes the *N*-methyl-*D*-aspartate receptor antagonist memantine (Namenda).

The combination of a CI + memantine appears to be better than a CI alone, especially for advanced AD.

The CIs produce a small improvement in cognition and, sometimes, in neuropsychiatric instability. Data is conflicting on their long-term effects. Not every patient benefits. Note that these drugs are for dementia only; do not use to treat MCI. The best results with CIs are achieved in mild-to-moderate Alzheimer's, but other types of dementia (e.g., multiinfarct and DLB) sometimes also improve. Treatment effects with these medications are modest only.

Dose escalations for each of these medications must be carried out over 4–6 weeks to minimize side effects. The main side effects are anorexia, nausea, and occasionally diarrhea or bradycardia (cholinergic symptoms). Rivastigmine is available as a patch that has fewer GI side effects and is useful in patients who will not swallow medications.

Neuropsychiatric instability in late-stage AD is common and difficult to treat. Mild-to-moderate depression in the early stages may respond to SSRIs, trazodone, or CIs; definitely avoid tricyclic antidepressants because of the anticholinergic symptoms, particularly short-term memory impairment and confusion.

Atypical antipsychotics (e.g., olanzapine, quetiapine, risperidone, clozapine) have been used to treat the agitation, insomnia, delusions, aggression, and wandering. However, in 2005, the FDA published a boxed warning that these drugs can cause increased mortality in the elderly with dementia (any cause but especially in the elderly with DLB), and in 2017, the FDA issued a formal warning about the increased risk of associated falls and fractures.

Vascular Dementia

Dementia with cognitive deficits associated with vascular factors (a.k.a. vascular dementia) is the 2nd most common form after AD. Vascular dementia results from infarction or ischemia of 3 major structures: large arteries, small arteries (e.g., lacunar), and small arteries in the white matter. The Hachinski ischemic score can help differentiate vascular (≥ 7) from AD (≤ 4), and is based on several features including a history of atherosclerosis, hypertension, prior stroke, focal deficits, and rate of onset.

Chronic hypertension is the most common cause of dementia due to lacunar infarcts and diffuse nonspecific white matter changes, which are visible on MRI. The changes result from chronic ischemia mediated by occlusive disease of small, penetrating cerebral arteries and arterioles. Diabetes is also a common cause of this condition.

Early symptoms include mild confusion and impairments in memory, perception, and executive functions. Marked difficulties in judgment and orientation develop later, along with dependence on others for ADLs. Neuropsychiatric symptoms (e.g., apathy, anxiety, psychosis, euphoria, depression, aggression) also develop as the deep white matter changes and infarcts accumulate. Pyramidal and cerebellar signs can be seen. With advanced disease, patients frequently present with urinary incontinence and dysarthria with or without other pseudobulbar features (e.g., dysphagia, emotional lability).

Frontotemporal Dementia

Frontotemporal dementia (FTD; previously Pick disease) is quite similar in presentation and course to Alzheimer disease, but it is characterized by a more rapid and significant change in personality and behavior, often with disinhibition, language deficits, or both. Onset is in the 5th to 6th decades (relatively young, compared to Alzheimer's), and the incidence in males exceeds females.

Common behavioral features include apathy, disinhibition, weight gain, food fetishes, compulsions, and loss of empathy.

Cognitive testing usually reveals spared memory but impaired planning, judgment, or language. Patients often show an absence of insight into their condition.

The naming of FTD subtypes is based on their primary manifestations; e.g., behavioral variant vs. progressive, nonfluent vs. semantic. Patients with FTD have more focal atrophy of the frontal and temporal lobes on CT or MRI, compared with the diffuse atrophy of Alzheimer's or a medial temporal/parietal distribution with Alzheimer's.

Currently, there are no effective treatments for FTDs but the serotonin selective reuptake inhibitors and the atypical serotoninergic agent trazodone have been shown to result in some behavioral improvement, mainly in irritability, agitation, depressive symptoms, and eating disturbances.

Creutzfeldt-Jakob Disease

Creutzfeldt-Jakob disease (CJD) is one of the very rare (1 per million people) prion diseases. Based on observations of causes, CJD is divided into sporadic (sCJD; most typical at 90%), familial (fCJD; about 10%); iatrogenic (iCJD; < 1%), and variant (vCJD). Usually, sCJD presents around 55–65 years of age, and we have no idea what causes it. fCJD has genetic associations. When you see CJD in younger patients, think either iCJD or vCJD. iCJD is caused by receipt of infected human tissues, hormones (e.g., growth hormone, gonadotropins, dural grafts, corneal or liver transplants), or exposure to contaminated surgical instruments. Current safety practices have essentially eliminated iatrogenic cases, though long incubation periods of former exposures can still present today. vCJD is believed to be caused by the prion that causes mad cow disease (bovine spongiform encephalopathy) in cattle. It is believed that the prion jumped species and now infects humans.

Regardless of cause, CJD develops as a rapidly progressive dementia (weeks as opposed to years) with characteristic startle myoclonus (response to loud noises or startle). The early stages of the neurologic disease are characterized by changes in behavior, emotional response, and intellectual function, often followed by ataxia and visual distortions, confusion, hallucinations, delusions, and agitation. Dementia and muteness quickly follow the early symptoms. Younger patients with vCJD tend to have dementia with predominantly psychotic features. The disease involves the cerebral cortex, basal ganglia, and spinal cord.

The diagnostic gold standard is brain biopsy. Supportive studies include:

- **MRI** of the brain with diffusion-weighted images shows abnormal diffusion in thalami, basal ganglia, or the cortical ribbon (helps also to differentiate sCJD from vCJD)
- **EEG** (characteristic pattern of periodic sharp wave complexes on a diffusely slowed background)
- **14-3-3 protein** in an otherwise bland CSF (Only the National Prion Disease Pathological Surveillance Lab does this test, at Case Western, and sensitivity/specificity is < 80%.)

Creutzfeldt-Jakob disease is fatal within 1 year in > 90% of patients. There are no known treatments.

Parkinson Disease Dementia

Parkinson disease (PD) is caused by a loss of dopaminergic neurons in the substantia nigra. (See discussion under Movement Disorders on page 12-17.)

Dementia in PD (PDD) is common, eventually affecting as many as 80% of patients. Its frequency increases with aging and, in contrast to Alzheimer disease, primarily affects executive functions and attention in its earlier stages, with relative sparing of language, memory, and calculations until later in the disease course. When dementia precedes or develops within 1 year after the onset of motor dysfunction, it is referred to as dementia with Lewy bodies (DLB). Neuropathology in both PDD and DLB shows Lewy bodies mixed with amyloid plaques and neurofibrillary tangles. Lewy bodies are spherical eosinophilic inclusions within the neuron (Figure 12-2). Remember that Alzheimer disease also has the characteristic findings of amyloid plaques and neurofibrillary tangles but without Lewy bodies (Figure 12-3).

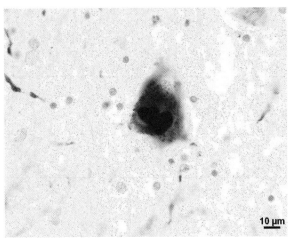

Figure 12-2: Lewy body

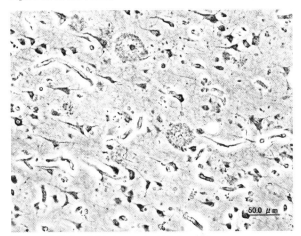

Figure 12-3: Amyloid plaques in Alzheimer disease

The core clinical features of DLB (besides dementia) are spontaneous motor features of parkinsonism (although this may not be present in every case); recurrent, vivid visual hallucinations; and prominent fluctuations of attention and cognition. Other supportive clinical features include hallucinations in nonvisual senses (e.g., tactile, olfactory, or auditory), delusions, REM sleep behavior disorder (dream enactment), unexplained falls or loss of consciousness, and depression.

Both the dementia and psychosis may be at least partially responsive to acetylcholinesterase inhibitors and memantine. Clozapine (which spares the D_2 dopamine receptor) can be helpful. Quetiapine is another option.

Patients with DLB have poor responses to the older antipsychotic drugs that block the D_2 dopamine receptor, including haloperidol and chlorpromazine—and even to some of the more recent "atypical" neuroleptics. With these drugs, patients have a dramatic and severe worsening of symptoms with extreme sedation, increased confusion, and postural instability (with falls). Avoid all antipsychotics other than clozapine and quetiapine in those with DLB.

As described in the Alzheimer's discussion above (see Treatment of AD on page 12-12), antipsychotic drugs are under an FDA boxed warning because they are associated with an increased risk of death when used in elderly patients with dementia, and especially so in those with DLB.

Progressive Supranuclear Palsy

Onset of progressive supranuclear palsy (PSP) usually occurs in the 6th decade of life and is a type of parkinsonian syndrome with ocular features. Clinical features include difficulty in balance, abrupt falls, visual and ocular disturbances, slurred speech, dysphagia, and personality change with prominent apathy. Difficulty in voluntary vertical movement of the eyes, typically downward initially but sometimes upward, and later paresis of voluntary saccades in all directions are characteristic. Patients can also have apraxia of eyelid opening (resembling blepharospasm) and eyelid closing. Cognitive slowing and dementia are prominent features. Buzzwords for PSP: dementia with gaze palsy and falls.

Huntington Disease

Huntington disease (HD) causes both a dementia and a movement disorder. (More movement disorders are discussed starting under Movement Disorders on page 12-17.) The gene responsible for HD is the *HTT* gene on chromosome 4p, which codes for a mutant huntingtin protein that is probably toxic. (Note: The protein is spelled with an **i**, while the disease is spelled with an **o**.) It is inherited in an autosomal dominant fashion with complete penetrance. Problems commonly begin in those who are in their late 30s. Of those diagnosed, 7% commit suicide.

HD causes dementia, chorea, and psychiatric disturbances, including personality changes, depression, and psychosis. Memory is relatively spared. Chorea is usually the heralding symptom. The emotional disturbances and changes in personality can be so severe that they can manifest as psychosis with persecutory delusions or hallucinations.

Disease is progressive with death (typically from pneumonia) within 30 years after symptoms begin. Diagnosis is made in the setting of positive family history, clinical features, and genetic testing demonstrating the *HTT* gene.

Atrophy of the caudate nuclei on CT or MRI ("boxcar" ventricles) is characteristic and correlates with deterioration in cognition. No curative medication exists, and the disease is invariably fatal. Tetrabenazine is effective in controlling mild chorea. Side effects are significant and include depression, sedation, and bradykinesia. Other symptoms can be ameliorated with antipsychotics (neuroleptics), benzodiazepines (e.g., clonazepam), and antidepressants.

Genetic counseling prior to genetic testing is available for family members but is performed only ~ 15% of the time.

AIDS

AIDS is the most common cause of dementia in younger patients. Dementia affects half of all AIDS patients not on antiretroviral therapy (ART). The manifestations can be mild (minor cognitive-motor disorder) to severe (HIV-associated dementia). Impairment is related to the degree and duration of immunosuppression. Controlling the virus in a patient who has had AIDS for a prolonged period, with a low CD4 count, often does not reverse dementia.

HIV-associated dementia (HAD) is characterized by cognitive impairment, movement disorders, and depression. It starts with small comprehension problems and anhedonia, accompanied by tremor and gait abnormalities. Over time, patients develop slower movements with substantial cognitive impairment. Exclude opportunistic infections of the CNS (e.g., cryptococcosis, toxoplasmosis, neurosyphilis) as part of the workup.

Treatment includes treating the HIV with ART, focusing specifically on designing a regimen of medications that enter the CNS at higher levels. Also treat associated depression. See more on HAD under HIV on page 12-22.

Depression

Some patients with major depression present with significant cognitive dysfunction, known as depressive "pseudodementia." One differentiating feature is that frontal lobe release signs (grasp, suck, rooting, and palmomental reflexes) are common in patients with dementia, particularly if moderate or advanced, but they are not typically seen in isolated depression. Patients with depression-related pseudodementia tend to be concerned about their deficits but perform rather normally on office cognitive testing, whereas patients with dementia are more often brought to attention by family members and may not have insight into their cognitive impairment. In addition, immediate recall is usually poor in depression (due to attentional dysfunction) but good in dementia.

Depression can be reactive or endogenous. Symptoms are the same for both. In endogenous depression, patients, as expected, can have an abnormal response to the dexamethasone suppression test in which the cortisol is initially suppressed, but the duration of suppression is shortened (normal is > 24 hours).

DELIRIUM

PREVIEW | REVIEW

- What are the 2 clinical hallmarks of delirium?

Delirium is an acute, and often transient, onset of altered mental status, typically within hours to days. It is most commonly seen in hospitalized elderly patients, patients in hospice units, and patients in the ICU. It increases mortality. Diagnose based on the clinical hallmarks of decreased attention span and varying states of confusion. Aim treatment at identifying any underlying cause and supportive care. The risk factors are many and include: infection, restraints, older age, dementia, untreated pain, and medications (particularly benzodiazepines). Delirium is also discussed in Geriatric Medicine, Book 2.

CNS: BRAIN — SUBCORTEX

DEMYELINATING DISEASES

PREVIEW | REVIEW

- What are 2 ocular presentations of MS?
- Which findings in CSF are helpful for the diagnosis of MS?
- What is the treatment for an acute exacerbation of MS?
- Natalizumab can cause which neurologic disease?
- Aside from patients with AIDS, PML can occur in which patients? What are the symptoms of PML?
- What is the cause of osmotic demyelination syndrome? Which clinical findings are seen in this condition?

MULTIPLE SCLEROSIS

Overview

Know all the following! Multiple sclerosis (MS) is a demyelinating disease of the central nervous system that usually begins between 20 and 30 years of age. Women are affected more often than men (about 2:1). The incidence is higher in northern latitudes, possibly because of reduced sun exposure. It is recognized that adequate vitamin D levels may have a protective effect and an important role as a modifiable nutrient risk factor. MS is a chronic condition with episodes of focal disorders of the optic nerves, spinal cord, and brain, which remit and recur over a period of many years.

The disease process is thought to be autoimmune, although no specific antibodies have been found and the disease may not always respond to immunomodulators. Infections as an etiology have not been excluded either. One theory is that there is an initial infectious insult and an autoimmune reaction acts as a secondary trigger. Another is that MS is a result of T-cell sensitization to myelin. A familial aggregation of MS has also been reported.

The neurologic symptoms depend on the region of brain that is affected.

There are 3 types of MS:

1) Relapsing-remitting (RRMS)
2) Secondary progressive (SPMS)
3) Primary progressive (PPMS)

The relapsing-remitting type (initially normal between spells but later presents with residual deficit between spells) can slowly transform into the progressive type (which classically is slowly progressive from onset). Although 85% of cases are initially RRMS, most transform to the progressive type after several years.

Patients with a 1st episode and ≥ 2 lesions on brain MRI have a 90% risk of developing MS in 10 years—as opposed to a 28% risk if no lesions are found on brain MRI.

Clinical Manifestations of MS

Paroxysmal symptoms make up the usual course of early disease (except in chronic progressive cases). Weakness or numbness in ≥ 1 limbs is the initial symptom in about 1/2 of the patients. Tingling of the extremities and tight band-like sensations around the trunk or limbs are commonly associated symptoms.

Although strict criteria are used to diagnose MS (discussed a little later), place MS in the differential anytime you encounter the following characteristic syndromes (especially if recurrent!).

Optic neuritis (ON) is the most common presentation of MS eye disease and the 1st manifestation in about 25% of patients. It occurs at some time in 50% of all MS patients. There is swelling of the optic disc, but with progression, the disc becomes pale. ON presents as a rapid loss of vision in one or both eyes, often accompanied by slight pain, especially on eye movement. The vision loss is usually central, but a variety of field defects can be seen. With unilateral involvement, the Marcus Gunn pupil (a.k.a. relative afferent pupillary defect) is typically seen. Light shone into the eye with ON produces slower and incomplete constriction of both pupils than light shone into the healthy eye. On the swinging flashlight test, when the flashlight is swung to the affected eye, both pupils dilate; however, when light is presented to the healthy eye, both pupils constrict briskly. More than 90% of these cases recover completely.

Internuclear ophthalmoplegia (INO) is caused by a lesion in the medial longitudinal fasciculus, and, although it presents as difficulty in moving the eyes horizontally, convergence is normal. (Remember that normal convergence means the patient can turn each eye inward slightly as they follow your finger to their nose, so that they continue to see a single object.) There is adduction paresis ipsilateral to the lesion, with the deficit ranging from complete medial rectus paralysis to slight slowing of an adducting saccade. Gaze-evoked horizontal jerk nystagmus is present in the abducting eye contralateral to the eye with adduction weakness. (Remember: Adduction means "toward the midline" and abduction means "away from the midline.") Think multiple sclerosis whenever you hear of a relatively young patient being diagnosed with INO. In older patients, however, it is more commonly due to cerebrovascular disease. The presence of bilateral INO in a young adult is virtually diagnostic of MS.

Acute myelitis causes a rapidly evolving (several hours or days) symmetrical or asymmetrical paraparesis or

NEUROLOGY

paraplegia, ascending paresthesia, loss of deep sensibility in the feet, a sensory level on the trunk, sphincteric dysfunction, and bilateral Babinski sign (upturning big toe with firm stroking of sole of foot).

Other symptoms of MS can include generalized fatigue, nebulous sensory abnormalities (e.g., pain, paresthesias, itching, feeling of coldness or swelling, numbness [especially of the face]), vertigo/diplopia, lower-extremity motor weakness/paralysis, ataxic gait, and bowel/bladder dysfunction. Flexion of the neck may induce a tingling, electric-like feeling down the shoulders and back known as the Lhermitte sign.

Young women with bilateral trigeminal neuralgia and/or bilateral INO have MS until proven otherwise!

Dementia is not a typical feature of MS, especially in the earlier stages, but substantial cognitive impairment may occur in some patients with advanced chronic progressive disease. If your patient presents with dementia and gait abnormalities, a more likely diagnosis is Parkinson disease, PSP, or NPH.

All symptoms of MS tend to worsen in the heat, called Uhthoff phenomenon. This is because heat increases conduction block in demyelinated pathways.

Diagnosis of MS

Diagnosis of MS is no longer based solely on the history and neurologic exam. The traditional (Posner) criteria incorporated signs and symptoms indicating 2 CNS lesions separated in time and space that were not caused by other CNS disease and included CSF findings. The fact that MS lesions disseminate over time and space remains an essential component of making the diagnosis: MS develops slowly over time with new lesions occurring in different parts of the brain, thereby causing different neurologic signs and symptoms. Current criteria incorporate CNS imaging as a diagnostic tool.

MRI has become an essential tool in the workup of MS. T1-gadolinium MRI shows the characteristic enhancement or "plaques" of patchy myelin loss (white matter disease) with 90% sensitivity. T2-weighted MRI shows MS lesions as hyperintense areas. Many non-MS lesions can show up as hyperintense, so the specific location where these lesions are found has diagnostic weight. Dawson fingers refers to MS lesions around the veins that radiate out from the ventricles.

The McDonald criteria consider time- and space-specific MRI findings. CSF findings are not included. MS lesions and their dissemination over time and space are the main diagnostic criteria:

- Time
  - Presence of asymptomatic enhancing and nonenhancing lesions
  - New T2 lesion

- Space
  - At least one T2 lesion in ≥ 2 of the 4 MS CNS regions (periventricular, juxtacortical, infratentorial, or spinal cord)

In addition, consider MRI of the spinal cord, especially if brain imaging does not reveal plaques and the patient's presentation is very suspicious for MS. The diagnostic criteria equate certain cord lesions to certain brain lesions. MRI is also essential to rule out conditions that can mimic MS. White matter disease due to ischemia (elderly) and vasculitis both have a very different pattern of distribution from that seen with MS.

CSF analysis is particularly useful during acute exacerbations when IgG immunoglobulins to myelin can be found in the CSF. When these globulins are processed using electrophoresis, a few "bands" appear; thus, the term oligoclonal bands. 90% of MS patients have increased IgG index and oligoclonal IgG bands in the CSF. CSF protein and cell count is generally normal—on occasion, a small CSF lymphocytosis may be present, but should be ≤ 50 cells/μL.

Evoked potentials (visual, brainstem auditory, and somatosensory evoked potentials) can help to establish the diagnosis of MS by identifying a clinically silent 2nd lesion.

So, the workup for MS includes an MRI, an LP, and evoked potentials. Ultimately, the diagnosis is made using a combination of clinical history, physical exam, laboratory, and imaging data.

Treatment of MS

There is no cure for MS. Treatment is very specialized and managed by neurologists. As a result, general internists are expected to know that the treatment of acute exacerbations is to rule out a possible triggering infection (e.g., UTI, pneumonia), then treat with **high-dose corticosteroids** (as opposed to the myriad treatment options for both intermittent and progressive disease). If an infection, like UTI, is causing a pseudoexacerbation or worsening of old deficits, then it is sufficient to treat the infection alone. If the patient has new neurologic deficits, then treat for an inflammatory flare; if needed, an MRI with and without contrast can help clarify whether a patient is experiencing a new flare. For treatment of a flare, glucocorticoids may shorten the duration of exacerbations but do not alter the natural course of MS. Treat with IV methylprednisolone, 1 g/day for 3–5 days.

Other drugs used to treat chronic MS: immunomodulators (beta interferons and monoclonal antibodies), glatiramer acetate (Copaxone, Glatopa), and other immunomodulatory drugs.

Other examples of drugs include fingolimod (Gilenya) and dimethyl fumarate (Tecfidera), which are oral medication options rather than the injection therapy options with glatiramer acetate or beta interferons. Be aware that patients taking natalizumab have an increased incidence of progressive multifocal leukoencephalopathy (PML)—discussed next. For interferons, monitor CBC and LFTs every 6 months because they cause flu-like symptoms, fatigue, and depression.

Interferons and glatiramer reduce relapses by 30%, while natalizumab reduces relapses by ~ 60%. Note: You are not expected to know detailed information about the pharmacological treatment of MS on exams.

PROGRESSIVE MULTIFOCAL LEUKOENCEPHALOPATHY

Progressive multifocal leukoencephalopathy (PML), which affects white matter only, is a progressive demyelination seen in patients with severe T-cell immunodeficiencies (e.g., HIV/AIDS), monoclonal antibodies, and chronic neoplastic diseases. An example of the monoclonal antibodies is natalizumab, used in the treatment of MS and moderate-to-severe Crohn disease. Natalizumab is an antibody to the VLA-4 antigen expressed on activated T cells and monocytes. Most cases of PML of this type have occurred with the combination of natalizumab and other immunomodulators.

Other cases of PML can be seen in patients taking a number of immunosuppressants (e.g., rituximab, fludarabine, mycophenolate, chronic corticosteroids) for treatment of rheumatologic, hematologic, post-transplant, and inflammatory bowel diseases.

It is caused by the polyomavirus JC virus.

Symptoms are varied and typically start with abnormal mentation (personality changes and intellectual impairment) and then slurred speech. Initial symptoms can be followed by hemiparesis progressing to quadriparesis, visual field defects, cortical blindness, aphasia, ataxia, dysarthria, dementia, confusional states, and/or coma. Some patients have a predominantly cerebellar syndrome.

A definitive diagnosis can be made with brain biopsy. Alternatively, follow up a suggestive MRI with a PCR analysis of spinal fluid. Finding JC virus in spinal fluid is strongly supportive of PML, although sensitivity of the PCR test decreases as the immune system is reconstituted on antiretroviral therapy (ART). ART has improved mortality in patients with PML, but many patients have persistent neurologic deficits because the nerves are unable to remyelinate. Standard antiviral drugs are ineffective for treatment.

The course is subacute and progressive, often leading to death in 3–6 months.

OSMOTIC DEMYELINATION SYNDROME

Osmotic demyelination syndrome (previously central pontine myelinolysis) occurs in patients with severe hyponatremia that is corrected too quickly with hypertonic saline. The risk increases as the following factors increase: length of time the patient is hyponatremic before correction is started, severity of the hyponatremia, and the rate of hypertonic saline infusion.

These patients can present with quadriparesis, mutism, pseudobulbar palsy, chewing and swallowing dysfunction, and/or locked-in syndrome. Paralysis is initially flaccid, but spasticity develops within a few days. See Hyponatremia in Nephrology & Urology, Book 2, for more discussion.

MOVEMENT DISORDERS

PREVIEW | REVIEW

- What are the 4 motor features of parkinsonism?
- Name some common drugs used to treat Parkinson disease.
- What is a potential side effect of anticholinergic drugs when used to treat Parkinson's? Ropinirole has which side effects?
- Selegiline can cause serotonin syndrome when combined with which other drugs?
- What is the clinical presentation of serotonin syndrome?
- What is a potential complication of an L-dopa dose reduction in a patient with Parkinson psychosis?
- What is the classic eye finding of progressive supranuclear palsy?
- What is the clinical presentation of essential tremor? What improves it?
- What causes TD? How is TD treated?
- What is the clinical presentation of neuroleptic malignant syndrome?
- Which comorbidities are associated with Tourette syndrome?
- Which antihypertensive drug is used to treat tics in Tourette syndrome?

PARKINSONISM

Know this topic well. Parkinsonism (a.k.a. secondary Parkinson's or Parkinson syndrome) is a neurological syndrome. Parkinsonism signs and symptoms have the characteristic set of 4 motor features (the **4 Rs**):

1) **R**esting tremor

2) **R**igidity and flexed posture

3) **R**etarded movement (bradykinesia and hypokinesia)

4) Loss of postural **R**eflexes

Resting tremors at a rate of 4–5 Hz (cycles per second) occur in the distal extremities. Tremor is usually the 1st symptom noticed. Sometimes the tremor is present with use, with dramatic worsening at rest.

Patients with parkinsonism have diffusely increased muscle tone, which, combined with the tremor, causes the "cogwheeling" seen with passive range of motion of the limbs. The rigid, flexed posture can include the entire body; ultimately, the spine, elbows, hips, and knees may become flexed. The classic hand position is flexed metacarpophalangeal joints with straight interphalangeal joints.

Hypokinesia/bradykinesia is the primary feature. With hypokinesia, the patient has decreased amplitude of voluntary movements—especially with repetitive tasks. This may manifest as micrographia (progressive reduction in amplitude of writing). Bradykinesia is difficulty initiating movement, slowness of movement, and decrease or loss of spontaneous movement (e.g., masked facies, tendency to sit motionless, decreased blinking).

Loss of postural reflexes contributes to the festinating gait; the patient walks progressively faster to remain under the forward center of gravity caused by truncal flexion. This eventually leads to falls and then to the inability to stand or walk without assistance.

There are many causes of parkinsonism. These range from Parkinson disease to drugs, toxins, metabolic disease, infections, repeated head trauma, and cerebrovascular disease.

The most common cause of parkinsonism is Parkinson disease ([PD]; discussed next).

Many drugs can cause secondary parkinsonism. The usual culprits are:

• Dopamine-depleting drugs (e.g., reserpine)
• Dopamine antagonists, such as phenothiazines or butyrophenones
• Antiemetics, such as metoclopramide

Drug-induced parkinsonism is typically much more symmetric than PD.

Common toxins: carbon monoxide, manganese, and organic solvents. Repeated head trauma can also cause parkinsonism (punch drunk syndrome). Parkinsonism also occurs in some forms of Huntington disease (rigid form, typically seen in younger patients), frontotemporal dementia, and spinocerebellar ataxia.

PARKINSON DISEASE

Overview

The pathologic findings in Parkinson disease (PD) are loss of pigmented cells in the substantia nigra of the midbrain and in other pigmented nuclei (i.e., locus ceruleus, raphe, dorsal motor nucleus of the vagus). Many of the remaining cells contain eosinophilic cytoplasmic inclusions, surrounded by a faint halo, called Lewy bodies.

The motor features of PD are caused by a dropout of dopamine-producing cells in the substantia nigra. Normally, dopamine from these cells is released in the basal ganglia, where it has a complex effect on the motor system,

facilitating voluntary movement. When there is a decrease in dopamine from deterioration of the substantia nigra, the motor symptoms of PD emerge.

Diagnosis

Know! PD is a clinical diagnosis, and diagnosis is easy to miss in the early stages.

The core features of PD are the tetrad of:

1) hypo- and bradykinesia,
2) resting tremor,
3) postural instability, and
4) rigidity.

These are manifested as an expressionless face, slowness, and a lack of voluntary movement, "resting" tremor, stooped posture, axial instability, rigidity, and festinating gait. For unknown reasons, symptoms always start on one side of the body and spread to the other side after a few years.

Consider causes of secondary Parkinson's. Look for signs that might suggest other neurodegenerative disorders, such as multiple systems atrophy, Lewy body dementia (more under Parkinson Disease Dementia on page 12-13), or PSP (more under Progressive Supranuclear Palsy on page 12-19).

80% of patients with PD eventually develop dementia.

Treatment

Overview

As with MS, treatment for PD is very specialized. Focus on diagnosis, major treatments, and side effects of treatment. Staying active and exercising are important goals that keep patients independent as long as possible.

Drugs that stimulate the dopamine system are the mainstay of therapy to treat symptoms:

• Levodopa + carbidopa, with or without the catechol-O-methyltransferase (COMT) inhibitor entacapone (Comtan) or tolcapone (Tasmar)
• Nonergot direct dopamine receptor agonists
  ◦ Ropinirole (Requip)
  ◦ Pramipexole (Mirapex)
  ◦ Rotigotine (Neupro skin patch)
• Amantadine
• Anticholinergics
• Monoamine-oxidase (MAO)-B inhibitors
  ◦ Selegiline
  ◦ Rasagiline

Treatment of Mild PD

Anticholinergics, such as amantadine, benztropine (Cogentin), and trihexyphenidyl, are used to treat mild symptoms, especially tremor.

Anticholinergics can cause altered mental status, including psychosis, especially in patients > 70 years of age and in individuals with cognitive impairment.

Treatment of Mild-to-Moderate PD

Dopamine receptor agonists (ropinirole, pramipexole and rotigotine) can be useful as monotherapy for mild-to-moderate PD, but 60% of patients require adjunctive levodopa (L-dopa) after 4 years.

Know that these direct dopamine receptor agonists can cause impulse control disorders, such as hypersexuality, compulsive shopping, and pathological gambling.

The **MAO-B inhibitor** selegiline delays the need for L-dopa in patients with mild PD by approximately 9 months. There is evidence that rasagiline may also slow decompensation in early Parkinson disease. To date, however, no treatment for PD has been proven to be neuroprotective.

Know that combining selegiline with tricyclics or SSRIs can potentially cause serotonin syndrome. This problem is caused by excessive serotonergic activation of both CNS and peripheral receptors. Signs and symptoms include cognitive impairment ranging from confusions to hallucinations to coma; autonomic effects, such as hyperthermia, tachycardia, shivering, and sweating; and somatic effects, such as hyperreflexia and clonus, twitching, and tremors. Symptoms can be mild to rapidly fatal, depending on the amount of overstimulation.

Treatment of Severe PD

More severe symptoms are commonly treated with **L-dopa + carbidopa**. L-dopa acts as a precursor for dopamine synthesis in the basal ganglia. The carbidopa blocks conversion of L-dopa to dopamine in the periphery, a desirable effect because peripheral dopamine does not cross the blood-brain barrier. Additionally, peripheral dopamine causes side effects, such as postural hypotension and nausea. Carbidopa does not help with the central side effects of L-dopa that emerge after several years. Note that L-dopa absorption can be reduced by dietary protein.

Although L-dopa is the most effective drug for PD, its use is withheld as long as possible, especially in younger patients, to delay the onset of complications that are common with chronic use—especially dyskinesias (drug-induced involuntary movements, choreiform, or dystonic) and motor fluctuations (periods of good symptom control alternating with periods of re-emergent parkinsonism).

Direct dopamine receptor agonists (ropinirole, pramipexole, and rotigotine) and COMT inhibitors (entacapone or tolcapone) are added to reduce the overall daily dose of L-dopa, to even out the serum levels of this drug, and to provide more continuous dopamine receptor stimulation.

The older dopamine agonists (bromocriptine, cabergoline, and pergolide) can have ergot-related adverse effects, including a risk of valvular heart disease, and are no longer used in the U.S. to treat PD. Cabergoline remains available for treatment of prolactinomas.

Complications of PD therapy include the following:

- End-of-dose "wearing off" effects (due to short half-life of L-dopa)
- Unpredictable "on-off" fluctuations that are characterized by unpredictable loss of L-dopa treatment effect and dyskinesias (50% of patients after 3–5 years)
- Psychiatric symptoms develop in 30% of patients treated with L-dopa or dopamine receptor agonists. These symptoms include agitation, confusion, hallucinations, and delusions. Older patients with cognitive impairment are especially at risk. Approximately 17% of patients treated with a dopamine agonist develop an impulse control disorder.

Know that patients who develop psychosis with L-dopa treatment sometimes require a reduction or a switch in their medications to control their behavior. These patients are especially susceptible to development of a neuroleptic malignant-like syndrome with the switch or dose reduction. This syndrome is sometimes termed Parkinsonism hyperpyrexia and presents with hyperthermia, delirium, muscular rigidity, high creatine phosphokinase (CPK) level, and autonomic instability. Drug holidays are no longer used in Parkinson patients for this same reason.

PROGRESSIVE SUPRANUCLEAR PALSY

Progressive supranuclear palsy (PSP) is similar to Parkinson disease in that patients have bradykinesia, abnormal gait, increased muscle tone, and later develop dementia.

The disease has its onset typically in the 6th decade of life (range: 45–75 years of age), with some combination of difficulty in balance, abrupt falls, visual and ocular disturbances, slurred speech, dysphagia, and changes in personality. Ultimately, the characteristic syndrome of supranuclear ophthalmoplegia, pseudobulbar palsy, and axial dystonia develops. Patients usually do not have a tremor.

Within 2 years, these patients develop the classic symptom of a vertical ophthalmoplegia, commonly with initial impairment of downgaze, progressing to complete ophthalmoplegia in all directions. Subsequently, patients have trouble reading, eating, and walking down stairs. There is a gradual stiffening and extension of the neck. Within another 2–3 years, they may be unable to walk because of marked imbalance.

The treatment is palliative, aimed to improve the quality of life. These patients commonly die of aspiration pneumonia due to severe dysphagia.

TREMORS

Overview

The type of tremor is based on when the tremor occurs:

- Static tremors occur at rest, or when the head and extremities are held in a fixed position (termed postural tremor).

- Kinetic tremors occur during voluntary movement.
- Action tremors persist unchanged throughout voluntary movement and generally disappear at rest.
- Intention tremors occur with target-directed movement and worsen as the movement unfolds.

Exaggerated Physiologic Tremor

Most people have a usually unnoticeable physiologic tremor that has a frequency of ~ 10 Hz. This normal tremor can be aggravated by anxiety, stress, fright, hyperthyroidism, and metabolic abnormalities, such as hypoglycemia, drug withdrawal states, and certain drugs (SSRIs, corticosteroids, tricyclics, theophylline, β-agonists, nicotine, and caffeine). This tremor can also be postural or seen with action.

Essential Tremor

Essential tremor is the most common type of nonphysiologic tremor. It is often familial. In familial cases, it seems to be transmitted as an autosomal dominant trait, with variation in age at onset and severity. It affects the hands as a postural and action tremor with a frequency of 4–8 Hz. It can also be a higher frequency and affect the head and chin as a "yes, yes" or "no, no" postural tremor. There can be an associated vocal tremor. Essential tremor is typically benign but sometimes results in functional disability. Note that a postural tremor of the head is very unlikely to be due to Parkinson's and is more often essential tremor. Parkinson tremors that affect the face commonly involve the lips, tongue, or jaw only.

The frequency of essential tremor is usually decreased transiently by drinking alcohol, and you can often diagnose an essential tremor when patients tell you that their tremor improves after an alcoholic drink. Propranolol and primidone are effective in reducing the limb tremors.

Gabapentin and topiramate reduce limb tremors a little and are 2nd line drugs. In severe cases, try botulinum toxin and deep-brain stimulation surgery.

TARDIVE DYSKINESIA

Tardive dyskinesia (TD) is mostly a result of long-term antipsychotic drug use or long-term or high-dose metoclopramide use. The only way to be certain to avoid TD is to keep patients off chronic antipsychotics, but this cannot be accomplished in many patients with chronic psychosis.

Some atypical antipsychotics (2nd generation drugs), particularly clozapine and quetiapine fumarate (Seroquel XR), are less likely to cause TD. Clozapine can cause bone marrow toxicity.

Tardive dyskinesia consists of many involuntary movements, including dystonia, chorea, athetosis, and tremor. The face, tongue, lips, eyelid, and bulbar muscles are most often involved, but you may also see neck, shoulder, and spine muscles with arching of the back.

Clonazepam is a useful benzodiazepine for patients with mild tardive dyskinesias and anxiety. Extract of ginkgo biloba significantly reduces tardive dyskinesia in patients with schizophrenia. More disabling cases can be treated with tetrabenazine, a dopamine depleter or botulinum toxin. Deep-brain stimulation surgery can be used in the most severe cases.

OTHER MOVEMENT DISORDERS

Neuroleptic Malignant Syndrome

Neuroleptic malignant syndrome is an unusual response to antipsychotics (both typical and atypical), resulting in hyperthermia, rigidity, diaphoresis, autonomic instability, and altered mental status with a risk of rhabdomyolysis-induced renal failure. Occasionally, other drugs, such as metoclopramide and promethazine, can also cause this syndrome. Labs often show leukocytosis, electrolyte disturbances, and elevated CPK levels.

This syndrome can occur days, weeks, or months after neuroleptic treatment is begun. It carries a mortality rate of 15–30% if not recognized and treated promptly. Know: Patients with Parkinson's who acutely discontinue their L-dopa therapy (or reduce dose) can develop neuroleptic malignant syndrome.

Treat neuroleptic malignant syndrome by discontinuing any offending drug; use of a direct dopamine agonist, such as bromocriptine or dantrolene; and supportive therapy, including adequate hydration and scrupulous pulmonary hygiene. If rigidity is sufficient to affect ventilation, sedate, intubate, and paralyze the patient. Pursue electroconvulsive therapy (ECT) in medically refractory patients. Patients can have recurrence of neuroleptic malignant syndrome if the drugs are restarted.

Hemifacial Spasm

Hemifacial spasm is a motor analog to trigeminal neuralgia. 80% of patients have a tortuous, dilated basilar artery (basilar dolichoectasia) that loops around and irritates the facial nerve! Other causes include aneurysm, acoustic neuroma, and, occasionally, MS.

Botulinum toxin injections are generally the best treatment. Some patients have benefitted from surgery to separate the facial nerve from direct contact with the basilar artery (microsurgical decompression). Occasionally, carbamazepine, baclofen, and gabapentin can be effective.

Tourette Syndrome

Tourette syndrome is a developmental neuropsychiatric disorder characterized by chronic (> 1-year duration) multiple motor tics and ≥ 1 vocal tics. Motor tics can be simple (including eye blinking or rolling, facial grimacing and head or limb jerking) or complex (including semi-purposeful movements, such as tapping, jumping, and copying the gestures of others [echopraxia]). Vocal tics can also be simple (such as sniffing, snorting, grunting, and coughing) or complex (including utterance of words or phrases, obscenities [coprolalia], or imitating the speech of others [echolalia]). Onset is commonly between 2 and 15 years of age. Many patients have comorbid attention-deficit/hyperactivity disorder (ADHD), obsessive-compulsive disorder, learning disorders, or conduct disorders.

Diagnosis is clinical and requires confirmation of both motor and vocal tics.

Milder tics and/or associated ADHD may respond to clonidine or guanfacine. More severe ADHD can be treated with stimulants, such as methylphenidate; data shows that these drugs may not exacerbate tics as previously thought, although close monitoring is necessary. Neuroleptics have been traditionally used to treat tics that are severe enough to interfere with daily functioning. However cost prohibitive, tetrabenazine is gaining traction as an effective agent and has fewer side effects. Treat focal motor tics with botulinum toxin.

Focal Dystonias

Focal or segmental dystonias are intermittent, brief, or prolonged spasms or contractions of a group of adjacent muscles that place the body part in a forced and unnatural position.

Know the following 4 focal dystonias:

1) Blepharospasm is bilateral, forceful, involuntary eye closure and can occur as an isolated syndrome or as part of Meige syndrome.
2) Meige syndrome is a combination of blepharospasm and oromandibular dystonia (involuntary jaw opening and jaw movements).
3) Spasmodic torticollis occurs when spasms of the neck and shoulder muscles turn the head to one side.
4) Writer dystonia (a.k.a. writer cramp) occurs when spasms of the hand and arm emerge with writing, limiting the ability to write legibly.

A few oral drugs may offer mild relief: benzodiazepines, baclofen, anticholinergics, and sometimes antidopaminergics. However, botulinum toxin is the treatment of choice, providing much more reliable but temporary relief when injected directly into the affected muscles. It requires repeat injections every 2–5 months.

CNS: BRAIN — VENTRICLES / CSF

INFECTIONS

PREVIEW | REVIEW

- What is the classic triad of symptoms observed in patients with a brain abscess?
- What is the diagnostic test for West Nile virus encephalitis?
- What is the treatment for CNS toxoplasmosis?
- What is the clinical presentation of neurocysticercosis?
- Characterize the CSF of a patient with cryptococcal meningitis.
- How useful is the CSF/serum cryptococcal antigen (sensitivity/specificity) in diagnosing meningitis?

BACTERIAL CNS INFECTIONS

Acute Meningitis

Headache, stiff neck, photophobia (due to meningeal inflammation), and lethargy are typically present with acute meningitis, but thought processes usually remain intact. Diagnose acute meningitis with analysis of the cerebrospinal fluid (CSF). If there are focal neurologic signs, mental status change, or papilledema, do a CT before the lumbar puncture (LP). CSF latex agglutination tests are no longer recommended in the initial evaluation of meningitis. With suspected meningitis, start antibiotics immediately after the LP and blood cultures; do not wait for any LP results. Also, if the LP is going to be delayed more than 30–60 minutes, go ahead and give antibiotics immediately (before the LP)! See Infectious Disease, Book 1, for a full discussion on bacterial meningitis.

Neurosyphilis also is discussed in Infectious Disease, Book 1.

Brain Abscess

The classic triad of brain abscess symptoms is headache, fever, and focal neurological deficit(s). Most abscesses arise from intracranial extension of cranial infections (i.e., sinuses, teeth) or after skull fracture or neurosurgical procedures. Much less often, they are due to bacteremic seeding. In adults, the most common organisms are *Staphylococcus* and *Streptococcus* species (e.g., *S. epidermidis* after a penetrating head injury), but do not forget about *Nocardia*. In the immunocompromised, consider toxoplasmosis.

VIRAL CNS INFECTIONS

CSF in Viral Encephalitis

With viral encephalitis, CSF has increased lymphocytes, normal to slightly increased protein, and normal glucose. EEG is almost always abnormal with diffuse slowing or focal temporal changes. MRI is more sensitive than CT and may show hemorrhagic changes.

Herpes Simplex Encephalitis

Altered mental status (due to parenchymal inflammation) is the hallmark of an encephalitis. Herpes simplex encephalitis is the most common type of non-epidemic viral encephalitis and presents with fevers, headaches, and focal seizures. In adults, it is usually due to a reactivation of the HSV-1 virus, although 25% are due to primary HSV-1 infection. HSV-2 is sexually transmitted and can cause aseptic meningitis during primary infection. HSV-2 less typically causes encephalitis but can cause polyradiculitis and myelitis. HSV encephalitis has a predilection for the temporal lobe; immunomodulators increase risk (i.e., natalizumab, TNF alpha inhibitors).

Varicella-zoster virus (VZV) can also cause encephalitis, especially in the immunocompromised; and it can cause vesicular lesions that can be confused for herpes simplex.

See Infectious Disease, Book 1, for treatment of HSV and VZV.

Mosquito-Borne Arboviruses

Mosquito-**BO**rne **AR**boviruses are **Ar**thropod-**BO**rne viruses. Mosquitoes are the main vector but ticks, fleas, and gnats may also be carriers. Neuroinvasive disease caused by arborviruses presents as encephalitis, meningitis, or flaccid paralysis. We'll go over mosquito-borne arboviruses here.

In the U.S., the West Nile virus is by far the main cause of neuroinvasive disease. Per the CDC, there were 2,240 reported cases in 2016; the breakdown of reported arboviruses was:

- West Nile virus (95%)
- La Crosse virus (1.5%)
- Powassan virus (1.0%)
- Jamestown Canyon virus (0.7%)
- St. Louis encephalitis virus (0.35%)
- Eastern equine encephalitis virus (0.3%)

West Nile virus (WNV; genus *Flavivirus*) causes fever with no neurologic symptoms in otherwise healthy patients. Encephalitis is more likely to occur in the immunocompromised and in older patients with comorbidities, such as hepatitis C, diabetes mellitus, and chronic alcohol use. West Nile encephalitis can additionally present with a flaccid paralysis; it is considered a modern-day mimicker of polio.

Flaviviruses that cause neuroinvasive disease in non-U.S. areas include the West Nile, yellow fever, Zika, and dengue viruses. Read more about these viruses in Infectious Disease, Book 1.

Diagnosis of Viral Encephalitis

Polymerase chain reaction (PCR) DNA amplification of the herpes viruses allows for an easy, rapid, and accurate diagnosis of herpes simplex and zoster. Initiate IV acyclovir in all encephalitis patients until herpes simplex is ruled out. This is the most important management principle in encephalitis patients.

Draw acute and convalescent serum titers to diagnose most arboviruses. West Nile diagnosis requires finding antibody in spinal fluid. Enterovirus may cause encephalitis, draw PCR if indicated.

Viral Myelitis

Myelitis (focal or segmental) is infection of the spinal cord—a classic focal viral cause is poliomyelitis affecting the anterior horn cells of the spinal column. Additional focal causes are other enteroviruses (coxsackievirus and enterovirus) and flaviviruses (e.g., West Nile). Reflexes are usually decreased and weakness is typically asymmetric with preserved sensation. Segmental viral forms of myelitis can cause a transverse myelitis (e.g., herpes simplex, varicella zoster, cytomegalovirus, Epstein-Barr). Motor weakness and sensory changes occur below the lesion. Autonomic dysfunction can also occur.

Slow Viruses and Prions

Slow viruses:

- Subacute sclerosing panencephalitis (SSPE) is caused by the measles virus; most cases occur around 10 years of age, many years after the initial infection.
- PML (discussed more under Progressive Multifocal Leukoencephalopathy on page 12-17 and under Progressive Multifocal Leukoencephalopathy on page 12-23)
- Prion: CJD (more under Creutzfeldt-Jakob Disease on page 12-12)

HIV

Infection with HIV can result in dysfunction of any part of the nervous system. Patients get subacute encephalitis, vacuolar myelopathy, aseptic meningitis, and peripheral neuropathies (including mononeuritis multiplex).

HIV-associated cognitive impairment is common. It ranges from asymptomatic to mild to what is called HIV-associated dementia (HAD). In adults, it takes the form of a slowly or subacutely progressive dementia with loss of retentive memory, inattentiveness, language disorder, and apathy.

Know that the differential diagnoses for HAD includes PML, toxoplasmosis, and lymphomas.

Since the use of ART began, the incidence (new cases per year) of HAD in the U.S. has dropped by half. Patients are getting a different type of dementia post-ART; this dementia is associated more with deficits in complex reasoning and less with global impairment. In addition, even though the incidence is dropping, HAD is occurring in patients with higher CD4 counts, even in patients who have had long-term viral suppression on antiretroviral agents.

Zidovudine myopathy can be seen and has mitochondrial features on muscle biopsy.

Peripheral HIV neuropathy has 3 forms:

1) Guillain-Barré syndrome (GBS) or chronic inflammatory demyelinating polyneuropathy (CIDP) phenotype may be seen. GBS is seen at seroconversion, and CIDP is seen in more moderate-to-severe HIV. Usually with GBS or CIDP there is cytoalbuminologic dissociation of the CSF (high protein and normal white blood cells), but if the clinical case is consistent with GBS or CIDP and there is an unexpectedly high number of white blood cells in the spinal tap, then consider HIV.

2) Distal symmetric polyneuropathy is common in AIDS patients (1/3 get it). Symptoms are paresthesias of the feet and distal weakness in the legs. Treatment typically includes tricyclic antidepressants or gabapentin.

3) A painful mononeuritis multiplex thought to be due to focal vasculitis also occurs.

Progressive Multifocal Leukoencephalopathy

Progressive multifocal leukoencephalopathy (PML) affects white matter only. PML is caused by the human JC polyomavirus, resulting in a progressive demyelination of the CNS white matter. (See a larger discussion of Progressive Multifocal Leukoencephalopathy on page 12-17.)

AIDS Myelopathy

Advanced HIV infection can cause a vacuolar myelopathy (see Infectious Myelopathies on page 12-39) and causes progressive weakness, incontinence, hyperreflexia, and ataxia. There is vacuolation and deterioration of the dorsal and lateral spinal columns. It is found in about 50% of AIDS patients at autopsy. This myelopathy must be differentiated from B_{12} deficiency, copper deficiency, human t-cell lymphotropic virus (HTLV), and from spinal cord compression due to some other cause, such as lymphoma.

PARASITIC CNS INFECTIONS

Toxoplasmosis

Toxoplasma gondii is an intracellular protozoan parasite that infects 30–50% of the world's population. Seropositivity ranges from 11% in the U.S. to > 80% in many warm, humid, low-altitude regions of the world. In immunocompetent hosts, initial infection is either asymptomatic or has flu-like symptoms (especially fever, headache, muscle aches, and tender lymphadenopathy), which can last from weeks to months then fully resolve. The parasite remains in the body but becomes dormant. If the infected host then becomes immunocompromised, the parasite can reactivate and cause a much more severe form of toxoplasmosis disease with brain lesions.

If a mother gets an active infection while pregnant, the child may get congenital toxoplasmosis, which can cause cognitive problems, blindness, and seizures—even later in life.

AIDS-related brain lesions: If you see multiple ring-enhancing lesions, the most likely cause is toxoplasmosis. CNS lymphoma, TB, and bacterial infections are less likely causes.

Because toxoplasmosis is a reactivation infection, patients typically have *T. gondii* IgG antibody, but not IgM antibody. But remember that many people are infected and only a few become immunocompromised, so finding a positive IgG *T. gondii* antibody is supportive of the diagnosis of toxoplasmosis but not diagnostic. Also know that an absent toxoplasmosis IgG does not exclude toxoplasmosis as the cause of a brain lesion in a patient with AIDS.

Treat with sulfadiazine, pyrimethamine, and leucovorin. Add dexamethasone if there is midline shift or rapid deterioration.

Do a brain biopsy if there is no improvement after empiric treatment, if there is a mass effect, or if there is only 1 lesion. Relapses occur often.

Neurocysticercosis

Neurocysticercosis is the most common worldwide parasitic CNS infection. It is caused by ingesting food or water contaminated with *Taenia solium* (a tapeworm). It forms cysts in the brain, which initially cause no symptoms. But when the cyst walls break down several years later, it causes cerebral edema, usually with seizures as the 1st symptom. In some patients, a large subarachnoid or intraventricular cyst can obstruct the flow of CSF. In a more malignant form of the disease, the cysticerci are located in the basilar subarachnoid space, where they induce an intense inflammatory reaction leading to hydrocephalus, vasculitis, and stroke as well as cranial nerve palsies.

MRI is the preferred imaging modality—when worms are still viable, MRI shows multiple, nonenhancing, hypodense lesions. As the worms die, they are surrounded by edema and flair. When dead, they calcify and shrink. Support the diagnosis with *T. solium* antibody testing on serum.

Treatment of CNS infection is controversial because of the lack of randomized studies and the propensity of dying worms to cause symptoms. Most experts treat with high-dose praziquantel or albendazole +/- corticosteroids. Give AEDs to patients at high risk for seizures. See more about neurocysticercosis in Infectious Disease, Book 1.

FUNGAL CNS INFECTION

Consider cryptococcal meningitis when working up a progressive headache, cognitive impairment, and/or meningeal signs in patients with AIDS or on chronic corticosteroids.

CSF pressure is usually very elevated. Standard CSF studies can be entirely normal, so always check the cryptococcal antigen titer in the blood and CSF (in HIV patients, sensitivity/specificity is > 95%). In HIV-negative patients, the CSF antigen is still 93–98% sensitive.

Treat with amphotericin B deoxycholate or liposomal amphotericin B and flucytosine × 2 weeks, then change to oral fluconazole × 8 more weeks (minimum). Lower doses of oral fluconazole are used for secondary prophylaxis in immunocompromised patients. Manage elevated ICPs with daily taps to keep CSF pressure < 200 mm H_2O, or patients can lose their vision. Shunts are appropriate if daily taps are needed. Do not use mannitol, acetazolamide, or corticosteroids.

See more about fungal CNS infections in Infectious Disease, Book 1.

HEADACHE AND FACIAL PAIN

PREVIEW | REVIEW

- Name some triggers of migraine headaches.

- What is the main difference between a complicated migraine and a migraine with aura?

- Which migraine patients should not receive a triptan drug?

- Which migraine prophylactic drug causes kidney stones?

- Are cluster headaches more common in men or women?

- What are the clinical features of a cluster headache?

- How do you treat a cluster headache?

- Which agent is 1st line to prevent cluster headaches?

- What is the most common variety of headache?

- What are the high-risk factors indicating the need for a CT scan after head trauma?

- Name a risk factor that is associated with IIH.

- What is the clinical presentation of IIH?

OVERVIEW

The history and examination of the patient are crucial in diagnosing the type and etiology of headache, including the quality of pain (dull, sharp, throbbing, and constant), location, duration, exacerbating or ameliorating factors, and associated symptoms. Also important are the mode of onset of pain and variation over time. Headaches can be classified as primary or secondary, and the 1st step is to determine the classification:

- Primary headaches
  - Migraine
  - Cluster headache and other trigeminal autonomic cephalgias
  - Tension-type headache
  - Other primary headaches
  - Tend to be chronic, recurrent, and without signs of neurologic disease
- Secondary headaches
  - Headache due to hemorrhage (i.e., subarachnoid hemorrhage)
  - Headache due to head and/or neck trauma, benign intracranial hypertension, brain tumors
  - Headache due to cranial or cervical vascular disorders (e.g., carotid dissection, sinus venous thrombosis, giant cell arteritis)
  - Headache due to a substance or its withdrawal (e.g., nitrates, EtOH, caffeine)
  - Headache due to infection (e.g., meningitis, encephalitis)
  - Headache due to disorders of homeostasis (e.g., HTN, hyperviscosity)
  - Headache of facial pain (e.g., cranium, neck, eyes, sinuses, teeth; trigeminal neuralgia; herpes zoster)
  - Headache due to psychiatric disorders

MIGRAINE

Presentation

Know: Migraines are a typically unilateral, periodic pulsatile (throbbing) headaches that run in families; begin in early adult life or childhood; and tend to occur less frequently as patients get older. Migraines are more common in females. 90% of patients who present to emergency departments with recurrent headaches have migraines. These headaches are typically unilateral (~ 60%) but not consistently on the same side (unlike vascular headache secondary to arteriovenous malformation [AVM]). They last several hours, usually 4–72 hours. They are considered episodic if < 15 episodes per month and chronic if > 15 episodes per month for 3 months. Yearly, < 5% of episodic sufferers progress to chronic sufferers.

Triggers include emotional stress, certain foods (e.g., chocolate, aged cheese, and other foods that are rich in tyramine), alcohol (particularly red wine or port), menstruation, exposure to glare or other strong sensory stimuli (including perfumes), and rapid changes in barometric pressure. In women, they often occur in the premenstrual period and can be worsened by oral contraceptives. Migraines are frequently associated with nausea, vomiting, sensitivity to smell, photophobia, and phonophobia. Movement of the head exacerbates the pain, while sleep and darkness may help lessen the pain.

Migraine with aura (previously called classic migraine) makes up 25% of all migraine headaches. It is preceded by an aura—most commonly visual symptoms, such as sparkling lights (scintillating scotomata) or jagged zigzag lines (fortification spectra), that move slowly across the visual fields for several minutes—and may leave scotomatous defects. Migraine auras last for 5–60 minutes with longer auras representing prolonged auras (complicated migraine) or concern for stroke.

Migraine without aura (previously called common migraine) occurs without an aura and is ~ 5× more typical than migraine with aura.

Other migraine auras (less common) include focal sensory disturbance or weakness (usually unilateral) or dysphasic speech. If sensory symptoms spread from one part of the body to another or evolve over time, they do so relatively slowly, over several minutes (not seconds, as in seizures), and not acutely as with concern for a transient ischemic attack (TIA).

Basilar migraine affects the brainstem. Patients are typically young women or children with a family history of migraine.

Patients with basilar migraines may experience:

* Visual phenomena that occupy both visual fields (temporary cortical blindness may occur)
* Vertigo
* Dysarthria
* Staggering
* Incoordination of the limbs
* Diplopia ("seeing double")
* Tingling (may occur in both hands and feet and sometimes around both sides of the mouth)

These symptoms last 10–30 minutes and are usually followed by an occipital headache. In exceptional cases, coma or transient quadriplegia can develop.

Acephalic migraine (migraine without headache) can present with abnormal transient neurologic dysfunction, such as visual symptoms, focal sensory deficits, transient aphasia, or hemiparesis. These spells are stereotyped and evolve over minutes, again unlike acute symptoms from a vascular etiology.

Status migrainosus is characterized by multiple or virtually continuous headaches with persistent scalp tenderness, over a period of 72 hours or longer.

Diagnosis of Migraine

Diagnosis is most often done with history alone. For patients who present with typical migraine symptoms, first give a trial of treatment (as follows) before neuroimaging or any other studies.

Atypical symptoms, including change in headache pattern, seizure, or focal neurologic symptoms, warrant further workup, including imaging studies; the initial study is usually a head CT with and without contrast.

Acute Treatment of Migraine

Acute treatment refers to any treatment that is given within the 1st hour of the headache. Acetaminophen, aspirin, and NSAIDs are effective in some patients, especially if the migraine is mild and infrequent.

Triptans are the 1st line drugs for migraine therapy. Triptans are more effective and are very safe to use even in patients with infrequent migraines. Under-dosing and less effective drugs are associated with failure to control migraines.

The triptans:

* Sumatriptan
* Zolmitriptan (Zomig)
* Rizatriptan (Maxalt)
* Naratriptan (Amerge)
* Almotriptan (Axert)
* Eletriptan (Relpax)
* Frovatriptan (Frova)

Know the following about the triptans:

* Rizatriptan, almotriptan, and eletriptan have the highest consistent success rates.
* Rizatriptan interacts with propranolol and requires that you adjust the rizatriptan dose downward (propranolol increases the levels).
* Sumatriptan has 3 methods of delivery: injection, intranasal, and oral.
* Combination tablet of sumatriptan + naproxen works synergistically and is better than taking either agent as monotherapy.
* Naratriptan and frovatriptan have the slowest onset but the fewest side effects.

Because of the risk of inducing ischemia, do not use triptans for any of the following conditions:

* Migraine with prolonged aura (> 1 hour), hemiplegic migraine, or basilar migraine
* Coronary vascular disease (CVD) or Prinzmetal angina
* History of stroke
* Uncontrolled blood pressure

Eletriptan, frovatriptan, and naratriptan can be used with monoamine oxidase inhibitors; the others are contraindicated. All triptans should not be used within 24 hours of ergot drugs.

Instead of the triptans, IV prochlorperazine or metoclopramide in addition to intravenous fluids are effective for termination of migraine in patients who present to the emergency department with vomiting. Diphenhydramine 25 mg IV helps prevent the unusual dystonic reaction of the antiemetic.

Dihydroergotamine (DHE) can be effective in some patients, but it also must be avoided in patients with CVD, HTN, pregnancy, history of peripheral arterial disease, and liver or kidney disease. You can try narcotics, but restrict their use to 2 days/week. You can use oral or IV corticosteroids to terminate status migrainosus, as well as IV valproic acid or IV ketorolac.

Increased use of any medication, including triptans and NSAIDs, to treat frequent headaches can incite a rebound, called a medication overuse headache. Instruct patients not to take analgesics more than 10 days/month. If a patient needs medication this often, then prescribe prophylactic treatment.

Prophylactic Treatment of Migraine

The American Heart Association/American Stroke Association 2014 Guidelines for the Prevention of Stroke in Women recommend prophylaxis for women with frequent migraines with aura if < 55 years of age, especially if they are taking oral contraceptives (OCPs). These guidelines also recommend aggressive smoking cessation efforts in women with migraine with aura.

Generally, avoid the use of OCPs in women who have migraine with aura (increased risk of stroke). For other patients, the frequency of headache determines whether prophylaxis is needed; normally, the threshold is > 2–3 headaches per month. There is usually a lag of 2–4 weeks between the start of prophylaxis and its effect.

The following are major categories of migraine prophylaxis agents:

- Beta-blockers: Propranolol and timolol are FDA-approved for migraine, but atenolol, metoprolol, and nadolol are also used; not recommended in patients > 60 years of age and/or smokers.
- Tricyclic antidepressants: amitriptyline; side effects include oversedation, dry mouth, palpitations, orthostasis, blurry vision, weight gain, constipation, and short-term memory impairment or confusion—especially in the elderly or in those with baseline cognitive impairment.
- Anticonvulsants: valproic acid, topiramate; topiramate can cause kidney stones, paresthesias, and word-finding difficulties. It also can cause weight loss, which is a positive side effect in many cases. Avoid use of these antiepileptic medications during pregnancy.
- Calcium channel blockers: verapamil, nimodipine; may develop tolerance
- ACE inhibitors and ARBs: lisinopril and candesartan
- NSAIDs
- Botulinum toxin injection: approved by the FDA in 2010 for refractory chronic migraine (i.e., migraine occurring ≥ 15 days/month with headaches lasting ≥ 4 hours/day). Thirty-one injections are delivered into 7 specific head and neck sites. The treatment usually needs to be repeated every 12 weeks, on average.

Definitely use prophylactic agents to treat migraine with prolonged aura and basilar migraines. Relaxation techniques also may be helpful for patients to prevent headaches.

CLUSTER HEADACHE

Cluster headache is a distinct syndrome that frequently responds to treatment with oxygen. The term "cluster" is derived from the periodicity of the headaches: They can occur up to several times/day for a few weeks before remitting. Cluster headache becomes chronic in 10% of patients.

Cluster headaches are more common in men (5:1). They tend to occur in the 20–50-year-old age group. 70% of patients find that alcohol triggers their headache.

The daily attacks may occur at the same hour each day (in 50% of patients). The pain is unilateral, severe (described as an "ice pick" or "hot poker"), and peri- or retroorbital. It peaks quickly, in 5–10 minutes, and resolves in 1–2 hours.

Another characteristic feature is nightly recurrence, about 1–2 hours after the onset of sleep or several times during the night. The cluster headache period may last 6–12 weeks, followed thereafter by complete freedom for many months or even years.

Associated vasomotor phenomena include ipsilateral blocked nostril, rhinorrhea, lacrimation, miosis, and flush and edema of the cheek that last about 45 minutes.

Patients with cluster headaches tend to be restless during attacks, as opposed to most migraine sufferers who prefer a dark, quiet room and stillness.

Treatment: The best acute treatment for cluster headaches is oxygen. Inhalation of oxygen at 6 L/minute × 15 minutes is usually rapidly abortive, acting to inhibit neuronal activation in the trigeminocervical complex. However, this is not always practical or available. Subcutaneous and intranasal triptans are effective and can be combined with oxygen; but remember, do not use triptans in patients with a history of or strong risk factors for CVD and stroke. For patients who do not get better with O_2 and cannot take triptans, octreotide and intranasal lidocaine are options.

Once a patient experiences the 1st of what will become a cluster episode, prophylactic treatment can be instituted. Verapamil is the drug of choice (outpatient oral titration up to 480 mg), but monitor the patient's pulse and ECG for bradycardia and heart block when titrating higher than 240 mg. Other drugs sometimes used include lithium, methysergide, prednisone, and topiramate. Use corticosteroids as acute drugs while waiting for verapamil to work. Taper off the medication once the cluster is over.

TENSION HEADACHE

Tension headache, the most common variety of headache, is characterized by pain that is chronic, bilateral, constant, nonthrobbing, squeezing, and devoid of migrainous or cluster features. It can be intermittent or chronic. Unlike most other headaches, it can be present throughout the day for long periods of time. The onset is slow with gradual increment in intensity, typically at the end of the day. Sleep is normally undisturbed, but headache returns upon awakening. It is more common in women. 1/3 of patients with chronic tension headaches have symptoms of depression.

Use aspirin, acetaminophen, or NSAIDs to treat acute attacks.

Consider preventive medication when attacks occur > 2 days/week—this can help prevent medication overuse, which can predispose to chronic headache. Limiting treatment to 9 days/month (2 doses of meds/day) helps prevent this complication. Effective prophylactic drugs include amitriptyline and other tricyclics (see Prophylactic Treatment of Migraine on page 12-26) and gabapentin. Relaxation, biofeedback, and behavioral therapy are helpful in dealing with the tension that brings about the headaches.

BENIGN SEXUAL HEADACHE

Benign sexual headache (a.k.a. coital headache) occurs more often in men than women (4:1). The headache occurs either as a tension-type headache as sexual excitement increases or as a severe, throbbing headache at the time of orgasm. These headaches can persist for several minutes or hours; they are benign. If the headache does not resolve after 2 hours or is accompanied by neck stiffness, vomiting, and/or neuro deficits, rule out an underlying vascular AVM, such as an aneurysm with subarachnoid hemorrhage. Evaluate with urgent neuroimaging. Treatment with NSAIDs before sexual activity may prevent the headache.

CONCUSSION

A concussion is transient neurologic symptoms in the setting of a head trauma. It is classified as a mild traumatic brain injury, usually without structural findings on imaging. With nearly 2–4 million sport-related concussions per year, there is growing awareness and interest in this clinical condition.

Common concussion symptoms include transient confusion, amnesia, headache, dizziness/vertigo, nausea/vomiting, behavioral changes, photophobia, imbalance, and loss of consciousness.

Though transient loss of consciousness may be seen, it is not mandatory for the diagnosis. Focal neurologic findings or a seizure require a CT head to evaluate for intracranial pathology of concern, as well as other risk factors identified by the Canadian CT Head Rule study. This study identified risk factors that would merit a head CT for evaluation:

- High-risk factors
  - Failure to reach Glasgow Coma Scale (GCS) of 15 within 2 hours
  - Suspected open skull fracture
  - Any sign of basal skull fracture
  - Vomiting > 2 episodes
  - > 65 years of age
- Medium-risk factors
  - Amnesia before impact > 30 minutes
  - Dangerous mechanism of injury

Most concussive symptoms resolve over hours to 7–10 days. The 2017 Berlin Concussion in Sport Group Consensus Statement—5th International Conference discusses the **11 Rs** of concussion:

1) **R**ecognize
2) **R**emove
3) **R**eevaluate
4) **R**est

5) **R**ehabilitation
6) **R**efer
7) **R**ecovery
8) **R**eturn to sport
9) **R**econsider
10) **R**esidual effects and sequelae
11) **R**isk reduction

Utilize the SCAT5 tool (sports concussion assessment tool, 5th edition) for sideline field assessment after concussion. The SCAT5 is designed to be a sideline rapid assessment tool. It includes symptom evaluation and cognitive screening with orientation, memory, concentration, balance, and delayed recall testing. The score determines if a concussion was suffered. The Concussion in Sport Group (CISG) also recommends the CCMI baseline testing battery to compare cognitive differences if present.

Recovery follows a 6-day graded return to play protocol that begins with complete physical and cognitive rest followed by graded increase in activity. Rehabilitation level 1 is no activity, and level 6 is return to normal play. Each stage lasts a minimum of 24 hours, and only when the patient achieves full recovery at a level can you move them to the next level of activity. The minimum recovery time for return to play is 6 days.

A minority of patients have persistent concussive symptoms, termed postconcussive syndrome that may last for months or longer. This may require symptomatic treatment for persistent migraines, anxiety/depression, and cognitive dysfunction.

Finally, some patients who have had repeated mild traumatic brain injuries may develop chronic traumatic encephalopathy, which is a chronic dementia-like syndrome associated with tau deposition in the brain. There is increasing awareness of this syndrome, as well. Chronic behavioral/cognitive decline is a hallmark, but other neurologic sequelae may be seen, such as Parkinsonism, tremor, and gait disturbance.

POSTTRAUMATIC HEADACHE

Posttraumatic or postconcussion headache can occur even after a minor head injury. It can present similarly to migraine clinically; however, some have proposed that the headache is due to abnormal neurotransmission within the brain. Accompanying symptoms include dizziness, fatigue, insomnia, nervousness, irritability, and inability to concentrate. Symptomatic treatment is usually effective, and the headache often spontaneously remits. Patient reassurance is important.

GIANT CELL ARTERITIS

Giant cell arteritis (GCA; a.k.a. temporal arteritis) typically occurs in patients > 55 years of age. History commonly includes a recent onset of headache. Jaw claudication, fatigue, weight loss, and low-grade fever can also occur. Up to 50% of patients have a history of polymyalgia rheumatica. Do not miss the diagnosis of GCA; if untreated, ischemic optic neuropathy can cause irreversible vision loss. Diplopia occurs in 10–15% of patients. On physical exam, look for a palpable temporal artery with associated tenderness.

The erythrocyte sedimentation rate (ESR) and the C-reactive protein (CRP) tests (for inflammation) are elevated. (So, if ESR and CRP are normal, it is not GCA.) Do a temporal artery biopsy if you suspect the diagnosis. Yield of bilateral artery biopsy (~ 2 inches of tissue) in expert centers is about 85%. See more on this topic in Rheumatology, Book 3.

TRIGEMINAL NEURALGIA

Trigeminal neuralgia (TN) is neuralgia occurring in ≥ 1 branches of the 5th cranial nerve (usually V2 or V3). The 3 branches of the trigeminal nerve cover the anterior upper (ophthalmic), middle (maxillary), and lower (mandibular) areas of the face. Even though TN occurs rarely, it is one of the most common causes of facial pain. TN most often affects people > 50 years of age and women somewhat more than men (~ 1.5:1).

The pain of TN is characteristically abrupt in onset, with the most intense pain at onset. It can be extremely severe and has a shock-like or burning quality—typically in the maxillary distribution. Sporadic episodes are usually triggered by innocuous activities, such as chewing, eating, or brushing teeth.

Start treatment with antiepileptic drugs, such as carbamazepine, phenytoin, gabapentin, or pregabalin.

IDIOPATHIC INTRACRANIAL HYPERTENSION / PSEUDOTUMOR CEREBRI

Idiopathic intracranial hypertension (IIH; a.k.a. pseudotumor cerebri) is a set of signs and symptoms—headaches, papilledema, and loss of vision—caused by increased intracranial pressure (ICP). IIH ordinarily occurs in obese, premenopausal women (90%) and can occur during pregnancy. It rarely occurs in children or in men.

Obesity is strongly correlated with IIH (90–95% of patients) and causal; with the increasing obesity of the U.S. population, the incidence of IIH is also increasing.

Drugs that can cause IIH include vitamin A (especially in the form of isotretinoin, used for the treatment of severe acne), tetracycline, and corticosteroids; but the condition can also be precipitated by steroid withdrawal.

Severe, irreversible vision loss is the major morbidity. It occurs in > 6% of patients and is 2× as common in men as in women. Perform magnetic resonance venography in at-risk patients to exclude venous thrombosis.

The cardinal symptom of IIH is a morning headache described as dull or as a feeling of pressure (90%) made worse by coughing or straining. There is almost always (90–100%) a peripheral visual field loss accompanied by blind spots that may be noticeable only with formal visual field testing. Pulse-synchronous tinnitus (60%) may be present. Transient visual obscurations (seconds of transient visual blackouts) can be another hallmark sign. Diplopia is less commonly seen.

On exam, papilledema is a hallmark finding. 6th nerve palsy may be obvious either unilaterally or bilaterally. CT/MRI is typically normal, with absence of deformity, displacement, or obstruction of the ventricular system—but may show slit-like ventricles. The CSF pressure is elevated, usually in the range of 250–450 mm H_2O. (Normal CSF pressure is generally 50–180 mm H_2O.)

Treatment of IIH includes a low-Na^{2+}, weight-reducing diet; symptomatic treatment for headaches; carbonic anhydrase inhibitors (acetazolamide); prevention of vision loss; and discontinuation of isotretinoin.

Repeat LPs, with drainage of sufficient fluid to maintain CSF pressure < 200 mm H_2O, is helpful in ~ 25% of cases.

Prednisone works acutely but is not recommended for chronic cases of IIH because of side effects, not the least of which is increasing ICP. Unilateral optic nerve sheath fenestration may preserve vision in the acute setting.

Consider ventriculoperitoneal (VP) shunt in refractory cases, especially if there is vision loss.

CNS: BRAIN — CORTEX, SUBCORTEX, AND BRAINSTEM

STROKE AND TIA

PREVIEW | REVIEW

- Which viral infection increases risk of strokes?

- In addition to exercise, smoking cessation, and control of diet, blood pressure, and lipids, which other interventions should be offered to certain patient groups in order to prevent stroke?

- Which imaging study would you do for a patient with a suspected SAH?

- Which imaging studies are recommended for evaluation of vasculature in patients with TIA or stroke?

- How does a patient with an ACA stroke typically present?

- How does a patient with an MCA stroke usually present?

- How does a patient with a PCA stroke typically present?

- How do you distinguish a central vs. peripheral 7th cranial nerve palsy on physical exam?
- What is the clinical presentation of lateral medullary syndrome? What type of stroke causes it?
- Which tests are recommended in the initial evaluation of ischemic stroke?
- What is the timeframe for prescription of tPA in patients with ischemic stroke?
- Which patients with a stroke between 3 and 4.5 hours are excluded from tPA?
- What are the recommendations for lowering blood pressure in patients with ischemic stroke who do not receive tPA?
- Why should you keep a patient with an ischemic stroke in the posterior fossa under close observation?
- What are the recommended antiplatelet regimens postischemic stroke?
- What are the most common causes of an intracerebral hemorrhage?
- What are the recommendations for treatment of blood pressure in a patient with an intracerebral hemorrhage?
- What is the most common cause of SAH?
- If imaging for SAH is negative and suspicion is high, what are alternative tests?
- What causes mycotic aneurysms?
- Which further evaluation is indicated in cocaine users who present with a cerebral bleed even if hypertensive?
- Which patient groups are prone to subdural hematomas?
- Describe the differences between subdural and epidural hematomas.

OVERVIEW

Stroke (a.k.a. cerebrovascular accident), after heart disease and cancer, is the 3rd most common cause of death in the U.S. The term stroke is applied to a sudden focal neurologic syndrome caused by cerebrovascular disease. Cerebrovascular disease refers to an abnormality of the brain caused by pathology of blood vessels, such as:

- Occlusion by embolus or thrombus
- Vessel rupture
- Altered permeability of the vessel wall
- Increased viscosity or other change in the quality of the blood flowing through the cerebral vessels

The primary vascular disorder may be atherosclerosis, hypertensive arteriosclerotic change, arteritis, aneurysmal dilatation, or a developmental malformation. The secondary parenchymal changes in the brain resulting from the vascular lesion can include ischemia (especially in the penumbra or periphery of infarcted tissue), infarction, and hemorrhage.

Important risk factors for stroke include familial predisposition, age, hypertension, diabetes mellitus, smoking, hypercholesterolemia, and atrial fibrillation (AF). Know that a rare cause is varicella-zoster infection, which increases risk of ischemic and hemorrhagic strokes and TIA by 30%. There is an even higher risk with the presentation of herpes zoster ophthalmicus. This risk is highest within 3 weeks of the appearance of the rash.

TIA

A transient ischemic attack (TIA) is brain ischemia without infarction. When brain infarction occurs, it is termed an ischemic stroke.

Note that the latest guidelines (2014) on TIA from the American Stroke Association has removed all references to duration of symptoms. The definition was changed because infarctions sometimes occur even when symptoms last < 24 hours, making the previous time-based definition of TIA occasionally incorrect.

COMPLICATIONS OF TIA

Patients with TIA are at risk for the following:

- Stroke
  - 10% have ischemic stroke within 3 months; 50% of this group do so within 48 hours.
- Cardiac events
  - 3% have cardiac events within 90 days.
  - Acute myocardial infarction (AMI) risk is increased.
  - Mortality in AMI after TIA is increased.

Risk stratification of TIA, **ABCD²** score:

- **A**ge: ≥ 60 = 1 point, < 60 = 0
- **B**P: ≥ 140/90 mmHg = 1, < 140/90 mmHg = 0
- **C**linical: weakness = 2, isolated speech = 1, other = 0
- **D**uration: ≥ 60 min = 2, 10–59 min = 1, < 10 min = 0
- **D**iabetes: present = 1, absent = 0

Score	2-Day Risk of Stroke
0–1	0%
2–3	1.3%
4–5	4%
6–7	8%

The 2014 AHA/ASA (American Heart Association/American Stroke Association) guidelines recommend hospitalization within 72 hours of an event if:

- ABCD² score ≥ 3
- ABCD² score 0–2 and unable to complete workup within 48 hours

- ABCD² score 0–2 and other evidence that events were caused by ischemia

Have patients with TIA imaged within 24 hours, or ASAP after their symptoms begin, to determine if any infarction is present. Also order CT or MR angiography of intracranial and neck vessels versus carotid duplex, echocardiogram, and blood work, including chemistries, blood glucose, lipids, and CBC. Order an ECG to rule out AF. See more under Evaluation of Ischemic Stroke on page 12-33.

CLASSIFICATION OF STROKES

Strokes are classified as ischemic or hemorrhagic. Ischemic strokes can be thrombotic or embolic.

Ischemic strokes (87% of all strokes):

- 20% are due to large artery atherosclerosis.
- 20% are due to cardiac emboli.
- 20% are due to lacunar/small vessel infarcts.
- 5% are due to vascular disorders (e.g., vasculitis, dissection).
- 35% are cryptogenic.

Hemorrhagic strokes are of 2 main types:

1) Intracerebral hemorrhage (ICH)
2) Subarachnoid hemorrhage (SAH)

PRIMARY PREVENTION OF STROKE AND TIA

The 2014 AHA/ASA guidelines for primary prevention of stroke and TIA include:

- Treatment of blood pressure and lipids
- Smoking cessation
- Antiplatelets or anticoagulation
- Diet and exercise
- Treatment of AF (See more on AF in Cardiology, Book 4.)
- Carotid endarterectomy if > 70% stenosis in selected patients, and if perioperative morbidity and mortality is < 6%
- Prophylaxis for migraine (previously discussed under Prophylactic Treatment of Migraine on page 12-26)
- Evaluation and treatment of obstructive sleep apnea
- Screening for aneurysms with CTA or MRA for the following:
  ◦ Patients who have ≥ 2 first-degree relatives with SAH/aneurysm (But screening is not recommended in patients who have only 1 affected first-degree relative.)
  ◦ Patients who have autosomal dominant polycystic kidney disease (ADPKD) and ≥ 1 relatives with ADPKD + SAH/aneurysm

IMAGING OF STROKES

A main reason to do neuroimaging is to determine whether a patient is eligible for tissue plasminogen activator (tPA), but there are other uses:

- Exclude intracranial bleeding
- Detect ischemia
- Exclude other illnesses that mimic stroke
- Image the vessels
- Assess possible viability of infarcted tissue

Imaging with CT: A nonenhanced CT (NECT) scan can be performed as a basic form of stroke imaging (Figure 12-4). Its main role is to rule out hemorrhage in the acute setting, though large strokes may have early ischemic signs, such as a hyperdense middle cerebral artery (MCA) sign showing the clot or sulcal blurring.

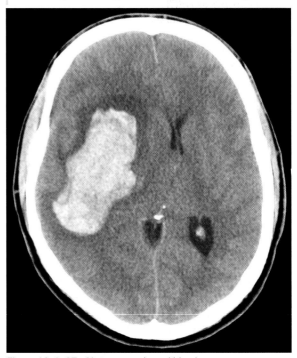

Figure 12-4: CT of intraparenchymal bleed

IV tPA can be given to patients with duration of stroke symptoms < 4.5 hours, a CT scan negative for hemorrhage, and no hemorrhagic risk contraindications.

The NECT can be enhanced by adding either of the following:

- Angiography (CTA)
- Dynamic perfusion studies (computed tomography perfusion [CTP])

When adding angiography, evaluation of source images (SI) helps to interpret the study (CTA-SI).

Imaging with MRI:

- Diffusion-weighted imaging (DWI)
- Fluid-attenuated inversion recovery (FLAIR)

NEUROLOGY

MRI can also be enhanced using additional imaging sequences:

- Perfusion (magnetic resonance perfusion [MRP])
- Angiography (MRA)
- Gradient-recalled echo (GRE)

Now that you know the abbreviations and acronyms, we'll go over which imaging to use in particular situations:

- Intracerebral hemorrhage (ICH): MRI-GRE is equivalent to NECT for finding blood. MRI is also better for detecting hemorrhagic transformation of ischemic stroke (occurs in about 5% ischemic CVAs).
- Subarachnoid hemorrhage (SAH): Use NECT.
- There is some data showing MRI with FLAIR is as sensitive as NECT. No matter which test you choose, an LP is still mandatory if the CT or MRI is negative.
- Ischemia: MRI-DWI is best. CTA-SI is comparable, but it is not as good for imaging of the posterior fossa/brain stem and for discovering small infarcts. MRI is also better than NECT to detect an occluded vessel.

Because of the above, unless your patient has signs and symptoms of SAH, MRI + DWI and MRI + GRE sequences (at minimum) are the best imaging for possible ischemic stroke because they both exclude ICH and identify areas of infarction—provided you can get the test without delay. Remember that time from symptom onset > 4.5 hours precludes use of tPA (< 3 hours is best). If you cannot get an MRI in a reasonable time frame, then get a CT with CTA-SI.

CTA or MRA is recommended to evaluate the intra- and extracranial vasculature of patients with TIA or stroke symptoms. Both imaging modalities are significantly more sensitive and specific than carotid Doppler ultrasound for diagnosing extracranial vascular stenosis. Carotid ultrasound also tends to over diagnose lesions and leads to unnecessary surgery in some patients, so only utilize that for screening purposes. CTA is better than MRI at identifying intracranial aneurysms.

If performing CTA or MRA does not extend the time from symptom onset out past 4.5 hours maximum (< 3 hours is best), either is recommended as part of the initial evaluation of stroke because, sometimes, clotted vessels can be treated with urgent intraarterial therapy or stents. Patients with a large clotted vessel—often the MCA—do not respond as well to IV tPA as they do to direct arterial intervention (intraarterial tPA or mechanical thrombectomy options).

Although assessing viable brain tissue after infarction is one of the main purposes for imaging a stroke patient, we are still in the beginning stages of learning how to incorporate the data into treatment plans. Dynamic CTP and MRP are the leading imaging techniques.

At this point, the standard of care has been at least a CT brain to exclude hemorrhage for tPA candidacy, which can be performed urgently to assess for the IV tPA window, but advanced imaging techniques for endovascular candidacy is increasingly becoming the standard of care at stroke centers. (See further information on Acute Treatment of Ischemic Stroke on page 12-34.)

ISCHEMIC STROKES

Thrombotic vs. Embolic Strokes

Thrombotic strokes: Atherosclerotic occlusion most commonly occurs in the internal carotid, middle cerebral, vertebral, and basilar arteries.

The initial neurologic symptoms often occur in a slow, stepwise progression ("stroke in evolution"). Often patients have a history of TIAs in the same distribution as the presenting symptoms of their stroke. If the patient has not had TIAs, a clear differentiation between thrombotic and embolic stroke can be difficult to detect. Other, rarer causes of thrombotic occlusion are lupus anticoagulant, polycythemia, meningovascular syphilis, dissecting aortic aneurysm, and thrombocytosis.

Embolic strokes: Neuro deficit is commonly worst at onset. Embolic strokes are not typically preceded by a TIA. Emboli from the heart, due to large particle size, usually go to the middle > posterior > anterior cerebral arteries. Emboli can also be multiple. Obtain an echocardiogram or transesophageal echocardiogram to evaluate left atrial size, valvular structure, and global ventricular function assessment.

Anterior Circulation

Anterior Cerebral Artery Strokes

When the anterior cerebral artery (ACA) is affected distal to the anterior communicating artery, the weakness and sensory loss primarily affect the contralateral leg.

Urinary incontinence and gait abnormalities can also be present. If the corpus callosum is affected, patients can develop tactile agnosia, which is an inability to recognize objects by touch.

Occlusion of the stem of the ACA proximal to the anterior communicating artery is generally well tolerated because collateral flow is provided by the contralateral ACA. When both ACAs arise from one occluded stem, there is resulting paraplegia, incontinence, lack of motivation (abulia), and frontal lobe personality changes.

Buzz phrase: The patient with ACA stroke typically presents with contralateral leg weakness that is opposite to the side of the stroke.

Middle Cerebral Artery Strokes

Most middle cerebral artery (MCA; Figure 12-5) stem occlusions are from emboli. MCA strokes result in:

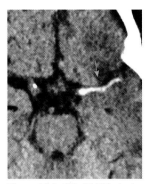

Figure 12-5: CT of MCA stroke

- contralateral weakness (hemiplegia), which is denser if the internal capsule is involved;
- contralateral sensory loss (hemianesthesia); and a
- contralateral homony-mous hemianopia.

The weakness pattern follows a lateral homunculus pattern: The face and arm are more affected than the leg on the contralateral side of the body compared to the brain lesion.

If the dominant hemisphere is involved (the left side in most people, even left-handed individuals), these patients experience aphasia. Examples of dominant hemisphere MCA strokes and their presenting signs:

- A lesion that affects the lower part of the left frontal lobe (Broca area) causes expressive (a.k.a. Broca) aphasia. These patients understand language, but they have trouble forming words and sentences, so their speech is nonfluent and effortful.
- A lesion at the boundary of the temporal and parietal lobes causes a fluent or sensory aphasia, called Wernicke aphasia. These patients cannot comprehend written or spoken language and have errors in their spontaneous speech, often speaking in invented words, called neologisms.
- An extensive infarction can produce global aphasia, which is both expressive and sensory.

If the nondominant hemisphere is involved, patients may experience changes in spatial perception and can develop hemineglect syndrome.

With parietal lesions of either hemisphere, cortical sensory signs are often present:

- Contralateral loss of 2-point discrimination
- Failure to perceive tactile stimuli on the opposite side of the involved hemisphere when stimuli are presented to both sides simultaneously (sensory inattention)
- Inability to recognize objects through touch (tactile agnosia)
- Inability to recognize letters drawn on their palm (agraphesthesia)

If the lesion involves the frontal lobe, patients may have a gaze preference or gaze deviation—they look toward the side of the lesion for 1–2 days after the stroke.

Buzz phrase: The patient with MCA stroke typically presents with face/arm > leg weakness that is opposite to the side of the stroke and a language deficit if the dominant hemisphere is involved.

Posterior Circulation

Posterior Cerebral Artery Stroke

Posterior cerebral artery (PCA) strokes typically occur from an embolic source.

PCA stroke syndromes can be categorized by which area of the brain is affected. The PCA supplies the occipital cortex, occipitoparietal cortex, medial temporal lobe, midbrain, and thalamus.

Depending on the area affected, there can be mild contralateral sensory loss, inability to name colors (color anomia), failure to see to-and-fro movements, inability to count objects, inability to control eye movements (oculomotor apraxia), inability to see > 1 object at a time if the dominant occipital lobe is involved (simultanagnosia), visual hallucinations, and/or memory loss.

The finding of a visual field defect can give you an idea of where the stroke is located (see Figure 12-10 on page 12-54 for reference). Visual field defects will be contralateral. You can find:

- a homonymous hemianopia with strokes affecting the medial occipital lobe,
- an inferior quadrantanopia with strokes affecting optic radiations through the parietal lobe, or
- a superior quadrantanopia with strokes affecting optic radiations through the temporal lobe.

Bilateral cortical blindness can result from simultaneous or successive PCA occlusion but may also be due to anoxia related to surgery, especially cardiac surgery. Rarely, patients with cortical blindness deny their visual defect (Anton syndrome).

If the patient has color anomia, the posterior aspect of the corpus callosum (splenium) may have been affected. Lesions that affect the dominant hemisphere's occipital lobe (which is most commonly the left) along with the splenium of the corpus callosum cause alexia without agraphia (inability to read but able to write).

If disruption of blood flow occurs bilaterally, the memory loss is severe and persistent.

Buzz phrase: The patient with PCA stroke commonly presents with visual field defects + color anomia + paresthesias without any motor findings.

Single Hemisphere Strokes

Single hemisphere strokes typically do not affect paraspinal muscles or muscles of the pharynx, jaw, and forehead. If these muscles are affected, think bilateral hemispheric involvement or brainstem stroke (see next). Remember: Upper motor neuron lesions of cranial nerve 7 do not affect eye closure or forehead wrinkling, which helps you to distinguish clinically between a central lesion and Bell's palsy (peripheral 7th nerve involvement).

Vertebral / Basilar Artery Occlusion

Vertebral and/or basilar artery occlusion in the posterior circulation is the usual cause of brainstem (posterior fossa) strokes. Consider this when you see any of the following:

- Bilateral extremity motor and sensory dysfunction (quadriplegia in severe cases)
- Crossed sensory findings (e.g., right face, left arm)
- Horner syndrome
- Cerebellar signs
- Stupor and coma
- Cranial nerve dysfunction not usually seen with single hemisphere strokes, such as diplopia, pharyngeal weakness, jaw weakness, and deafness
- Crossed hemiplegias (e.g., ipsilateral cranial nerve deficit and contralateral arm or leg weakness)

Know: A vertebral stroke can cause **lateral medullary syndrome** (a.k.a. Wallenberg syndrome), which has a mixed bag of symptoms:

- Ipsilateral cerebellar signs and symptoms (due to involvement of the inferior cerebellar peduncle and cerebellum)
- Nausea, vomiting, nystagmus (vestibular nuclei)
- Ipsilateral Horner syndrome (due to involvement of the descending sympathetic fibers)
- Ipsilateral palate and vocal cord weakness (involvement of the nucleus ambiguus)
- Crossed sensory loss (ipsilateral face and contralateral body, due to involvement of the trigeminal nucleus and tract and spinothalamic tract, respectively)

Buzz phrases: The patient with posterior circulation stroke typically presents with:

- Vertigo and diplopia if due to vertebrobasilar artery, sometimes with antecedent TIA symptoms
- Lateral medullary syndrome
- Vertigo + nystagmus + nausea + ataxia (if cerebellar)

Lacunar Infarcts

Small artery disease, usually due to chronic hypertension or diabetes, can lead to small vessel occlusion with resultant necrosis of small areas of the brain. Over time, resorption of these necrotic regions causes small infarcts, or lacunae, to develop.

Although most are silent, hallmarks of symptomatic lacunar infarcts are:

- Pure hemiplegia (with no sensory dysfunction)
- Pure hemisensory stroke (with no motor dysfunction)
- Sensorimotor stroke
- Ataxic hemiparesis (ataxia ipsilateral to hemiparesis)
- Clumsy hand-dysarthria syndrome

Multiple bilateral frontal lobe lacunae can result in pseudobulbar palsy—emotional lability with uninhibited crying or laughter and evidence of upper motor neuron signs, such as brisk jaw jerk, hyperreflexia, and Babinski sign.

Evaluation of Ischemic Stroke

Assess the patient with a neurologic deficit like any other emergency, using the **ABCs** first: stabilize **a**irway, **b**reathing, and **c**irculation.

If the patient is stable, take a good history. The most important element is the time of symptom onset because that determines eligibility for an IV thrombolytic. If the patient awoke with deficits, then the last time they remember having normal function is the time of symptom onset. Remember that complicated migraines, postictal states, and subdural hemorrhages can resemble a stroke; therefore, ask about headaches, seizure activity, and falls.

Physical exam focuses on possible sources and alternative diagnoses. Look for evidence of seizures (tongue biting), trauma, myocardial ischemia, carotid and vertebral artery bruits, heart murmurs, and arrhythmias.

The National Institutes of Health Stroke Scale (NIHSS) score is a standardized instrument incorporated as part of a physical exam at most stroke centers. The general concepts of the scale are presented in Table 12-3 on page 12-34.

The NIHSS helps to quantify neurologic deficits, communicate with neurologists, possibly identify the occluded vessel, make an early prognosis, and identify a patient's suitability for thrombolytics. Patients get points for their inability to complete the various parts of the assessment.

The AHA/ASA 2013 Guidelines for the Early Management of Acute Ischemic Stroke recommend the following immediate diagnostic tests at presentation:

- NECT or MRI of the brain (discussed under Workup on page 12-2) is done to rule out hemorrhage. If negative for hemorrhage, then do a CT angiogram or MRA (if CTA is contraindicated) to evaluate vessels—but do not allow this to delay any necessary reperfusion therapy.
- Blood glucose level
- Oxygen saturation measurement
- Serum electrolytes and renal function tests
- CBC with platelets
- Prothrombin time (PT), partial thromboplastin time (PTT), INR
- 12-lead ECG +/− telemetry monitoring for arrhythmias
- Optional tests in selected patients
  - Thrombin time (TT) and/or ecarin clotting time (ECT) or chromogenic anti-Xa assay if on direct thrombin inhibitors (but not readily available)
  - Hepatic function test
  - Toxicology and alcohol screen
  - Pregnancy test
  - Again, do an LP with CSF assessment if SAH is a concern and NECT (or MRI with FLAIR) does not show blood.

NEUROLOGY

- EEG if you suspect the patient has seizures
- ABG if hypoxic

Acute Treatment of Ischemic Stroke

Critical Times

Always refer patients via 911 to a primary stroke center (PSC) or a comprehensive stroke center (CSC).

The AHA/ASA 2013 guidelines recommend these goals:

- Door to physician should be ≤ 10 minutes
- Door to stroke team should be ≤ 15 minutes
- Door to CT initiation should be ≤ 25 minutes
- Door to CT interpretation should be ≤ 45 minutes
- Door to drug (≥ 80% compliance) should be ≤ 60 minutes
- Door to stroke unit admission should be ≤ 3 hours

If the stroke occurred < 4.5 hours ago and the NIH stroke scale rating is > 4, tPA is effective in decreasing severity or reversing neurologic deficits, provided that the patient fits inclusion/exclusion criteria (2013 AHA/ASA stroke treatment guidelines).

tPA Criteria for < 3 Hours

< 3 hours tPA inclusion criteria:

- Diagnosis of ischemic stroke causing measurable neurologic deficit
- Onset of symptoms < 3 hours before beginning treatment
- ≥ 18 years of age

< 3 hours tPA exclusion criteria:

- Minor or rapidly improving stroke symptoms
- Significant head trauma or prior stroke in last 3 months
- Symptoms suggest SAH
- History of prior intracranial hemorrhage
- Intracranial tumors or arteriovenous malformation (AVM) or aneurysm
- Arterial puncture at noncompressible site
- Infarct in last 7 days
- Recent intracranial or intraspinal surgery
- SBP > 185 mmHg or DBP > 110 mmHg
- Active internal bleeding
- Platelets < 100,000/mm^3
- Anticoagulation with INR > 1.7 or PT > 15 seconds
- Used direct thrombin inhibitors or direct factor Xa inhibitor with abnormal INR/aPTT/PT/ECT/TT/Xa activity assay
- Blood glucose < 50 or > 400 mg/dl (< 2.77 or > 22.20 mmol/L)
- CT with multilobar infarction (hypodensity > 1/3 cerebral hemisphere)

Relative exclusions:

- Seizure with postictal deficits
- Major surgery or serious trauma in prior 14 days
- GI or GU hemorrhage within last 21 days
- AMI within 3 months

Additional tPA Criteria for 3–4.5 hours

Inclusion criteria (3–4.5 hours):

- Diagnosis of ischemic stroke causing measurable neuro deficit
- Onset of symptoms within 3–4.5 hours before beginning treatment

Table 12-3: NIH Stroke Scale	
Category	**Clinical Response**
Consciousness: Level	Choose a response: alert, arousable by minor stimuli, requires repeated or painful stimuli, unresponsive or reflexes only, or areflexic.
Consciousness: Questions	Ask month and age; no partial credit. Aphasic and stuporous patients score 2. Intubated patients score 1.
Consciousness: Commands	Ask patient to open and close eyes, then to grip and release nonparetic hand.
Gaze	Test horizontal eye movements.
Vision	Test visual fields by confrontation with finger counting.
Facial Palsy	Ask patient to show teeth or raise eyebrows and close eyes.
Motor: Arm and Leg	Test for pronator drift.
Ataxia	Perform finger-nose-finger and heel-shin tests.
Sensation	Assess for sensation or grimace to pinprick or withdrawal from noxious stimulus.
Language	Describe what is happening in a picture, name items printed on paper, and read a sentence.
Speech	Read words from a list.
Extinction and Inattention	Assess previous tests to determine if patient orients only to one side.

For the full scale with scoring, go to www.ninds.nih.gov/sites/default/files/NIH_Stroke_Scale.pdf.

Relative exclusion criteria (3–4.5 hours):

- Age > 80
- Severe stroke (NIHSS > 25)
- On anticoagulation regardless of INR
- History of both DM and prior ischemic stroke

Endovascular Interventions

Intraarterial fibrinolysis or mechanical thrombectomy is a consideration for patients who have contraindications to IV fibrinolytics.

Other Aspects of Acute Ischemic Stroke Care

Management that emphasizes supportive care and treatment of complications:

- Give airway support to stroke patients with reduced consciousness or airway compromise; oxygen prn.
- Monitor with telemetry for the first 24 hours after a stroke to assess for arrhythmias.
- Treat hypertension cautiously, so as not to extend infarct size. If the patient meets criteria for tPA except for BP, go ahead and treat to reduce BP to ≤ 185/110 mmHg, then give tPA. If not giving tPA, withhold meds for BP < 220/120 mmHg and allow the patient to gradually drop their pressure on their own. If BP > 220/120 mmHg, then treat with the goal of reducing the BP ~ 15% in the first 24 hours. Recommended medications include IV labetalol, nitroprusside, and nicardipine infusion.
- Restart antihypertensives for patients with longstanding hypertension after 24 hours (if not treated already for BP > 220/120 mmHg).
- Maintain normoglycemia 140–180 mg/dL (7.77–9.99 mmol/L).
- Look for and treat sources of fever. Give antipyretics to reduce fever.

Know: In patients who are ineligible for treatment with tPA, and who are not taking anticoagulation for any other underlying disease, give 325 mg aspirin once, followed by aspirin 150–325 mg/day while hospitalized. The optimal dose is not yet clear. The risk of hemorrhagic transformation of an infarct is not high enough to offset the benefits of aspirin therapy, so treat all eligible patients, even if a small hematoma is present within the infarcted area. Heparin or low-molecular-weight heparin (LMWH) is generally discouraged in the acute setting of stroke due to bleed risk. Use anticoagulation with oral agents in cardioembolic settings for secondary prevention (i.e., AF and other subtypes, outlined further below). If the ischemic stroke is large, hold off starting anticoagulation for the first 1–2 weeks due to bleed risk; if the stroke size is minimal, then starting after the first 24 hours is reasonable. Of note, cardiac embolism from endocarditis is an absolute contraindication to anticoagulation because of increased risk of CNS hemorrhage.

If the stroke occurs in the posterior fossa, admit the patient for close observation. Expansion of the contents of the posterior fossa can cause either upward or downward herniation; these patients then decompensate quickly and without warning.

Chronic Treatment of Ischemic Stroke

Reduce the patient's risk factors for stroke by treating hypertension, diabetes, and lipids according to 2014 AHA/ASA national guidelines, and add aspirin 50–325 mg/day.

Equally acceptable alternatives to aspirin are clopidogrel and the combination of ASA + dipyridamole. These provide a small amount of increased benefit compared to aspirin alone. Consider using these agents as 1st line therapy based on a financial cost discussion or if the patient has had a recurrent stroke and was already on aspirin. Use clopidogrel in patients with aspirin allergy. Know that aspirin + clopidogrel does not offer additional benefit in general and does increase risk of bleeding. Nevertheless, a specific indication for dual therapy is for the first 90 days following a stroke due to large artery intracranial disease.

Headache is a common side effect of dipyridamole, which sometimes causes patients to self-discontinue the drug. Normally the headaches can be treated symptomatically with acetaminophen.

Anticoagulate the patient who has AF if the patient meets guidelines. (See more on AF in Cardiology, Book 4.) Newer agents are available and becoming widely utilized for anticoagulation in nonvalvular AF and do not require blood test monitoring (i.e., apixaban, rivaroxaban, dabigatran) Warfarin is still used for other indications for anticoagulation for secondary prevention, such as prosthetic valves, rheumatic mitral valves, DVT with patent foramen ovale (PFO), cerebral venous thrombosis, and LV thrombus. It is sometimes considered for low ejection fraction or extracranial dissection. Refer for carotid endarterectomy if the patient has > 70% occlusion and an expected lifespan of > 5 years and the anticipated operative morbidity and mortality is < 6%.

Blood pressure control is paramount in secondary prevention of stroke. Control of lipids, glucose, diet, and exercise remains important, as is treatment of underlying sleep apnea.

Cerebral Venous Thrombosis

Thrombus in the cerebral venous system prevents drainage of blood flow from the brain and can have protean clinical presentations (i.e., headaches, seizures, focal deficits, altered mental status). It is 3× more common in women and is associated with OCPs, pregnancy, hypercoagulable states, infection, and previous head trauma. MRI with MR venography are the best imaging modalities. Treatment is with anticoagulation.

CEREBRAL HEMORRHAGE

Overview

The primary forms of cerebral hemorrhage are **intracerebral** and **subarachnoid**. The secondary forms, usually caused by trauma, are **subdural** and **epidural**.

Intracerebral Hemorrhage

Overview

Intracerebral hemorrhagic stroke is generally due to the rupture of small arteries, especially when the small artery branches off at a 90° angle from the parent vessel and the blood pressure is very high. The most common causes are hypertension, AVM rupture, amyloid angiopathy, and ischemic strokes (especially post thrombolytics). Warfarin use is a risk factor, especially when the INR is > 3.

Some patients have preexisting evidence of intermittent, small bleeds on MRI of the brain. It is possible that these MRI-visible microbleeds are indicators denoting which patients are prone to future intracerebral hemorrhage. Because the bleeding arises from small arteries, the symptoms of microbleeds typically evolve gradually but continuously. See (Figure 12-6) for a CT of an acute intracerebral hemorrhage with leakage into the lateral ventricles.

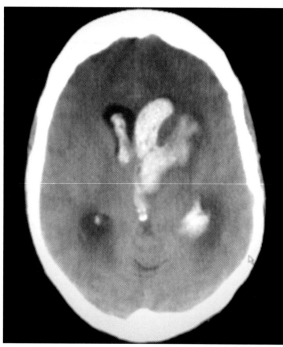

Figure 12-6: CT of acute intracerebral hemorrage

Signs and Symptoms / Diagnosis

Intracerebral hemorrhagic stroke occurs in the following 4 areas of the brain (from most common site to least common):

1) **Putamen** and the adjacent **internal capsule** (50%): If the hematoma involves the internal capsule, there is contralateral hemiparesis and usually sensory loss and hemianopia. This type of hemorrhage can be difficult to distinguish from a middle cerebral artery infarct (one of the reasons to do the enhanced NECT or MRI to look for blood at presentation). For central white matter of the temporal, parietal, or frontal lobes, symptoms are based on the lobe affected.

2) **Thalamus**: contralateral hemianesthesia without cortical sensory signs. Some motor signs may be present if the adjacent internal capsule is involved.

3) **Pons**: coma, pinpoint pupils, and quadriplegia. There can be decerebrate posturing bilaterally.

4) **Cerebellum**: acute dizziness, ataxia, and vomiting with no change in mentation and no loss of consciousness

Amyloid angiopathy is a typical cause of intracerebral hemorrhagic stroke after the 5th decade of life. The hemorrhage tends to be lobar and subcortical and there can be multiple instances. It rarely involves the deep structures (as does a hypertensive bleed). These hemorrhages can recur within months or years. Dementia occurs in 30% of patients. Other clinical features include acute reactive hypertension, vomiting, headache, and nuchal rigidity.

Other causes of intracerebral hemorrhage include:

- Bleeding diatheses
- Trauma
- Bleeding into a tumor mass
- Cocaine use

Treatment of Intracerebral Hemorrhage

Treatment includes the basic supportive care given to ischemic stroke patients. (See Other Aspects of Acute Ischemic Stroke Care on page 12-35.)

Immediately reverse any anticoagulant effects with both vitamin K and replacement of clotting factors, no matter the reasons for anticoagulation. Give protamine sulfate for any hemorrhage associated with unfractionated heparin. Also, stop any antiplatelet agents.

Control of ICP is important, and mannitol is usually used.

The 2015 AHA/ASA Guidelines for the Management of Spontaneous Intracerebral Hemorrhage state that acute lowering of systolic blood pressure to 140 mmHg is safe in patients who present with SBP 150–220 mmHg. For patients who present with SBP > 220 mmHg, the guidelines state that a continuous IV infusion (e.g., labetalol, esmolol, nicardipine, enalapril) can be considered for aggressive BP lowering. Be sure to maintain frequent BP monitoring while instituting this strategy.

Neurosurgeons are consulted. The neurosurgeon considers clot removal depending on the site and for cerebellar hematomas > 3 cm. Also consider surgery for lobar clots > 30 ml within 1 cm of the surface. In patients with minor deficits or deeply comatose patients, surgery is generally not done. Interventional radiologists can perform coil embolization for AVMs.

Subarachnoid Hemorrhage

Overview

Subarachnoid hemorrhage (SAH) usually results from bleeding from an intracranial aneurysm. Aneurysms are most common at the bifurcation of vessels in the circle of Willis or its major branches. This most likely occurs between 40 and 60 years of age, and it occurs in women more often than in men.

The majority occur in the anterior circulation: 40% of aneurysms affect the internal carotid artery, 35% involve the anterior cerebral artery, and 20% the middle cerebral artery.

SAH can also occur after a parenchymal bleed, when there is rupture into the ventricular system. Nonaneurysmal causes of SAH are rare but include AVMs, sickle cell disease, bleeding diatheses, pituitary apoplexy, trauma, cocaine abuse, and intracranial arterial dissection. Among persons with saccular aneurysms, there is an increased incidence of congenital polycystic kidneys, fibromuscular dysplasia of the extracranial arteries, Moyamoya disease, AVMs of the brain, and coarctation of the aorta.

Signs and Symptoms

Ruptures typically occur when the patient is active rather than at rest. More than 1/3 of patients report a history of sentinel bleed symptoms days or weeks earlier.

The characteristic symptoms of SAH are the acute "thunderclap" or "worst headache of my life" sensation in combination with neck stiffness. Common associated symptoms include loss of consciousness, nausea/vomiting, and photophobia. Systemic manifestations of SAH can include ECG changes of giant inverted T waves (cerebral T waves), hyponatremia, and diabetes insipidus.

The most important determinant of outcome is the neurological condition of the patient upon arrival at the hospital. 10% die before getting to hospital, 25% die within the first 24 hours. If comatose, the prognosis is poor.

Diagnosis of SAH

NECT is the best test to identify blood in the subarachnoid space. The NECT in Figure 12-7 shows a massive SAH in which all the white in the brain tissue is due to blood in the subarachnoid space. If the NECT shows no SAH and no mass, then do a lumbar puncture (LP). The CT misses progressively more subarachnoid bleeds as time passes from initial rupture—picking up only about 50% of bleeds after 5 days. In an SAH, CSF is bloody with xanthochromic supernatant (pink or yellow tint); however, even clear CSF does not preclude the diagnosis because it may take hours after onset of the bleed before you find red cells at the level of the spine where you draw the CSF sample. Nevertheless, most cases have many thousands of red blood cells without sufficient clearing from tube 1 to tube 4 (indicating this is not a traumatic tap). Additionally, in some cases you can have an elevation of white blood cells due to an aseptic meningitis reaction to the blood, so do not mistake that for meningitis when the primary issue could still be an SAH.

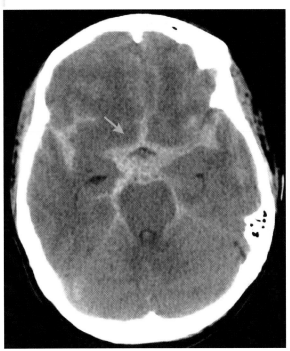

Figure 12-7: Massive subarachnoid hemorrhage

If a bleed is still suspected in the setting of a normal NECT and LP, then angiography is the procedure of choice. CTA and MRA are alternatives to invasive angiography, and their sensitivity and specificity are close to the standard angiogram.

Complications of SAH

After a sentinel bleed, rebleeding is common. The risk is highest in the first 24 hours, but the risk remains high for at least 1 month.

Vasospasm can occur in up to 70% of patients and begins 3–5 days after the hemorrhage. It reaches a peak at 5–14 days and resolves in 2–4 weeks.

Communicating hydrocephalus is the 3rd major complication. It occurs in 15–20% of patients after SAH. The likelihood of hydrocephalus depends on the volume of intraventricular and subarachnoid blood.

Seizures occur in 5–10% of patients; 2/3 begin within the 1st month after the hemorrhage, while the remaining occur within the 1st year.

Treatment of SAH

If the patient is on an anticoagulant or antiplatelet agent, stop the drug before performing any interventions. Surgical clipping and endovascular coil insertion into the bleeding vessel are the major interventions used to prevent the aneurysm from bleeding again. Remaining treatment focuses on preventing complications, such as calcium channel blockers to prevent vasospasm.

Control of ICP and blood pressure is important as well, although recommendations are less clear-cut than with intracranial hemorrhages. Refractory vasospasm may need angiographic interventions.

Know that 1st degree relatives of patients who experience an SAH have a 2–5× increased risk of an SAH. The AHA/ASA 2014 Guidelines for the Primary Prevention of Stroke recommend aneurysmal screening, as discussed previously under Primary Prevention of Stroke and Tia on page 12-30.

Note on other aneurysms: Mycotic aneurysms are caused by septic emboli, most often from infected heart valves. They are commonly small and occur in the distal vasculature. This is in contrast to saccular aneurysms that occur more proximally at the branch points of the arteries (at the point where the middle cerebral artery branches off of the internal carotid artery).

Cocaine Use

Know that cocaine use can cause AVMs and aneurysms that rupture during episodes of severe drug-induced hypertension. These can cause either intracerebral or subarachnoid strokes. Evaluate all active cocaine users with an intracranial bleed with angiography.

Subdural Hematoma

Subdural hematoma (SDH) is usually due to direct trauma, but deceleration forces can also cause it. Consider SDH in patients with a history of falls, blows to the head, alcoholism, a recent motor vehicle accident, and in the elderly. Subdural bleeds are usually of venous origin.

SDH can be acute or chronic, and each type manifests differently. In acute SDH, 1/2 of the patients immediately become comatose, but the other 1/2 remain lucid for a period of hours to days, after which cognition becomes gradually and progressively impaired until coma develops.

Symptoms can also be fluctuating. Other signs of increased ICP are often present; e.g., headache, nausea/vomiting, neck stiffness, and gait abnormalities.

In chronic SDH, the trauma is often forgotten. Over a period of weeks, patients may develop headache, lightheadedness, slowness in thinking, apathy, drowsiness, unsteady gait, and occasionally seizure. Initially, they may be diagnosed as having a vascular lesion, brain tumor, drug intoxication, a depressive illness, or Alzheimer disease.

NECT is used in triage of these patients, but MRI with FLAIR is the most sensitive test. NECT in Figure 12-8 shows a subdural hematoma with a skull deformity.

Treatment for SDH is typically surgical—except for very small bleeds without any neurologic symptoms, which are observed closely.

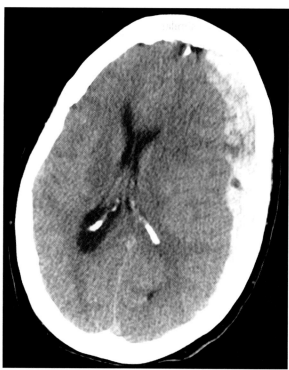

Figure 12-8: Subdural hematoma

Epidural Hematoma

Epidural hematomas, because of their arterial origin, evolve more rapidly than subdural hematomas. These are commonly caused by temporal trauma that damages the middle meningeal artery—in association with temporal bone fractures. Symptoms of increased ICP are usually rapidly progressive. However, a short period of lucidity can occur, followed by rapid obtundation.

As with SDH, you can diagnose epidural hematomas with NECT, but MRI with FLAIR is most sensitive.

Treatment consists of early evacuation of the hematoma via a craniotomy. If untreated, herniation occurs, with mortality ranging from 15–40%.

TRANSIENT GLOBAL AMNESIA — STROKE AND TIA MIMIC

Transient global amnesia (TGA) is characterized by abrupt onset of global anterograde amnesia, with a variable impairment of retrograde memory not associated with any other major neurologic signs or symptoms. Except for amnesia during and around the event, patients recover completely in 2/3 of cases within 2–12 hours and in almost all cases within 24 hours. TGA is considered benign, and the condition recurs infrequently.

Patients are commonly between 50 and 80 years of age and suddenly develop an inability to make new memories. They act disoriented, asking multiple questions repeatedly. The amnesia can even extend back to years, although more typically just days to weeks. Some patients have accompanying nausea and dizziness. Consider TIA, which can present similarly.

Precipitating events are seen in many cases and include strenuous exercise, intense emotion, sexual intercourse, mild head trauma, pain, temperature extremes (e.g., swimming in cold water), cervical manipulation, coughing spells and other Valsalva-like activities, and medical procedures that require anesthesia (e.g., colonoscopy). The etiology is unknown, although migraine can be a predisposing factor.

NECT and brain MRI with DWI are usually normal. PET and SPECT studies have shown hypoperfusion and hypometabolism in the hippocampi and associated mesial temporal lobe structures during the attack, with resolution following the attack. The attacks self-resolve. No treatment is necessary.

CNS: SPINAL CORD

MYELOPATHIES

PREVIEW | REVIEW

- Describe the findings in subacute combined degeneration due to B_{12} deficiency.

- Which other mineral deficiency can present like the subacute combined degeneration due to vitamin B_{12}?

- What are risk factors for an epidural abscess? What is the most common cause?

- What causes Pott disease?

- Describe the clinical presentations of neurosyphilis.

- What is the clinical presentation of transverse myelitis?

- What is neuromyelitis optica? Which autoantibody is the culprit?

- What are the symptoms of cervical myelopathy?

- What is lumbar spinal stenosis? What are the classic exacerbating and relieving body positions and movements?

- From the patient's history, which clues help you differentiate lumbar spinal stenosis from vascular claudication?

- What is the clinical presentation of syringomyelia?

- What is the clinical presentation of ALS?

- Which conditions can cause UMN and LMN signs in the same patient?

OVERVIEW

Myelopathies are diseases of the spinal cord. Typical manifestations are gait ataxia, spasticity, and hyperreflexia. Bowel and bladder incontinence arise as disease worsens. There are many subcategories.

METABOLIC MYELOPATHY — SUBACUTE COMBINED DEGENERATION OF SPINAL CORD

Subacute combined degeneration of the spinal cord due to B_{12} deficiency is the prototype for metabolic myelopathy. Severe B_{12} deficiency causes segmental loss of myelin, especially in the dorsal and lateral columns. Clinical presentation is gradual weakness with paresthesias and loss of proprioception with development of ataxia. Severe cases end in extensive bilateral lower extremity weakness, spasticity, and urinary incontinence +/– cognitive impairment. These cognitive changes include confusion, apathy, delusions, paranoia, and mental deterioration.

Tip: Think of B_{12} deficiency in a patient with brisk knee jerks (due to pyramidal tract dysfunction) and absent ankle jerks (due to peripheral neuropathy).

Know that the neurologic changes can occur without any associated macrocytosis, megaloblastosis, or anemia! The CSF is typically normal and electromyography (EMG) shows slowing of sensory conduction.

Diagnose by measuring serum B_{12}, methylmalonic acid (MMA), and homocysteine levels. MMA and homocysteine are more sensitive tests that are included to make a diagnosis in patients who have low-normal or normal B_{12} levels. In states of B_{12} deficiency, both MMA and homocysteine are increased.

Treat the B_{12} deficiency as early as possible with vitamin B_{12} supplementation, usually by injections, which must continue indefinitely to prevent symptom recurrence.

Of note, copper deficiency can present with symptoms similar to myeloneuropathy due to B_{12} deficiency; therefore, consider it in cases of GI absorption issues (i.e., gastric bypass) or excess zinc ingestion.

INFECTIOUS MYELOPATHIES
AIDS

Advanced AIDS patients can get vacuolar myelopathy with vacuolation and deterioration of the dorsal and lateral spinal columns (seen on pathology, usually autopsy) that presents as ascending paresis with a sensory component (loss of vibration and proprioception) and urinary incontinence. MRI is normal, but CSF may have elevated protein and sensory evoked potentials are abnormal. Clinical presentation is very similar to subacute combined degeneration of the cord. It commonly accompanies HIV-associated dementia but occasionally occurs alone. Many other conditions can do this in a patient with virtually no immune system, but be sure to exclude a cord lesion with MRI.

Epidural Abscess

Spinal epidural abscess is a medical emergency that requires rapid diagnosis and treatment. The abscess can develop from bacteremic seeding from any source or from contiguous infection after spine surgery but also, rarely, from LP. Risk factors include immunodeficiency states (e.g., diabetes, HIV/AIDS), alcoholism, and any conditions or behaviors that cause transient bacteremia (e.g., injection drug use, boils). The abscess can start as a spinal osteomyelitis and progress to an abscess, causing cord compression. *S. aureus* is the most common etiology of epidural abscess.

Remember: The main symptom of epidural abscess is back pain. Suspect epidural abscess in anyone with back pain and fever. For example, rule out epidural abscess in the postpartum patient who had an epidural during delivery—the cause is almost always some type of nosocomial *Staphylococcus* species.

Initial symptoms include a few days to 2 weeks of fever and backache with localized tenderness, radicular pain, and neurological deficits. Not all patients have all of the symptoms, and the diagnosis can be easily missed.

Abscess is best diagnosed with immediate contrasted MRI with FLAIR (contrasted CT is a less sensitive alternative). Perform myelography if the abscess is not clearly seen by MRI (or CT, if that is the only option).

Treatment: immediate decompression with laminectomy and drainage, particularly if there is any associated neurologic deficit, and with appropriate antibiotic treatment.

Tuberculosis

Pott disease is tuberculous osteomyelitis of the spine that sometimes causes cord compression. Usually, this form of TB is due to reactivation disease (rarely is it primary tuberculosis). Less than 40% of affected patients have constitutional symptoms (fever, night sweats, and weight loss). Most commonly they have back pain, but neurologic deficits and/or radicular symptoms are also possible.

Diagnosis is confirmed by biopsies for pathology and culture. A positive TB skin test or serum interferon-gamma release assay (IGRA) supports the diagnosis. Treatment is with standard 4-drug TB therapy (see Pulmonary Medicine, Book 2, for details).

Syphilis

Neurosyphilis is a potential complication if syphilis is untreated and may present earlier in patients with HIV/AIDS. Both secondary and tertiary syphilis can affect the spinal cord. The secondary manifestation of meningovascular syphilis can present as stroke or as infarction of the spinal cord (rare). Tertiary syphilis presents as cognitive impairment, tabes dorsalis, and/or aortitis.

Remember cognitive impairment by the mnemonic **PARESIS**: **p**ersonality, **a**ffect, **r**eflexes, **e**yes (Argyll Robertson pupil), **s**ensorium, **i**ntellect, **s**peech. The Argyll Robertson pupil is constricted and reacts to accommodation but does not react to light.

Tabes dorsalis is syphilitic involvement of the posterior columns that causes deficits in proprioception, manifesting as ataxia and paresthesias. Tabes dorsalis is diagnosed with physical examination, along with the following:

- Screening tests for syphilis (RPR [rapid plasma reagin] or VDRL [venereal disease research laboratory])
- *Treponema pallidum*-specific testing (MHA-TP [microhemagglutination assay for *T. pallidum*])
- +/- LP and biopsies with routine path and cultures

Read more about diagnosis and treatment of syphilis (including neurosyphilis) in Infectious Disease, Book 1.

INFLAMMATORY MYELOPATHY — TRANSVERSE MYELITIS

Transverse myelitis (TM) is a rare condition in which there is inflammation of both sides of 1 or 2 segments of the cord (usually thoracic). The exact cause is uncertain, but it appears to be an autoimmune reaction. Onset may follow a viral infection, rarely a vaccine, or be idiopathic, but it is also seen with multiple sclerosis and several other autoimmune disorders (systemic lupus erythematosus, mixed connective tissue disease, Sjögren's, sarcoidosis, scleroderma, and rheumatoid arthritis). A partial lesion, multiple spinal cord lesions, or associated lesions on an MRI of the brain suggests MS rather than an idiopathic transverse myelitis. Additionally, longitudinally extensive myelitis (over > 3 contiguous vertebral segments) is more suggestive of a recurrent process from defined etiologies, such as neuromyelitis optica (see below), neurosarcoidosis, a connective tissue disease (e.g., lupus, Sjögren's), or a dural arteriovenous fistula.

Clinical presentation is most often acute and progressive over a few days, with early paresthesias, bilateral leg weakness, and numbness with a sensory deficit below the level of the lesion. Sphincteric disturbances and backache are also common. Urinary incontinence, a sensory level over the trunk, or a Babinski sign differentiate it from a rapidly progressive polyneuropathy, such as Guillain-Barré syndrome.

MRI of the spinal cord with contrast shows the inflammation of the cord. CSF analysis shows increased protein, lymphocytosis, and normal glucose.

MRI of the brain is always done to exclude lesions consistent with MS.

Neuromyelitis optica (NMO; a.k.a. Devic disease): This variant of myelitis manifests primarily by attacking the optic nerves and/or longitudinally extensive segments of the spinal cord. The presence of serum NMO-IgG antibodies, also known as antiaquaporin antibodies, is associated with increased risk of recurrent myelitis. NMO antibodies also have a sensitivity of 73% and specificity of 91% for the diagnosis of Devic disease.

TM Treatment: The 2011 AAN guidelines on transverse myelitis recommend empiric steroids and even plasmapheresis if there is no response to steroids, although the level of evidence for these is weak.

COMPRESSION-INDUCED MYELOPATHIES

Cervical Spondylosis with Myelopathy

Cervical spondylosis is age-related wear and tear on the cervical spine. It begins with changes in the intervertebral discs, which occur gradually and accumulate with age. Neck pain is common. If the disc herniates, it will compress a nerve root, causing a radiculopathy at that level. Note: Radiculopathy manifests by numbness, paresthesias, weakness, and hyporeflexia in the corresponding region that is supplied by the compressed nerve root. The area affected is referred to as dermatome (sensory) or myotome (muscle groups).

When the spondylosis becomes more severe, it can result in compression of the spinal cord itself (myelopathy), causing spasticity, hyperreflexia, and gait abnormalities. Gait abnormalities may be attributed incorrectly to increasing age of the patient. A quick test is to check reflexes; in patients > 65 years of age, a brisk ankle reflex can be the sole clue to cervical myelopathy.

If a rheumatoid arthritis patient presents with a post-op focal neuro deficit, suspect C1–C2 spinal cord trauma induced by intubation. This is likely if the patient has chronic asymptomatic C1–C2 subluxation. Anesthesiologists are generally well aware of this susceptibility and may order C-spine flexion and extension views preoperatively to assess for any signs of cervical subluxation. Of course, other mechanisms can cause similar injury in these patients.

Thoracic Myelopathy

Thoracic sensory levels: T4/T5 disease is at nipple line and T10 disease is at umbilicus.

In thoracic myelopathies, think tumor, vertebral compression fracture, or transverse myelitis—not compression from spine osteoarthritis.

Lumbosacral Myelopathy

The cord ends at L1–2. Lumbosacral disease affects the cauda equina and nerve roots, and may cause L4, L5, or S1 radiculopathy with the following presentations:

Affected dermatomes:

- L4 = medial aspect of leg
- L5 = anterolateral aspect of leg and dorsum of foot, including great toe (**L**5 = **l**arge toe)

- S1 = lateral side of foot by the small toe and plantar aspect of foot

Affected myotomes:

- L5 = weakness of the great toe extensor and ankle dorsiflexion (Patients have trouble standing on the heel and present with foot drop.)
- S1 = weakness of ankle plantar flexion (Patients have trouble standing on the toes.) Ankle reflex is absent.

Lumbar spinal stenosis is a congenital narrowing of the spinal canal, affecting the conus medullaris or cauda equina. Patients are more susceptible to myelopathy caused by impingement of the cauda equina secondary to disc disease, ligamentous degeneration, and arthritis.

Lumbar spinal stenosis can result in neurogenic claudication, characterized by a deep, progressive ache in the legs, sometimes causing lower extremity numbness, paresthesias, or weakness, which is precipitated by standing or walking for a few minutes. These symptoms are aggravated by upright posture, which extends the spine, and relieved by sitting or squatting (i.e., flexing the hips and spine).

Buzz phrases that help diagnose spinal stenosis include "gets better when bending over" or "improves when walking uphill." These activities curve the vertebral bodies and open space in the canal.

Differential diagnosis for spinal stenosis includes vascular claudication, which also causes symptoms when walking or exercising leg muscles but not when standing upright (Table 12-4).

Table 12-4: Spinal Stenosis vs. Vascular Claudication			
	Change in Symptoms		
	Walking	Standing	Sitting
Lumbar Spinal Stenosis	Worse (except when walking uphill)	Worse	Better
Vascular Claudication	Worse	Better	Better

A presumptive diagnosis of spinal stenosis is made clinically. Neuroimaging (usually MRI) before treatment is not necessary for patients < 50 years of age with no neurologic deficits. In this group of patients, MRI is done only if there is worsening of symptoms during the 1st month of treatment or no improvement by the end of this 1st month. In patients > 50 years of age and in those with neurologic deficits, imaging is often done immediately to confirm the diagnosis before determining treatment.

Treatment is conservative—physical therapy and analgesics. Surgery is a last resort for patients who have debilitating pain not relieved with conservative measures. Surgery is indicated urgently, however, in patients with progressive neurologic deficits or incontinence.

NEUROLOGY

MISCELLANEOUS MYELOPATHIES

Ischemic Myelopathy

Ischemic myelopathy is caused by decreased perfusion or infarction of the anterior spinal artery that supplies the anterior 2/3 of the spinal cord. The clinical presentation is bilateral leg weakness (often complete paraplegia) and leg sensory loss but with preservation of vibration and position sense (posterior columns). This can be seen after aortic trauma or dissection, aortic aneurysm repair, and revascularization procedures involving the iliofemoral vessels, but it can also occur spontaneously, typically in patients with severe generalized vascular disease. Diagnosis is with MRI, and treatment is often supportive, but there are some strategies available if they occur following vascular procedures.

Syringomyelia

Syringomyelia is a progressive myelopathy caused by cavitation of the central spinal cord, usually in the cervical region but sometimes extending into the thoracic region. It can be idiopathic, developmental, or acquired. About 2/3 of cases are associated with Arnold-Chiari (a.k.a. Chiari II) malformation—a congenital malformation in which there is a downward shift of the cerebellar tonsils and medulla through the foramen magnum into the cervical area of the spine, sometimes with syrinx (cyst) formation.

Syringomyelia causes a painless weakness and wasting of the hands and arms (brachial amyotrophy) and segmental sensory loss of dissociated type (i.e., loss of thermal and painful sensation with sparing of tactile, joint position, and vibratory sense). Symptoms of syringomyelia typically occur as a "suspended" or "cape-like" sensory deficit across the shoulders and proximal upper limbs.

The loss of pain and temperature, with initially preserved light touch and vibration sensation, indicates involvement of the crossing spinothalamic fibers in the central part of the cord. When the anterior horn cells are affected, with lateral expansion of the syrinx, weakness and atrophy of the upper limbs occur, starting in the hands and moving proximally to include the arms and then shoulder muscles. Occipital and nuchal headaches are also very common.

Diagnose syringomyelia with MRI.

Surgical decompression or shunt placement can be tried for ongoing pain or neurologic deterioration.

Anterior Horn Cell Disorders

Anterior horn cell problems cause motor deficits only. **Amyotrophic lateral sclerosis** (ALS; a.k.a. Lou Gehrig disease) is the most common cause of anterior horn cell disorder. The hallmark of ALS is marked, simultaneous upper and lower motor neuron signs. Men are affected more often than women.

A patient with ALS presents with some variation of:

- hyperreflexia and spasticity (upper motor neuron), along with
- fasciculations, weakness, and atrophy (lower motor neuron).

Consider ALS in a patient with weakness or difficulty with fine motor skills as well as fasciculations and/or atrophy on exam. Additionally, consider it with progressive dysarthria or dysphagia, particularly when tongue fasciculations and atrophy are seen. Patients report muscle cramping. Shortness of breath becomes apparent as disease progresses with worsened shortness of breath while lying flat due to weakness of the diaphragm. Exaggerated laughing or crying (pseudobulbar affect) can be another clinical clue. Some cases may start with weakness of a limb progressing to other limbs first, whereas others may start with earlier swallowing, speech, or breathing dysfunction with progressive weakness ensuing (bulbar onset). Cognitive dysfunction is not a main feature, though an association with frontotemporal dementia may be seen.

ALS is relentlessly progressive, involving upper and lower extremities, respiratory, truncal, and bulbar musculature, and it is terminal usually within 3–5 years after diagnosis. Management of these patients includes determining how to proceed with respiratory and nutritional support as the disease progresses. Riluzole is typically used, but extends life by only about 3 months.

Polio used to be the most common cause of anterior horn cell disorder; now **postpolio syndrome** must also be considered. Postpolio syndrome is typified by areflexia and progressive weakness without upper motor neuron signs. Spinal muscular atrophy is a set of hereditary disorders of the anterior horn lower motor neurons. Recent genetic therapy breakthroughs have been made for spinal muscular atrophy with recent FDA approval. A polio-like presentation today is more likely to be due to West Nile virus encephalitis.

Examples of conditions that cause upper motor neuron (UMN) and lower motor neuron (LMN) findings in the same patient include:

- ALS (motor)
- B_{12} deficiency with subacute combined degeneration of the cord (motor + sensory)
- Cervical myelopathy (motor + sensory)
- Syringomyelia (LMN = arms, UMN = legs, motor + sensory)
- Friedreich ataxia (ataxia + motor + sensory)
- Syphilis (motor + sensory)

PERIPHERAL NERVOUS SYSTEM

RADICULOPATHIES

A radiculopathy is a peripheral nerve injury at the level of the nerve root, just as the nerve exits the spinal cord.

Problems caused by the radiculopathy occur along the nerve pathway. Radiculopathy presents with motor or sensory problems anywhere along the nerve path, such as weakness, loss of motor control, pain, and numbness.

NEUROPATHIES

PREVIEW | REVIEW

- Where are the main points of compression for ulnar, median, and peroneal nerves?
- What frequently causes nocturnal awakening with hand pain? Which nerve?
- Mononeuritis multiplex is caused by which diseases?
- Which infection should you consider in a hiker who presents with new onset of foot drop?
- Name 5 disease processes that can cause facial palsy.
- What is the clinical presentation of Bell's palsy?
- Diabetes can cause which neuropathies?
- Which CSF findings are characteristic of Guillain-Barré syndrome?
- How does the treatment of CIDP differ from the treatment of Guillain-Barré syndrome?
- Name the drug used to treat diabetes that also can induce B_{12} deficiency and cause a severe peripheral neuropathy.

OVERVIEW

Neuropathies can be divided into several categories based on which nerves are affected.

If the process involves only 1 nerve, it is called **mononeuropathy**. Mononeuropathies are generally due to entrapment (as with carpal tunnel syndrome). Other causes include focal ischemia and trauma.

If ≥ 2 nerves are affected in a limited distribution, the term **mononeuritis multiplex** is used. Mononeuritis multiplex results from systemic disorders like diabetes or vasculitis.

The process may involve the plexuses—either the brachial or lumbosacral plexus. Involvement of multiple nerves within a plexus is referred to as **plexopathy**. The main symptoms are pain, weakness, and sensory loss in the distribution of the involved nerves. The most common causes are trauma, diabetes, and infections. MRI of the plexus may help to determine the etiology.

Neuropathies that symmetrically and diffusely involve the peripheral nerves are called **polyneuropathy** (or **peripheral neuropathies**). Typical axonal polyneuropathy involves distal segments more than proximal. There are many causes of peripheral neuropathy.

Inflammatory and hereditary neuropathies are the most frequently missed causes of polyneuropathy. So, consider inflammatory causes and include a careful family history in your evaluation of peripheral neuropathies!

The workup for any neuropathy includes glucose tolerance testing, free T_4 and TSH levels, vitamin B_{12}, creatinine, CBC, and serum and urine immunofixation.

Do an electromyography and nerve conduction study (EMG/NCS) regardless of whether the symptoms are mono- or polyneuropathy. EMG/NCS helps to identify any disease of muscle and nerve.

Do serum protein electrophoresis, immunoglobulin electrophoresis, and quantitative immunoglobulin assays if the patient is > 40 years of age, particularly if the EMG/NCS suggests a demyelinating neuropathy.

MONONEUROPATHIES

Focal / Compressive

Focal mononeuropathies are caused by localized peripheral nerve damage, usually from a compression injury (although ischemia can also cause damage, especially in autoimmune diseases associated with vasculitis). Single nerve involvement can be caused by leprosy, sarcoidosis, and herpes zoster.

The main sites of compression or entrapment are the ulnar nerve at the elbow, the median nerve at the wrist, the radial nerve at the spiral groove, and the peroneal nerve at the knee (discussed below). Because radiculopathies and mononeuritis multiplex can have presentations similar or identical to focal/compressive neuropathies, you must also consider them in the workup of patients presenting with focal neuropathic symptoms.

Radial neuropathy (acute wrist drop) is mostly from nerve compression but is occasionally seen as a result of diabetic neuropathy and can also occur with lead toxicity. It has been called "Saturday night palsy" in inebriated patients because it occurs after bouts of unconsciousness whereby the nerve becomes compressed in the radial groove of the humerus. This typically resolves slowly over several weeks or months—provided the patient does not continually reinjure the nerve! Physical therapy is the best treatment, using wrist splints.

Lower brachial plexus injury (from surgery/tumor/trauma) causes a claw-hand deformity, similar to that which may be seen with severe ulnar neuropathy.

Carpal tunnel syndrome (CTS) is median nerve entrapment at the wrist, commonly from repetitive stress, causing sensory loss, paresthesias, and weakness involving the first 3 or 4 digits of the hand, but patients can have pain anywhere in the arm or shoulder! Thumb muscle wasting may occur (Figure 12-9 on page 12-44). Median nerve entrapment at the wrist almost invariably causes nocturnal awakening due to hand pain or paresthesias. Prevalence of hypothyroidism is 1–10% in patients with CTS. Do not

NEUROLOGY

forget about the association of CTS with acromegaly. (See more on acromegaly in Endocrinology, Book 1.)

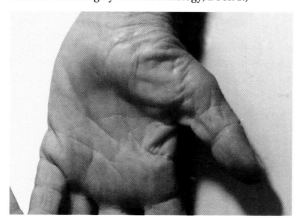

Figure 12-9: Thumb muscle wasting due to carpal tunnel syndrome

Initial treatment of CTS is neutral alignment with wrist splints and modifying behavior to avoid repetitive stress. If this is ineffective, steroid injection may help. The next step is surgical median nerve release.

Know: Pregnancy can cause an acute presentation of CTS, and symptoms typically improve after delivery. Splints are the best treatment for this patient group.

Ulnar neuropathy causes sensory loss and paresthesias in the little finger and ulnar aspect of the ring finger, as well as weakness of finger abductors and adductors in more severe cases. It is usually due to compression of the nerve at the elbow (cubital tunnel syndrome) but, much less commonly, can also result from a lesion at the wrist. Rarely, trauma to the heel of the hand can result in distal ulnar injury (bicyclists can get a distal ulnar neuropathy at Guyon canal). Elbow pads and splints help. Surgery (anterior transposition) is also an option for refractory cases of cubital tunnel syndrome.

Sciatic nerve compression (sciatic neuropathy) is uncommon but can occur from surgical procedures of the hip, iatrogenic injections, trauma (e.g., gunshot wound to the upper leg), and prolonged compression (e.g., from loss of consciousness). This can cause weakness of both ankle and toe dorsiflexion (peroneal nerve) and plantar flexion (tibial nerve), as well as hamstring weakness. Numbness is below the knee. Ankle reflex is lost on the affected side.

When you hear the term sciatica, it generally refers not to compression of the sciatic nerve but to radicular irritation from the back; i.e., L5 or S1 radiculopathies. Sciatica might just be painful sensations shooting down the leg from lumbosacral root impingement and might have a normal neurologic exam.

Peroneal nerve compression typically occurs at the proximal head of the fibula, causing foot drop. Remember that L5 radiculopathy also causes foot drop.

To distinguish between peroneal nerve compression and L5 radiculopathy: Patients with peroneal nerve compression cannot evert the foot well but can still invert it, while L5 radiculopathy prevents or hinders both eversion and inversion (Table 12-5). Also, it is useful to test proximal L5 innervated muscles, such as the hamstrings and thigh abductors, which is not affected with peroneal nerve compression.

Table 12-5: L5 Radiculopathy vs. Peroneal Nerve Compression			
	Foot Drop?	Able to Invert Foot?	Able to Evert Foot?
L5 Radiculopathy	Yes	No	No
Peroneal Nerve Injury	Yes	Yes	No

Know: CMT disease (discussed under Charcot-Marie-Tooth Disease on page 12-46) can cause symptoms similar to peroneal nerve compression, but it has a bilateral foot drop presentation with other features, such as distal atrophy and dysmorphic feet (high arches and hammer toes).

Mononeuritis Multiplex

Note that mononeuritis multiplex can present identically to the focal/compressive neuropathies above. Rather than being caused by nerve compression, mononeuritis multiplex is caused by a systemic disease. Vasculitis and vascular occlusion of the vasa nervorum (vessels that supply the nerves) are the main causes.

Consider any of the following as a possible cause of mononeuropathy +/– multiplex:

- Rheumatoid arthritis
- DM
- Connective tissue diseases
- Vasculitis
- Polyarteritis nodosa
- Lyme disease (Think of this in a hiker with new-onset foot drop.)
- Neuralgic amyotrophy

Neuralgic amyotrophy (a.k.a. Parsonage-Turner syndrome, brachial plexus neuropathy, acute brachial radiculitis) is temporary inflammation of the brachial plexus that is commonly idiopathic. Initially, it causes extreme pain in the shoulder with radiation to the arm, neck, and back. Within hours to days after the onset of pain, the shoulder muscles and proximal arm musculature become weak and then later atrophic. Bilateral involvement can occur. Commonly affected nerves are the suprascapular, long thoracic (causing winging of the scapula), axillary, musculocutaneous, and anterior interosseous nerves. The plexus pattern can be patchy, affect multiple individual nerves, or even just one nerve. Diagnosis is clinical, supported by EMG/NCS. It improves in 1–3 years with conservative management.

Bell's and Other Facial Nerve Palsies

Bell's palsy is caused by dysfunction of the external 7th cranial nerve. It is regarded as idiopathic, but herpes simplex (or its associated immune response) is the cause of most cases (definitively supported by finding evidence of the virus by PCR in the affected nerve roots).

Varicella zoster is also a cause and is diagnosed when vesicles involve the tympanic membrane and external auditory canal (Ramsay Hunt syndrome).

Important systemic diseases can also cause a facial palsy that presents identically:

- Lyme disease
- Acute HIV
- Neurosarcoidosis
- Guillain-Barré syndrome
- Diabetes mellitus

Some experts call these palsies Bell's, but others prefer to identify them as a systemic manifestation of underlying disease.

Other causes of facial palsy: schwannomas and parotid tumors.

Bell's palsy affects an entire half of the face, including the forehead. It causes ipsilateral facial muscle paralysis and occasionally results in no taste sensation on the anterior 2/3 of the tongue, loss of lacrimation, and hyperacusis. Pregeniculate lesions cause the loss of taste, salivation, and lacrimation, while more distal lesions spare these functions.

Note: For bilateral Bell's palsy, consider sarcoid, Lyme disease, HIV, or GBS.

To help differentiate Bell's palsy from other nerve damage, know that cortical lesions spare the muscles of the forehead and upper eyelid, whereas Bell's palsy affects them.

Diagnosis is clinical. Imaging of the head is reserved for patients who do not improve within 6 months or who continue to progress with facial weakness after 3 weeks.

Know that if the palsy is preceded by a period of facial twitching, the risk of tumor is higher. Perform urgent imaging of these patients.

Patients who begin to improve within 3 weeks commonly recover completely. If complete ipsilateral paralysis occurs, full recovery is less likely.

A week of prednisone shortens the course and improves function if started within 7 days of clinical onset. Studies assessing combined antiviral drugs (acyclovir or valacyclovir) + prednisone show conflicting results. Some experts give both; others do not unless obvious signs of herpes are present (i.e., vesicles). Lubricant eye drops and covering of the involved eye at night is important to prevent corneal ulceration. Eyelid surgery is reserved for patients with severe palsy, or when there is corneal anesthesia or xerophthalmia not amenable to eye lubricants.

Diabetic Mononeuropathies

Know: Diabetes can cause several cranial neuropathies. Neuropathies affecting cranial nerves 3, 4, and 6 present with eye pain, drooping eyelids, and double vision; those affecting cranial nerve 7 present with Bell's palsy. Isolated median, radial, ulnar, and peroneal neuropathies are also more common in patients with diabetes.

Note that diabetic involvement of the 3rd cranial nerve typically presents with diplopia and weak eye movements without any changes in the pupil.

Remember: A diabetic 3rd cranial neuropathy spares the pupil. If a patient has a 3rd cranial neuropathy with pupillary dilation, think compression of the 3rd cranial nerve by an aneurysm of the posterior communicating artery. This warrants an urgent MRI and MRA!

Diabetic lumbosacral plexopathy (amyotrophy) presents with leg pain (82%) followed by proximal weakness of the leg. It initially tends to be unilateral (88%) but eventually involves both legs. Autonomic dysfunction occurs in 50% of patients; weight loss > 10 lbs occurs in about 80%. Sensory symptoms and signs can also occur. The condition develops over months and so does partial or complete recovery. No specific treatment exists, although steroids may help the pain.

POLYNEUROPATHIES

Demyelinating vs. Axonal Polyneuropathies

Axonal polyneuropathies are usually a sensorimotor combination, with sensory abnormalities appearing first (paresthesias progressing to numbness), and distal motor weakness (often mild) appearing later. The nerve conduction velocity is normal in these conditions.

Demyelinating polyneuropathies affect motor fibers significantly more than sensory fibers and present with weakness out of proportion to the typical metabolic axonal polyneuropathies. Nerve conduction studies are diagnostic, with slowing of conduction, with or without conduction block, in affected nerves. Of the patients with demyelinating neuropathy, approximately 10% have a serum paraprotein. Although occasionally associated with a solitary plasmacytoma, the paraprotein is usually benign.

Autoimmune, Inflammatory Polyneuropathies — Guillain-Barré Syndrome

Guillain-Barré syndrome (GBS) is the most common autoimmune, inflammatory polyneuropathy. GBS is a syndrome with demyelinating (most common) and axonal variants.

In the vast majority of cases, a mild gastrointestinal or respiratory infection precedes the polyneuropathy. GBS was reported after influenza vaccination in the late 1970s and 1990s and after the meningococcal conjugate vaccine in 2005. Causality has not been established for

NEUROLOGY

either vaccine, and the subject is highly controversial. There is no requirement with these vaccines to warn patients about possible GBS, but patients with a history of GBS are cautioned to avoid vaccination for the 1st year after their illness and indefinitely for a specific vaccine that was given within 6 weeks of the onset of a patient's GBS.

Classic demyelinating GBS (termed acute inflammatory demyelinating polyradiculoneuropathy [AIDP]; 90% of U.S. cases) presents as an ascending paralysis (with distal and proximal weakness), including weakness of respiratory muscles, with areflexia. Patients may initially have some mild sensory abnormalities and paresthesias, but GBS is primarily a motor illness with absent reflexes. Disturbances in autonomic function and urinary retention may also be seen.

The Miller Fisher axonal variant (MFV; 5% of cases) is a type of GBS that includes only areflexia, ataxia, and ophthalmoplegia.

Two other axonal variants are even less commonly seen:

1) AMAN (acute motor axonal neuropathy),
   more associated with *Campylobacter* diarrhea

2) AMSAN (acute motor and sensory axonal
   neuropathy)

Paraparetic (partial paralysis), ataxic, Bickerstaff brainstem encephalitis, a cervical pharyngeal variant, and purely motor or purely sensory forms of the illness have also been observed.

In patients with any type of GBS, the CSF has a normal cell count and a high protein (albuminocytologic dissociation); suspect another diagnosis if the CSF has > 10 WBC/mm^3 (i.e., HIV). EMG/NCS helps to characterize the variant (axonal or demyelinating).

Anti-GQ1b IgG is a unique serum protein measurable in over 80% of MFV cases of GBS, and it assists with diagnosis of this variant.

The acute axonal variants are typically associated with preceding *Campylobacter jejuni* infections and also with development of many antibodies against the gangliosides found in peripheral nerves (especially anti-GQ1b).

Close respiratory monitoring and care are important. Measurement of vital capacity (VC), maximal inspiratory pressure (MIP), and maximal expiratory pressure (MEP) are used for the bedside estimation of diaphragmatic strength and respiratory function. The trend of these measurements is a guide to the likelihood of respiratory failure. Use the 20–30–40 rule to determine need for ventilator support: VC < 20 ml/kg, MIP less negative than –30 cm H$_2$O, and MEP < 40 cm H$_2$O.

Of note, significant neck flexion weakness (i.e., unable to raise head against gravity when lying flat) is another predictor of respiratory failure.

Plasmapheresis and IV immunoglobulin therapy (IVIG) are equally effective. Use one or the other if patient presents within 4 weeks of initial symptoms.

Steroids are not effective.

Complete recovery is the norm for about 80% of patients; however, 10% have a very prolonged course with or without significant residual weakness. Approximately 5% of patients do not survive the illness.

Chronic Inflammatory Demyelinating Polyneuropathy

Chronic inflammatory demyelinating polyneuropathy (CIDP) begins insidiously and evolves slowly, either in a steadily progressive or stepwise manner, progressing or relapsing over a period of > 8 weeks. In about 15% of cases, CIDP begins like a mild or moderate variant of GBS, but it slowly worsens or has a chronic relapsing course.

Chronic symmetric sensorimotor loss, EMG findings of demyelination, and elevated CSF protein define the illness.

CIDP cases are usually not traceable to an inciting event, such as an infection. (Still, it's useful to think of CIDP as "Guillain-Barré that won't go away.") Consider CIDP in the patient with a demyelinating polyneuropathy (by EMG/NCS) that extends beyond 8 weeks in duration.

LP and EMG results are identical to GBS (high protein, no pleocytosis, and demyelinating polyneuropathy). Exclude systemic disorders, specifically HIV, hepatitis viruses, Lyme, thyroid disease, diabetes, myeloma, sarcoidosis, and connective tissue disorders, such as lupus.

Unlike in Guillain-Barré syndrome, glucocorticoids hasten recovery and prevent relapse in CIDP. Plasmapheresis or IVIG are also standard treatments. (Pick 1 of the 3.) Several other immunomodulators are used chronically.

Charcot-Marie-Tooth Disease

Charcot-Marie-Tooth (CMT) disease is by far (90%) the most commonly inherited peripheral polyneuropathy. There are many "types" composed of > 50 separate gene associations under the general heading of CMT, all caused by mutations in myelin genes that are inherited variably (autosomal dominant [most common], autosomal recessive, or X-linked).

CMT diseases are demyelinating in the most common forms, but axonal or mixed in a sizable portion of the rest, and are differentiated based on genetic markers. All have both motor and sensory impairment and typically present within the first 2 decades of life. The neuropathy is symmetrical and progresses slowly. It is distal predominant with distal sensory loss and bilateral foot and, later, hand weakness. There tends to be dysmorphic feet (high arches and hammer toes) and a family history of neuropathy. Patients present insidiously, often with a long history of spraining ankles or having other minor symptoms before formal evaluation. Diagnosis is made with EMG to characterize the neuropathy subtype and genetic testing for confirmation. CMT1A (autosomal dominant, demyelinating form) is the most common and targeted genetic

NEUROLOGY

testing of *PMP22* and is ordered first for that; otherwise, gene panel testing has become the most cost effective and efficient way of trying to diagnose the genetic subtype. Treatment is supportive.

Diabetic Peripheral Neuropathy

Diabetes mellitus is the most common cause of polyneuropathy in general clinical practice. Diabetic peripheral neuropathy (DPN) is an axonal neuropathy that mainly causes sensory changes, including pain, paresthesias, and numbness in a length-dependent, stocking glove fashion.

Muscle weakness is generally mild. Some have distal loss of reflexes. In long-standing cases, trophic changes are noted. Some patients have predominant loss of joint position and vibration sensations.

Control of blood sugars is the most important therapy. Effective treatments for pain include the FDA-approved DPN drugs duloxetine (Cymbalta, Irenka) and pregabalin (Lyrica)—both are equally effective. Other drugs are used including tricyclic antidepressants, carbamazepine, gabapentin, lamotrigine, tramadol, and venlafaxine. Topical treatment with capsaicin cream and lidocaine also help. Alpha lipoic acid is a supplement that can be beneficial.

Be aware that metformin treatment of diabetes mellitus can occasionally result in malabsorption of vitamin B_{12} with subsequent peripheral neuropathy resembling DPN. This is an easily prevented serious side effect of metformin.

Alcoholic Peripheral Neuropathy

Alcohol is directly toxic to both nerves and muscles and causes many kinds of neuropathies (peripheral, autonomic, compressive [e.g., passing out on arm]). The polyneuropathy is typically axonal but is made worse if demyelination is superimposed (caused by nutritional deficiencies).

Symptoms of alcoholic axonal neuropathy start with pain and numbness in the feet in a stocking distribution. Over time, patients lose reflexes, proprioception, and strength.

Patients slowly recover with multivitamin therapy and abstinence from alcohol.

Other Causes of Axonal Neuropathies

Know other somewhat common causes of axonal polyneuropathy including:

- Toxins, such as heavy metals (e.g., lead, arsenic)
- Chemotherapy drugs (e.g., vincristine)
- Isoniazid
- B_6 (pyridoxine) overdose from nutritional supplements
- Organophosphates
- Systemic illnesses (myeloma, amyloidosis, porphyrias, thyroid disease, hepatitis viruses, amyloidosis, and HIV/AIDS)

Time of Onset

Time of onset helps to differentiate among the polyneuropathies:

- **Short** onset (days) is nearly always due to inflammatory, immunologic, toxic, or vasculitic etiology. Think porphyria, GBS, and a few of the toxic polyneuropathies.
- **Long** onset (over several years) is seen with the hereditary disorders, such as CMT.
- **Subacute** onset (several weeks to 2 years) occurs in the majority of patients:
  ◦ Toxicity (Lead and glue-sniffing cause mainly motor effects, while INH and vincristine cause sensorimotor effects.)
  ◦ Nutritional deficiencies (especially B_1, B_6, and B_{12})
  ◦ Paraneoplastic (See Lambert-Eaton Myasthenic Syndrome on page 12-48.)
  ◦ Rheumatologic disorders
  ◦ Diabetes
  ◦ Of note, CIDP presents rather subacutely over weeks and then progresses or relapses over > 8 weeks.

NEUROMUSCULAR JUNCTION

DISEASES OF THE NEUROMUSCULAR JUNCTION

PREVIEW | REVIEW

- What are the clinical presentations of MG?
- How is MG diagnosed?
- Which other tests should be done in patients with MG?
- Which cancers cause Lambert-Eaton myasthenic syndrome?
- What happens to deep tendon reflexes in MG and LEMS?

MYASTHENIA GRAVIS

Myasthenia gravis (MG) is an autoimmune disorder. Most patients have autoantibodies to:

- postsynaptic acetylcholine receptor (AChR; 85%) or
- muscle-specific tyrosine kinase (MuSK) receptor.

40% of those who test negative for acetylcholine receptor antibody (AChR-Ab) are MuSK antibody (MuSK-Ab) positive. A smaller group of MG patients has neither antibody (termed seronegative MG [SNMG]), though that proportion keeps getting smaller as newer commercial antibodies become available (most recently LRP4 antibody tests).

MG is associated with thymomas (~ 10% of patients) and thymic hyperplasia (~ 60%), although it is not understood exactly how the thymus is related to antibody formation.

There are 2 forms of MG:

1) **Generalized MG** presents as episodic weakness with repetitive movements (weakness—not tiredness, not soreness). Symptoms are worse at the end of the day. Common presenting complaints include weakness while brushing hair, putting away dishes or climbing stairs, and diplopia after a long day. Weakening with repetitive muscle stimulation during the physical exam (muscle fatigability) suggests the diagnosis. Ptosis is common. In addition to weakness of extraocular muscles, muscles of facial expression, mastication, swallowing, and speech are affected in 80% of patients at some time in the illness. Muscle atrophy is rare, and tendon reflexes are normal.

2) **Ocular MG** presents as weakness localized to the eyes (lids and extraocular muscles).

Practice pearls: Demonstrating fatigable ptosis (i.e., worsening of ptosis on 30 seconds of sustained upgaze) is a good way to differentiate myasthenic ptosis from other forms of ptosis. Of course, the pupil size is normal, unlike in Horner syndrome (with miosis, ptosis, anhydrosis). In addition, the pattern of extraocular muscle weakness often does not fit the distribution of a single oculomotor nerve, and may change from one examination to the next.

Diagnosis of MG is best confirmed by measuring AChR-Abs and MuSK-Abs. AChR-Abs are present in 85–90% of patients with generalized disease but only in ~ 60% of those with isolated ocular disease. Often, MuSK-Abs are present in patients who are negative for AChR-Abs (~ 50%). Antibody levels are not necessarily prognostic, but they do rise and fall with immunotherapy.

The classic edrophonium (Tensilon) test is not done much because results are not as reliable as antibody measurements.

The ice pack test can be used for patients with ptosis as part of their symptoms. Ice in a glove is applied to the closed eyelid for 2 minutes, which results in less ptosis. Sensitivity of this test is ~ 80%.

Electrodiagnostic studies, including repetitive nerve stimulation studies and single-fiber EMG, are useful in supporting the diagnosis.

Do thyroid function studies because 30% of patients with MG have chronic autoimmune thyroiditis. Look out for symptoms that suggest lupus or rheumatoid arthritis because there is considerable overlap. Image the chest with CT or MRI in all confirmed diagnoses to rule out thymoma.

Treatments used for MG:

- Anticholinesterase agents (e.g., pyridostigmine [Mestinon])
- Immunomodulators in patients uncontrolled on pyridostigmine (e.g., steroids, cyclosporine, mycophenolate)
- IVIG or plasmapheresis (for myasthenic crisis only because duration of action is very short)
- Thymectomy (This now has evidence-based support even without thymoma in patients with generalized MG < 60 years of age, but definitely perform in patients with thymoma.)

Myasthenic crisis is a rapid deterioration of myasthenia that can cause respiratory failure and severe weakness. Infections or certain medications (see below) can precipitate crises. Blood gases are poor predictors of respiratory failure in MG. The functional respiratory capacity is a better indicator of impending respiratory failure; monitor it closely. Besides respiratory support, patients respond to plasmapheresis and IVIG.

Know the few drugs that can precipitate myasthenic crisis in patients with either known or undiagnosed MG:

- Aminoglycosides
- Fluoroquinolones
- β-blockers
- Procainamide
- α-interferon
- Magnesium sulfate
- Penicillamine
- Quinidine

LAMBERT-EATON MYASTHENIC SYNDROME

Lambert-Eaton myasthenic syndrome (LEMS) is a paraneoplastic syndrome. About 60% of cases are seen in patients with small cell lung cancer; other associated cancers include prostate, breast, stomach, rectum, and lymphomas. It is also seen rarely in autoimmune diseases. LEMS is itself an autoimmune disease in which antibodies are produced that are specific for calcium channels in presynaptic peripheral nerve terminals, causing decreased release of acetylcholine from the nerve terminals.

Know the following about symptoms:

- Typical symptoms are gradually progressive proximal muscle weakness, ptosis, erectile dysfunction, aching thighs, dry mouth (autonomic dysfunction), and hyporeflexia, especially in the lower extremities.
- It looks like MG, except it rarely involves the ocular muscles and repetitive exercise may actually reverse the weakness for the first few contractions. Also, deep tendon reflexes are depressed in LEMS as opposed to MG where they are preserved.

Diagnose Lambert-Eaton's by measuring voltage-gated calcium channel (anti-VGCC) antibodies. Anti-VGCC antibodies are not 100% specific; they are sometimes found in patients who do not have Lambert-Eaton's. Therefore, measure them only in patients who have a high pretest probability of true disease. EMG can help distinguish between Lambert-Eaton's and myasthenia—with decremental response (weakening) in myasthenia in general to 3 Hz stimulation but incremental response (strengthening) to rapid stimulation in Lambert-Eaton myasthenic syndrome (50 Hz).

Look for malignancy in anybody diagnosed with Lambert-Eaton's—especially small cell lung cancer.

Treatment includes addressing any underlying malignancy along with drugs that increase the amount of acetylcholine in the synapse for mild symptoms (guanidine, 3,4-diaminopyridine, and pyridostigmine). For refractory or severe weakness, proceed to IVIG, plasmapheresis, azathioprine, cyclosporine, mycophenolate, rituximab, or prednisone.

MUSCLE

MYOPATHIES

PREVIEW | REVIEW

- Where is the muscle weakness that occurs with inclusion body myositis?

- Progressive limb girdle weakness in an adult patient who has a family history of the same is indicative of which diagnosis?

NOTE

Myopathy simply means muscle disease. Myopathies are typically classified under neuromuscular diseases (hence their discussion here). Symptoms can be muscle weakness, stiffness, cramps, and spasms.

INFLAMMATORY MYOPATHIES

Inflammatory myopathies are caused by chronic muscle inflammation, usually:

- Dermatomyositis
- Polymyositis
- Inclusion body myositis

Both dermatomyositis and polymyositis often cause:

- Elevated CPK
- Proximal muscle weakness

Both respond to corticosteroids.

Inclusion body myositis is a less common type of myositis in which patients present with:

- A slowly progressive, painless muscle weakness with involvement of proximal (initially) then distal muscles
- Hallmark signs are significant quadriceps and finger flexor weakness with some asymmetry.
- Elevated CPK
- Oculomotor muscle sparing

Inclusion body myositis does not respond well to corticosteroids. Muscle biopsy in inclusion body myositis shows vacuolar inclusions.

See more on dermatomyositis, polymyositis, and inclusion body myositis in Rheumatology, Book 3.

ENDOCRINE MYOPATHIES

Proximal muscle weakness of varying degrees may be seen in patients with thyroid and parathyroid disease, acromegaly, severe vitamin D deficiency, and conditions of steroid excess.

Hypothyroid patients have generalized muscle weakness, myalgias, and slowness of contraction and relaxation; they can have increased CPK. Muscle cramping is prominent in hypoparathyroidism.

METABOLIC MYOPATHIES

Consider a metabolic cause of muscle dysfunction in patients with muscle fatigue, pain, cramping, and, in more severe cases, contractures and myoglobinuria. These symptoms are precipitated by exercise in patients with disorders of carbohydrate metabolism and by fasting in those with disorders of lipid metabolism. The major categories are:

- Disorders of **carbohydrate metabolism** (e.g., myophosphorylase and phosphofructokinase deficiency): Myophosphorylase deficiency (McArdle's) presents with difficulty with intense exercise (i.e., sprinting), prolonged cramping (known as contractures), and a "second-wind" phenomena where moderate exercise capacity improves after about 10 minutes of exercising.
- Disorders of **lipid metabolism** (e.g., carnitine deficiency): Carnitine palmitoyltransferase 2 (CPT 2) deficiency is the hallmark aerobic defective metabolic myopathy, where prolonged exercise (e.g., long distance running), fasting, or illness can precipitate episodes of rhabdomyolysis.
- Disorders of **mitochondrial function**: Mitochondrial myopathies are distinguished by the presence of ragged red fibers on light microscopy of a muscle biopsy and a range of associated clinical features in addition to muscle disease, such as neuropathy, short stature, hearing loss, seizures, diabetes, and stroke.

MUSCULAR DYSTROPHIES

Duchenne muscular dystrophy is an X-linked disorder that causes progressive muscle weakness, starting at about 2 years of age, and progresses to death as a young adult due to cardiac or respiratory failure comorbidity. The weakness is more proximal than distal. Look for an elevated CPK.

Myotonic dystrophy consists of 2 types of inherited, adult-onset, neuromuscular disorders that have multisystem effects. Myotonic dystrophy Type 1 is caused by mutations in the *DMPK* gene, whereas Type 2 results from mutations in the *CNBP* gene. The genetic abnormalities result in weakened skeletal muscle, myotonia (prolonged contraction on muscle percussion), cardiac

NEUROLOGY

conduction defects, cataracts, hypogonadism, and insulin resistance. Patients characteristically have frontal balding and a "hatchet" face appearance as a result of jaw and temporal muscle wasting. Typically, patients complain of skeletal muscle weakness (limb girdle in Type 2 and more distal in Type 1) and have positive family history. Consider this disease in a patient who presents as an adult with symptoms of muscle dystrophy. Refer these patients to a neurologist who can make the diagnosis using genetic tests. Treatment is supportive only.

AIDS-RELATED MYOPATHY

AIDS-related myopathy is uncommon and typically thought to be due to zidovudine but some investigators attribute it to the direct effects of the virus (controversial). Patients present with a generalized (proximal > distal) weakness and an elevated CPK. Treatment: Stop the zidovudine. Of note, muscle biopsy shows mitochondrial pathology with this medication.

MISCELLANEOUS DISORDERS

CNS TUMORS

BRAIN TUMORS

The most common tumors that metastasize to the brain include lung cancer, breast cancer, melanoma, and renal cancer. There are a wide variety of adult primary brain tumors. The most common malignant primary tumor is the highest-grade glioma, glioblastoma multiforme (GBM; more in Oncology, Book 3), and the most common benign primary brain tumor is a meningioma. Neurofibromatosis Type 1 is autosomal dominant, sporadic, and associated with optic gliomas, soft tissue sarcomas, Lisch nodules, and café-au-lait macules. Neurofibromatosis Type 2 is associated with bilateral vestibular schwannomas, cataracts, and plaque-like or nodular skin lesions. Tuberous sclerosis is a benign giant cell tumor that causes symptoms based on location (i.e., obstruction of periventricular aqueduct of Sylvius). Medulloblastomas occur in the cerebellum and are associated with familial adenomatous polyposis and nevoid basal cell carcinoma. von Hippel-Lindau syndrome is associated with the capillary rich hemangioblastomas that appear as an enhancing nodule within a cyst anywhere in the CNS system.

Patients with brain tumors may present with a variety of focal neurologic deficits depending on the location of the tumor(s). Patients may also present with a first-time seizure or symptoms of increased ICP, such as headache, nausea/vomiting, papilledema, or visual changes.

Order brain imaging for individuals with these symptoms.

Brain metastases can be treated surgically for a single lesion or with stereotactic radiosurgery for a limited number of small lesions. A high number of lesions require treatment with whole brain radiation. For malignant primary brain tumors, a combination of radiation, surgery, and chemotherapy may be undertaken. Long-term prognosis is generally poor. Alternatively, benign primary brain tumors can be monitored clinically. If the tumors are compressing structures in a symptomatic or dangerous way, they can be surgically removed, in which case surgery can be curative.

For acute management of edema related to tumor, corticosteroid therapy can be employed, such as dexamethasone, which does help decrease vasogenic edema. Corticosteroid therapy does not help treat cytotoxic edema, as is seen with as stroke. Seizures related to malignant tumor are generally treated with an antiepileptic that has minimal reaction with other medications or chemotherapy agents, such as levetiracetam.

See Table 12-6 for further salient details about brain tumors.

SPINAL CORD TUMORS

Epidural metastases occurring at thoracolumbar regions are most commonly from breast cancer, multiple myeloma, lymphoma, prostate cancer, and lung cancer. Progressive back pain at the spinal level is usually the first symptom, followed by motor symptoms. Resulting spinal cord compromise is an acute neurological emergency, warranting a stat neurosurgery consultation for spinal

Table 12-6: Highlights for Selected CNS Tumors	
Type	**Description**
Glioblastoma multiforme	Butterfly lesion across corpus callosum, poor prognosis, necrosis on pathology Treat with surgery, radiation, and chemotherapy (temozolomide as mainstay; bevacizumab for continued progression).
Oligodendroglioma	"Fried egg" cells on pathology
Meningioma	Generally benign, dural tail on imaging, psammoma bodies on pathology
Acoustic neuroma	Think neurofibromatosis Type 2 with bilateral acoustic neuroma
Melanoma, renal cell carcinoma, choriocarcinoma, thyroid carcinoma	Metastatic lesions most likely to have hemorrhage
Primary CNS lymphoma	Treat with high dose methotrexate. AIDS-related primary CNS lymphoma is associated with Epstein-Barr virus.

decompression and/or radiation therapy to prevent loss of neurologic function. The most common primary spinal cord tumors are the glial tumors, ependymomas (can generally be resected) and astrocytomas (total resection success depends on tumor grade).

CNS METASTASES

PREVIEW | REVIEW

- A patient with history of prostate cancer or new onset of urinary incontinence should make you consider which diagnosis?

CNS metastases commonly cause a slow onset of symptoms (headaches, focal neuro deficits, impaired cognition, seizures, and/or stroke symptoms), although they can be abrupt if there is hemorrhage into a tumor.

Know the following main mets to the brain (Table 12-7):

Parenchymal brain metastases occur most commonly with lung, renal, and breast cancer, as well as with melanoma and lymphoma.

Dural metastases occur with breast and prostate cancer.

Epidural metastases at the level of the spinal cord cause back pain, usually worse when lying down. New onset of bladder or bowel dysfunction (i.e., incontinence, urgency) is very important and alerts you to consider spinal epidural metastases, especially in the setting of new back pain. In a patient with a history of cancer—especially prostate, breast, and lung cancer—and with cord compression symptoms (i.e., cauda equina), metastases must be ruled out!

Meningeal malignancy is most frequently seen with lymphomas, carcinoma of the breast, and melanoma. It is less commonly seen in cancers of the lung and the gastrointestinal tract, childhood leukemia, and systemic lymphoma.

MRI with contrast is the best imaging study.

Treatment of CNS metastases depends on how many metastases are present, the cancer prognosis, and the functional status of the patient. An approachable, single metastasis in a functional patient is treated with surgery and radiation. Small lesions (< 3 cm) and/or surgically inaccessible lesions can be treated with stereotactic radiosurgery. Less functional patients with numerous lesions are usually treated with whole brain radiation and chemotherapy +/– corticosteroids.

METABOLIC AND TOXIC DISORDERS

PREVIEW | REVIEW

- What is Wernicke encephalopathy? How is it treated?
- How does the presentation of the typical Wernicke patient differ from that of the typical Korsakoff patient?
- What effect does a hyponatremic state have on lithium resorption by the kidney?
- What are the symptoms of lithium toxicity?

WERNICKE'S / KORSAKOFF'S

Wernicke encephalopathy and Korsakoff syndrome are considered different presentations of the same disease process. Wernicke's is milder and reversible while Korsakoff's is more severe and only partially reversible. The cause is thiamine (B_1) deficiency.

Wernicke encephalopathy is most often associated with alcoholism, but it can be seen in cases of protein-energy malnutrition (i.e., extreme catabolic states, kwashiorkor, marasmus), malabsorption, and specific loss of thiamine during dialysis.

It is characterized by global confusion with inattention, apathy, disorientation, and memory loss that worsens over days to weeks. The major sites of brain involvement include the thalamus, hypothalamus, midbrain, floor of the 4th ventricle, and cerebellar vermis.

Abnormal eye movements are typical and include horizontal nystagmus and a disordered conjugate gaze that progresses to ophthalmoplegia (bilateral lateral rectus weakness, either in isolation or together with palsies of other extraocular muscles). The pupils may become sluggishly reactive to light. The person may have trouble standing or walking due to truncal ataxia.

Diagnosis is clinical. Recognize and treat the disease in the early stages or progressive loss of consciousness including stupor, coma, and death can rapidly follow within weeks.

Know the typical Wernicke's presentation: confused + staggering gait + trouble moving eyes.

Korsakoff syndrome is a chronic amnestic syndrome associated with alcoholism, malnutrition, and vitamin B_1 deficiency; it is often coincident with Wernicke's and may emerge as the symptoms of Wernicke's are treated.

NEUROLOGY

Table 12-7: Main Mets to the Brain						
	Breast	**Lung**	**Prostate**	**Melanoma**	**Lymphoma**	**Renal**
Parenchymal	+	+		+	+	+
Dural	+		+			
Epidural	+	+	+			
Meningeal	+			+	+	

The amnesia that occurs with Korsakoff's can be both retrograde and anterograde. Attention and mentation appear normal. Patients often confabulate because of the memory problems. The stories are frequently happy-go-lucky fantasies, termed "gleeful confabulation."

The typical Korsakoff's presentation: an underweight, poorly nourished, but very attentive alcoholic who tells fantastical stories that couldn't possibly be true and then has no memory of the discussion.

Other neurologic manifestations of Wernicke's and Korsakoff's are peripheral neuropathy, retrobulbar optic neuropathy, impaired olfactory discrimination, and postural hypotension.

Treatment: Immediate treatment with thiamine resolves the problem of Wernicke's and prevents Korsakoff syndrome. Once Korsakoff's develops, thiamine has only partial effect; in fact, the majority of patients who emerge from Wernicke's have some irreversible symptoms of Korsakoff's.

Treatment for Wernicke's is thiamine, at a minimum dose of 500 mg (in saline) by infusion 3×/day for 2–3 days, followed by 250 mg thiamine IV or IM daily for another 5 days. Thereafter, continue oral thiamine supplementation, typically at a dose of 100 mg/day. Also, correct deficiency in other vitamins and minerals, especially niacin and Mg^{2+}. Wernicke's usually improves within hours of thiamine replacement.

IV glucose can precipitate Wernicke's in alcoholics.

Remember: Give IV thiamine before IV glucose in any patient with a possible metabolic cause of coma.

LITHIUM TOXICITY

Lithium levels in the upper therapeutic range frequently cause tremor and asterixis. Remember: Hyponatremia causes increased lithium resorption from the kidney. Above a level of 1.5–2 mEq/L (1.5–2 mmol/L), the patient develops confusion, delirium, dizziness, nystagmus, ataxia, stammering, diffuse myoclonus, nephrogenic diabetes insipidus, vertical nystagmus, and opsoclonus. Toxic lithium levels cause seizures and coma; treat with hemodialysis.

The symptoms of toxicity can resemble Creutzfeldt-Jakob disease.

Note: Opsoclonus is rapid, involuntary, multivectorial (horizontal and vertical), unpredictable, conjugate eye movements.

ANTICHOLINERGIC TOXICITY

Classically, symptoms are:

- red as a beet (cutaneous vasodilation),
- dry as a bone (anhidrosis),
- mad as a hatter (hallucinations),
- blind as a bat (mydriasis),
- full as a flask (urinary retention), and
- hot as a hare (hyperthermia).

See General Internal Medicine, Book 5, for more detail on these and other toxicities and their treatments.

NARCOLEPSY

PREVIEW | REVIEW

- What 4 symptoms are associated with narcolepsy?

Narcolepsy is a rare disease caused by a selective loss of hypocretin in the hypothalamus, the etiology of which is unknown. More than 85% of Caucasian and Japanese patients with narcolepsy-cataplexy syndrome have a specific HLA haplotype that includes HLA-DR1501 (formerly called DR15 or DR2) and HLA-DQB1-0602 (formerly called DQ1 or DQ6).

Narcolepsy tetrad:

1) Daytime sleepiness
2) Cataplexy (60–75% of patients! With excitement, limbs become flaccid, often resulting in falls.)
3) Hypnagogic hallucinations (occurs as patient falls asleep)
4) Sleep paralysis (on waking)

Narcolepsy is treated with modafinil or armodafinil (non-amphetamine drugs), stimulants (such as methylphenidate or methamphetamine—many side effects and addictive potential), or sodium oxybate (especially in more severe cases with associated cataplexy). Scheduled daytime naps and avoidance of sleep deprivation is useful. Cataplexy can also be treated with tricyclics (e.g., imipramine, clomipramine, protriptyline) or the selective serotonin reuptake inhibitors (e.g., venlafaxine, fluoxetine).

VISUAL DISORDERS

PREVIEW | REVIEW

- What are causes of acute-onset unilateral blindness in older patients?
- What do flashes followed by decreased vision suggest?

ACUTE-ONSET UNILATERAL BLINDNESS

Know all of the following. See Table 12-8 for a summary.

In **older patients**, acute-onset of unilateral blindness is usually due to any of the following:

- Anterior ischemic optic neuropathy (AION), which may be:
  - Arteritic (especially giant cell arteritis; 5%)
  - Nonarteritic (thrombosis; 95%)

- Retinal vein occlusion (secondary to diabetic retinal vascular disease)
- Retinal artery occlusion (from thrombus or emboli from the carotid artery or heart)

In the **younger patient**, think optic neuritis, but sometimes it can be from migraine. Painful monocular visual loss in a young patient is concerning for optic neuritis. Migraine-induced blindness typically resolves rapidly, whereas blindness due to any of the other mentioned causes is prolonged or permanent.

Ischemic optic neuropathy, optic neuritis, and papilledema (e.g., from increased ICP) all can present with swollen discs with fundal splinter hemorrhages. Remember: Temporal (giant cell) arteritis also causes diplopia and jaw claudication.

Malingering as a cause of blindness (mono/bi) can be ruled out with evoked action potentials.

DIPLOPIA

Weak or paralyzed eye muscles cause ophthalmoplegia and manifest as diplopia. It can be a result of disease in the muscle itself, in the nerve that stimulates the muscle, or in the neuromuscular junction (myasthenia gravis).

A reminder of diseases that can present with diplopia (we have covered most of these separately):

- 3rd, 4th, and 6th cranial nerve palsies
- Myasthenia gravis
- Graves disease
- Wernicke encephalopathy
- Miller Fisher axonal variant of GBS
- Botulism
- Tick paralysis
- Mitochondrial disease
- Oculopharyngeal muscular dystrophy
- Infections/Masses that affect the cavernous sinus

If you see diplopia with pain:

- Think disease in the eyeball if pain is localized in the eye.

- Think myopathy or orbital processes if pain is present with movement of the eye. Influenza is a classic cause of orbital myopathy.

Optic neuritis may also cause pain on eye movement, but it does not cause diplopia!

VISUAL FIELD DEFECTS

Scotomas

Scotomas are alterations in an isolated area of the visual field with loss or dimness of vision. Do a complete ophthalmologic exam on any patient with any type of scotoma.

Acephalic migraine (migraine without headache) can cause fortification scotomas that constantly change in size and can be bilateral.

Moore lightning streaks occur in older patients upon entering a darkened area. They are caused by the vitreous pulling on the retina; they are benign.

Retinal detachment causes flashes followed by decreased vision (from blood) or increased floaters. This is an ophthalmological emergency.

Hemianopia and Quadrantanopia

Bitemporal hemianopia (see Figure 12-10 on page 12-54) is the term for blindness in the lateral half of both visual fields. It is a very specific finding caused by compression of the nasal retina nerve fibers in the optic chiasm as they cross over each other to the contralateral side.

The usual causes of bitemporal hemianopia are:

- Pituitary adenomas (the one we all remember)— most common (See Endocrinology, Book 1.)
- Pituitary hyperplasia
- Craniopharyngioma
- Meningioma

Rare causes are aneurysm of the circle of Willis, sarcoidosis, and metastatic carcinoma.

Table 12-8: Causes of Acute Transient Unilateral Blindness (Transient Monocular Vision Loss)					
Age	Disease	Etiology	Clinical Course	Exam	Outcome
Older (> 50)	Anterior ischemic optic neuropathy	Giant cell arteritis; nonarteritic (thrombotic)	Nonprogressive	Optic disc infarction	From normal to complete blindness
	Central retinal vein occlusion	Vascular disease or venous thrombosis	Nonprogressive	Hemorrhagic retinopathy	Usually some visual impairment
	Central retinal artery occlusion	Embolic or thrombotic	Nonprogressive	Cherry red spot	Only ~ 25% maintain useful vision
Younger (< 40)	Optic neuritis	Multiple sclerosis	Progressive (hours to days)	Marcus Gunn pupil; optic disc pallor	90% recover completely
	Migraine	Neurovascular	Resolves rapidly	Normal	Normal vision

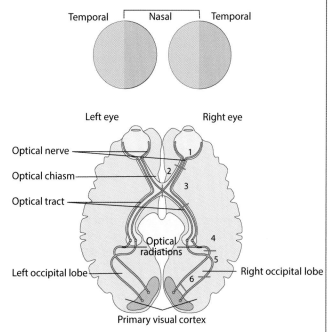

Visual Defects

1 Ipsilateral blindness

2 Bitemporal hemianopia

3 Left hemianopia

4 Left upper quandrantanopia

5 Left lower quandrantanopia

6 Left hemianopia with macular sparing

Temporal   Nasal   Temporal

Left eye   Right eye

Optical nerve
Optical chiasm
Optical tract
Optical radiations
Left occipital lobe   Right occipital lobe
Primary visual cortex

Figure 12-10: Visual field defects

Homonomous means the same part of the visual field is affected in each eye. **Homonomous hemianopia** is seen with:

- posterior cerebral artery (PCA) strokes affecting the medial occipital area,
- middle cerebral artery (MCA) strokes affecting all optic radiations between the optic chiasm and the occipital area, and
- internal capsule strokes also affecting all optic radiations.

Central sparing of the visual field (5° to 25°) means the stroke did not affect, or just partially affected, the posterior occipital lobe.

Quadrantanopia is when only a quadrant of the visual field is affected. Causes of quadrantanopia:

- an inferior homonomous quadrantanopia indicates a PCA stroke or lesion affecting optic radiations through the parietal lobe or
- a superior homonomous quadrantanopia indicates a PCA stroke or lesion affecting optic radiations through the medial temporal lobe.

NYSTAGMUS

PREVIEW | REVIEW

- Which brain lesion is suggested by upbeating jerk nystagmus? Downbeating?

Nystagmus is an involuntary oscillation of the eyes. The movements can be pendular (like a pendulum) or jerk. Jerk nystagmus has 2 components: slow and fast. The eyes drift (= slow component), and try to quickly recover (= fast component). The fast direction defines the direction of the nystagmus. Nystagmus is sometimes (but not always) associated with vertigo.

Jerk nystagmus is most common in vestibular disorders but does not indicate whether the lesion is within the central nervous system or if it involves the cranial nerve itself. Upbeating jerk nystagmus usually indicates a lesion in the pons but can be seen in lesions of the medulla or cerebellum (i.e., infratentorial). Downbeating jerk nystagmus indicates a lesion at the cervicomedullary junction.

Gazing in particular directions precipitates the abnormal eye movements in certain types of nystagmus. For instance, drugs (e.g., antiepileptic medications) can cause horizontal and vertical gaze-evoked nystagmus (occurring when the person looks right, left, or up)—in other words, it is present in all directions. Isolated vertical gaze-evoked nystagmus typically indicates disease in the posterior fossa.

DIZZINESS / VERTIGO

PREVIEW | REVIEW

- Name the maneuvers frequently employed to treat BPPV.
- What are the clinical features of Ménière disease?
- Which TIAs cause vertigo?

SIGNS AND SYMPTOMS

When the term dizziness is used by a patient, it is necessary to differentiate among the following:

- Vertigo = a sense of spinning or swaying.
- Lightheadedness = presyncope. ("I feel like I'm going to pass out.")
- Imbalance = unsteadiness.
- Vague = not one of the 3 above. It may be hard for the affected person to describe.

When we discuss dizziness here, we are considering only vertigo.

CAUSES OF VERTIGO

Benign Paroxysmal Positional Vertigo

Benign paroxysmal positional vertigo (BPPV) describes recurrent, brief episodes of vertigo caused by the motion of changing head position that generally lasts seconds at a time. It is thought to be due to loose otoconia (crystals that reside in the saccule and utricle) in the semicircular canal. When they escape this region, they can set up eddy currents in the endolymph, causing symptoms of vertigo. BPPV is also seen with head trauma, labyrinthitis, giant cell arteritis, migraine, hypertension, hyperlipidemia, stroke, and aging. Diagnosis is made by performing the Dix-Hallpike maneuver to elicit nystagmus and the patient's symptoms with positional movements.

Most BPPV resolves spontaneously over a couple of weeks or can be treated successfully with various repositioning maneuvers that move the otoconia to a position of the inner ear that is less likely to induce vertigo. These are the Epley and Semont maneuvers and their variations. In some patients, episodes recur periodically from several days to many months—rarely for years.

Meclizine does not cure BPPV, but it is sometimes used to control nausea. Nonvertigo causes of dizziness are discussed in General Internal Medicine, Book 5.

Vestibular Neuritis

Vestibular neuritis (e.g., vestibular neuronitis, acute peripheral vestibulopathy) causes a sudden onset of nonpositional vertigo that is self-limited but may last weeks to months and occasionally can recur. This disorder occurs mainly in young to middle-aged adults, without preference for either gender.

Vestibular neuritis is caused by an inflammatory process affecting the vestibular portion of the 8th cranial nerve and can be associated with viral infections. Pure vestibular neuritis does not affect hearing. If hearing is affected, it means it is no longer solely the nerve being affected but also the labyrinthine canals—and this is called vestibular labyrinthitis.

Usually the onset of vertigo is fairly abrupt, although some patients describe a prodromal period of several hours or days in which they felt off balance. Persistence of the symptoms for a day or more as a one-time event differentiates the disorder from Ménière disease, which is a paroxysmal disorder with vertigo that lasts for hours in discrete spells that also can be associated with aural fullness, hearing loss, and tinnitus.

Corticosteroids probably help recovery from vestibular neuritis. More studies are needed to confirm this effect. If steroids are not used, treatment is symptomatic only.

During the acute stage, antihistamines (i.e., meclizine), antiemetics (i.e., promethazine), clonazepam, or scopolamine may be helpful in reducing the symptoms.

Aminoglycoside Toxicity

Aminoglycoside toxicity can cause sensorineural hearing loss and transient intermittent vertigo followed by more chronic disequilibrium, gait imbalance, and oscillopsia. Onset can be unpredictable and hearing loss can be permanent. There is currently no known therapy available to treat or reverse the ototoxic damage once it occurs.

Ménière Disease

Ménière disease is characterized by recurrent attacks of vertigo and intermittent tinnitus that begins between 20 and 40 years of age. The characteristic triad is episodic vertigo (often associated with nausea and vomiting) and tinnitus, with development of low-frequency hearing loss after recurrent episodes. Another commonly reported symptom is aural fullness. It frequently begins unilaterally but can become bilateral in 20–30% of patients.

An increase in the volume of endolymph and distention of the endolymphatic system (endolymphatic hydrops), partly related to salt intake, drive the disease process.

Diagnosis is clinical. Audiometry can help determine if hearing loss has occurred. If hearing loss is present at diagnosis, exclude neurosyphilis as a cause by checking a serum VDRL or RPR.

Antihistamines, antiemetics, and sedatives are used in acute episodes. Chronic treatment includes eradicating caffeine and reducing the intake of salt, alcohol, nicotine, and monosodium glutamate. Thiazide diuretics are used when spells continue after dietary modification. 95% of patients get their disease under control and function normally. For medically recalcitrant Ménière disease, endolymphatic sac surgery, surgical labyrinthectomy, and vestibular nerve sections remain therapeutic options.

Vertebrobasilar TIAs or Stroke

Vertebrobasilar TIAs (transient ischemic attacks) may cause intermittent, recurrent vertigo. A posterior circulation TIA can be hard to diagnose because it may present with only vertigo and no other symptoms of vertebrobasilar insufficiency, but there typically are other clues, such as vision loss, diplopia, dysarthria, ataxia, and extremity motor or sensory dysfunction. Additionally, the patient usually has risk factors for stroke.

Workup of the posterior circulation requires special imaging. Know: Currently, the recommended testing for imaging of the posterior circulation is CT or MR angiography. CTA is preferred over MRA. Know that duplex Doppler ultrasound is not recommended for these vessels because of a lack of sensitivity, as it is assessing the anterior rather than the posterior circulation.

TINNITUS

Know these causes of tinnitus:

- Pulse synchronous tinnitus with idiopathic intracranial hypertension
- Intermittent tinnitus with Ménière's
- Aspirin overdose
- High noise levels
- Hearing loss

The tinnitus that occurs with hearing loss is thought to be a compensatory reaction to the hearing loss itself. Note that no tinnitus occurs with vestibular neuritis.

NEUROMA

PREVIEW | REVIEW

- How do you work up a patient with metatarsal pain?

Morton neuroma (a.k.a. Morton metatarsalgia) is a fairly common disease of the foot in which the patient has metatarsal pain. Palpation of the interspace and the metatarsal joint eliciting a clicking sound is called Mulder sign. Generally, Morton neuroma is diagnosed with MRI or ultrasound, which shows a small intermetatarsal ovoid mass. Differential diagnosis includes a metatarsal stress fracture. Treatment is with shoe inserts, local corticosteroid injections, and, at last resort, surgical excision.

COMPLEX REGIONAL PAIN SYNDROME

Complex regional pain syndrome (CRPS) is extreme tenderness, pain, swelling, dysesthesias, and vasomotor instability in an extremity after a traumatic injury.

Prevention is the best treatment. The best studied preventive treatment is giving vitamin C, which significantly reduces the chance of developing CRPS. The higher the dose (1,500 mg/day), the better the results.

Early mobilization is thought to be preventive, but there are no good studies proving this.

Management of CRPS is usually with a team approach, starting as early as possible and using a combination of physical therapy, occupational therapy, and medications (e.g., NSAIDs, topical lidocaine, gabapentin, bisphosphonates, amitriptyline). One combination of therapy has not been proven to be better than another.

THE MEDSTUDY HUB: YOUR GUIDELINES AND REVIEW ARTICLES RESOURCE

For both review articles and current internal medicine practice guidelines, visit the MedStudy Hub at

medstudy.com/hub

The Hub contains the only online consolidated list of all current guidelines focused on internal medicine. Guidelines on the Hub are easy to find, continually updated, and linked to the published source. MedStudy maintains the Hub as a service to the medical community and makes it available to anyone and everyone at no cost to users.

MedStudy

Cardiology

SECTION EDITOR

John P. Reilly, MD
Vice Chairman, Department of Cardiology
Section Head, Interventional Cardiology
Program Director, Fellowship in
  Interventional Cardiology
Ochsner Medical Center
New Orleans, LA

REVIEWERS

Matthew Sorrentino, MD
Professor of Medicine
Vice Chair for Clinical Operations
Department of Medicine,
  Section of Cardiology
University of Chicago Medicine
Chicago, IL

Mary Olsovsky, MD
Colorado Springs, CO

MEDICAL EDITOR

Sharon Maynard, MD
Associate Professor of Medicine
University of South Florida
  Morsani College of Medicine
Program Director, Nephrology Fellowship
Lehigh Valley Health Network
Allentown, PA

Table of Contents

PHYSICAL EXAM... 13-1
  PULSES.. 13-1
  MURMURS AND HEART SOUNDS 13-1
    Note.. 13-1
    Murmurs 13-1
    Heart Sounds..................................... 13-2
  JUGULAR VENOUS WAVEFORMS................. 13-3

CHEST X-RAYS..**13-4**

PROCEDURES AND LABS...........................**13-6**
  ECHOCARDIOGRAM 13-6
  CARDIAC STRESS TESTS........................... 13-7
    Overview... 13-7
    Exercise Tolerance Test 13-7
    Stress Imaging Tests 13-8
    Picking the Correct Cardiac Stress Test........... 13-9
  CARDIOPULMONARY EXERCISE TESTING........ 13-9
  CARDIAC CATHETERIZATION AND OTHER
    CARDIAC IMAGING TESTS 13-9
    Contrast Cardiac Catheterization 13-9
    Cardiac CT... 13-9
    Cardiac MRI 13-10
  PULMONARY ARTERY CATHETERIZATION..... 13-10
  CARDIAC BIOPSY.................................... 13-11

HYPERTENSION 13-11

CARDIAC MEDICATIONS............................. 13-11

ANGINA... 13-12
  OVERVIEW 13-12
  ANTIANGINAL DRUGS 13-13
  EVALUATION OF CHRONIC STABLE ANGINA
    (STABLE ISCHEMIC HEART DISEASE)........... 13-14
    Note... 13-14
    History and Physical Exam —
      Determine Probability of CAD................. 13-14
    Noninvasive Tests for Chronic Stable Angina —
      Diagnosis and Risk Stratification 13-14
    Determination of Further Workup in Chronic
      Stable Angina 13-15
  TREATMENT OF CHRONIC STABLE ANGINA... 13-15
  CARDIOVASCULAR DISEASE PREVENTION
    IN WOMEN... 13-15

ACUTE CORONARY SYNDROME..................... 13-16
  CLASSIFICATION OF ACS........................... 13-16
  NOTES.. 13-16
  MARKERS FOR AMI 13-16
  TREATMENT OF ACS 13-17
    Prehospital Management 13-17
    Evaluation of Patients with Symptoms
      Suggestive of ACS.............................. 13-17
  ACS — GENERAL MEASURES 13-19
    ECG, NTG, Morphine, Beta-Blockers, ACEIs,
      and Atropine 13-19
    Anticoagulant / Antiplatelet Therapy in ACS .. 13-19
    Fibrinolytic Therapy in ACS 13-20
  ACS — MANAGEMENT OF NSTE-ACS —
    THE ACUTE ISCHEMIA PATHWAY............... 13-20
    Early Invasive vs. Ischemia-Guided Therapy ... 13-20
    Early Invasive Therapy in NSTE-ACS 13-20
    Ischemia-Guided Therapy in NSTE-ACS........ 13-21
    Long-Term Antiplatelet Therapy
      after NSTE-ACS................................. 13-21

ACS — MANAGEMENT WITH STEMI OR
  NEW LEFT BUNDLE BRANCH BLOCK.......... 13-21
    Note... 13-21
    Immediate Reperfusion Therapies 13-22
    Cocaine and Methamphetamine Users with
      ST Elevation 13-23
    Additional Treatment Recommendations from
      the 2013 ACC / AHA STEMI Guidelines...... 13-23
    Complications of Myocardial Infarction......... 13-23
    Implantable Cardioverter-Defibrillators......... 13-24

CORONARY ARTERY DISEASE **13-24**
  NOTE 13-24
  RISK FACTORS FOR CAD 13-25
  HYPERLIPIDEMIA SCREENING 13-25
    Evaluation of Hyperlipidemia 13-25
    Review of Lipoproteins........................... 13-25
    Hereditary Dyslipidemias......................... 13-27
  TREATMENT OF HYPERLIPIDEMIA 13-28
    Overview... 13-28
    General Concepts of Primary Prevention 13-28
    2013 ACC / AHA Clinical Practice Guidelines
      on Blood Cholesterol to Reduce ASCVD
      Risk in Adults.................................... 13-29
    Dietary Therapy 13-29
    Drugs for Dyslipidemias.......................... 13-29
  LIPIDS IN ACUTE CORONARY SYNDROME 13-31
  GOAL LEVELS OF LDL IN PATIENTS
    WITH CAD.. 13-31
  REVASCULARIZATION 13-32
    Overview... 13-32
    CABG vs. PCI...................................... 13-32
    Stents 13-32
    Other PCI Techniques 13-33

PERIPHERAL ARTERIAL DISEASE.................... **13-33**
  CAUSES OF PAD AND
    INTERMITTENT CLAUDICATION 13-33
  DIAGNOSIS OF PAD................................. 13-34
  TREATMENT OF PAD 13-34
  ACUTE LIMB ISCHEMIA 13-34
  RENAL ARTERY STENOSIS.......................... 13-35

CAROTID ARTERY DISEASE.......................... **13-35**
  CAROTID ARTERY ATHEROSCLEROSIS 13-35
  INTERNAL CAROTID ARTERY DISSECTION..... 13-35

CEREBRAL EMBOLIC DISEASE....................... **13-35**
  OVERVIEW 13-36
  TRANSIENT ISCHEMIC ATTACK................... 13-36

AORTIC DISEASE **13-36**
  AORTIC ANEURYSMS............................... 13-36
    Overview... 13-36
    Thoracic Aortic Aneurysms 13-36
    Abdominal Aortic Aneurysm..................... 13-37
  COARCTATION OF THE AORTA................... 13-37

VALVULAR HEART DISEASE **13-37**
  SPECIFIC VALVE LESIONS 13-37
    Note.. 13-38
    Aortic Stenosis... 13-39
    Chronic Aortic Regurgitation 13-40
    Acute Aortic Regurgitation....................... 13-41
    Mitral Stenosis 13-41
    Chronic Mitral Regurgitation.................... 13-41
    Mitral Valve Prolapse 13-42
    Acute Mitral Regurgitation 13-42
    Tricuspid Stenosis 13-42
    Tricuspid Regurgitation............................ 13-42
    Pulmonic Stenosis.................................... 13-43
    Pulmonic Regurgitation 13-43
    Ebstein Anomaly...................................... 13-43
  INFECTIVE ENDOCARDITIS........................ 13-43
    Overview... 13-43
    Antibiotic Prophylaxis 13-44
  RHEUMATIC FEVER 13-44
  VALVE SURGERY 13-45
  FINAL PEARLS ABOUT MURMURS................ 13-45

ARRHYTHMIAS **13-46**
  MECHANISMS OF ARRHYTHMIAS............... 13-46
  BRADYARRHYTHMIAS................................. 13-46
  SICK SINUS SYNDROME 13-46
  HEART BLOCK.. 13-46
  TACHYARRHYTHMIAS 13-46
    Note.. 13-47
    Atrial Flutter 13-47
    Atrial Fibrillation...................................... 13-47
    MAT.. 13-50
    SVT... 13-50
    WPW 13-50
  VENTRICULAR ARRHYTHMIAS 13-51
    PVCs 13-51
    Ventricular Tachycardia 13-51
    Nonsustained Ventricular Tachycardia.......... 13-52
  PACEMAKERS... 13-52
  ANTIARRHYTHMIC THERAPY...................... 13-53
    Drugs 13-53
    Electrophysiologic Testing........................ 13-54
    Radiofrequency Ablation 13-54

SYNCOPE **13-55**

CARDIOMYOPATHIES................................ **13-56**
  NOTE 13-56
  DILATED CARDIOMYOPATHY...................... 13-56
  HYPERTROPHIC CARDIOMYOPATHY........... 13-56
  RESTRICTIVE CARDIOMYOPATHY................ 13-57
  ARRHYTHMOGENIC RIGHT
    VENTRICULAR CARDIOMYOPATHY........... 13-57
  UNCLASSIFIED CARDIOMYOPATHIES 13-57

HEART FAILURE...................................... **13-58**
  OVERVIEW.. 13-58
  LOW-OUTPUT HF 13-58
    NYHA Classification 13-59
    ACC / AHA Staging and Management.......... 13-59
    Determining Prognosis in HF.................... 13-60
    Mechanism of HF...................................... 13-60
    Treatment for HF 13-60
    Emergency Treatment for Severe HF........... 13-63
  HIGH-OUTPUT HF 13-63
  RIGHT VENTRICULAR FAILURE 13-64
  PULMONARY EDEMA 13-64

PERICARDIAL DISEASES............................. **13-64**
  NONCONSTRICTIVE PERICARDITIS 13-64
  CONSTRICTIVE PERICARDITIS..................... 13-65
  RECURRENT PERICARDITIS......................... 13-66
  PERICARDIAL EFFUSION 13-66
  TAMPONADE.. 13-66

CONGENITAL HEART DISEASES.................... **13-66**
  NOTE 13-66
  ASD.. 13-66
    Ostium Secundum ASD 13-66
    Ostium Primum ASD................................. 13-67
    Sinus Venosus ASD 13-67
  PDA 13-67
  PULMONARY STENOSIS.............................. 13-67
  VSD.. 13-67
  COARCTATION OF THE AORTA.................... 13-67
  ANOMALOUS CORONARY ARTERY 13-67
  TETRALOGY OF FALLOT.............................. 13-68
  SUDDEN DEATH IN EXERCISING
    YOUNG PEOPLE 13-68
  OTHER.. 13-68

PULMONARY HEART DISEASE **13-68**
  COPD AND SLEEP APNEA........................... 13-68
  EISENMENGER SYNDROME 13-68
  CHRONIC THROMBOEMBOLIC
    OBSTRUCTION.. 13-68
  PULMONARY HYPERTENSION..................... 13-68

PREGNANCY AND THE HEART **13-69**

The Electrocardiogram

THE 12-LEAD ECG **13-70**

AXIS DEVIATIONS.. **13-70**

RATES AND INTERVALS................................. **13-70**

INTERVALS **13-71**
  PR INTERVAL.. 13-71
  QRS DURATION... 13-71
  QT INTERVAL 13-71

WAVEFORMS AND SEGMENTS....................... **13-72**
  P WAVE.. 13-72
  R WAVE 13-72
  T WAVE.. 13-73
  U WAVE 13-73
  ST SEGMENT.. 13-73
  QRS COMPLEX 13-73

VENTRICULAR HYPERTROPHY...................... **13-73**
  LVH.. 13-74
  RVH 13-74

CONDUCTION DISTURBANCES...................... **13-74**
  AV BLOCKS... 13-74
  BUNDLE BRANCH BLOCK............................ 13-74
    Overview... 13-74
    LBBB... 13-75
    RBBB... 13-75
    IVCD.. 13-75
    LAFB.. 13-75
    LPFB.. 13-75
    Bifascicular Block...................................... 13-76
  WIDE QRS 13-76

ARRHYTHMIAS **13-76**
    ECTOPIC VS. ESCAPE............................... 13-76
    ATRIAL ARRHYTHMIAS 13-76
    VENTRICULAR ECTOPIC BEATS
      AND HEART BLOCK................................ 13-77

MYOCARDIAL INFARCTION......................... **13-77**
    COMMON FINDINGS................................ 13-77
    LOCATION OF MI VS. ECG CHANGES 13-77
    NOTES... 13-77

REMEMBER **13-77**

ANALYSIS SUMMARY **13-78**
    OVERVIEW... 13-78
    ECG CASE STUDIES 13-79
    FINDINGS FROM ECG CASE STUDIES........... 13-90

AMBULATORY ECG MONITORING **13-91**
    CONTINUOUS AMBULATORY ECG
      (HOLTER) MONITORS 13-91
    EVENT MONITORS.................................. 13-91

THE MEDSTUDY HUB: YOUR GUIDELINES
    AND REVIEW ARTICLES RESOURCE.............. **13-91**

PHYSICAL EXAM

PREVIEW | REVIEW

- True or false? Pulsus paradoxus can be seen in cardiac tamponade.
- What is pulsus bisferiens? What does it indicate?
- What does pulsus alternans indicate?
- True or false? Sustained handgrip increases the murmur of mitral valve prolapse but decreases the murmur of HCM.
- When is a persistently split S_2 heard?
- What causes a paradoxically split S_2?
- In which patient population is an S_3 usually pathologic?
- When are large *v* waves seen on the right side (jugular vein)? Left side (PA catheter tracing)?
- When is rapid *x* and *y* descent seen?
- When is the *y* descent absent?
- When are large, right-sided *a* waves seen?
- When are cannon *a* waves seen?
- When does a slow *y* descent occur?
- When are large, left-sided *a* waves seen?

PULSES

Pulsus paradoxus is an exaggeration of the normal decrease in systolic blood pressure with inspiration. It can be detected clinically using a manual (not automatic) blood pressure cuff. While deflating the cuff very slowly, note the systolic blood pressure where the 1st Korotkoff sound is heard only during inspiration. Slowly deflate the cuff and note the systolic pressure at which the Korotkoff sounds continue through both inspiration and exhalation. The difference between these 2 pressures quantifies the pulsus paradoxus. A difference of ≥ 10 mmHg is considered abnormal. It is present with:

- cardiac tamponade (especially),
- constrictive pericarditis,
- asthma, and
- tension pneumothorax.

Note: Korotkoff sounds are those heard during blood pressure determination with a cuff.

The paradox is that, when severe, the pulse palpated on examination is of variable strength, while precordial activity is regular.

Pulsus bisferiens (2 systolic peaks of the aortic pulse per cardiac cycle) is seen with aortic regurgitation (with or without stenosis!) and hypertrophic cardiomyopathy (HCM; see Hypertrophic Cardiomyopathy on page 13-56).

Pulsus alternans (varying pulse pressure with a regular pulse rate) is seen with severely depressed systolic function of any cause that leads to decreased stroke volume.

Pulsus parvus et tardus (parvus—low amplitude, tardus—slow upswing) = aortic stenosis.

Brachiofemoral delay, the femoral pulse occurring after the brachial pulse, is present in coarctation of the aorta.

Pulse asymmetry occurs in aortic dissection, with good upper extremity pulses, but with diminished or absent lower extremity pulses. The asymmetry can also occur between the left and right upper extremities.

Peripheral arterial disease (PAD, previously called peripheral vascular disease [PVD]), can cause decreased or absent peripheral pulses; a bruit may also be heard over the proximal arteries (such as the femoral artery).

MURMURS AND HEART SOUNDS

Note

Know heart sounds and murmurs! Know the differentiating maneuvers in Table 13-1 on page 13-2 and the heart sounds described in Table 13-8 on page 13-38 and in Valvular Heart Disease on page 13-37. Learn these topics so you can determine how 1 abnormal finding (e.g., a particular heart sound) correlates with certain findings on ECG and chest x-ray.

Murmurs

All valve murmurs increase in intensity when blood flow increases across the valve. Standing and the strain phase of Valsalva decrease right and left cardiac filling and cause the sound of most murmurs to decrease, but these actions increase the intensity of the murmurs of mitral valve prolapse (MVP) and hypertrophic cardiomyopathy (HCM). Squatting and lying down (or passive straight-leg raises if already supine) increase cardiac volume. This increased volume and afterload also increases intensity of all murmurs except, again, MVP and HCM (see Mitral Valve Prolapse on page 13-42 and Hypertrophic Cardiomyopathy on page 13-56).

Sustained handgrip (20–30 seconds) boosts systemic vascular resistance and left ventricular volume and therefore decreases the intensity of murmurs of HCM and aortic stenosis (AS). It delays the murmur of MVP by increasing left ventricular volume. Handgrip is most useful to differentiate between AS (murmur intensity decreases) and mitral regurgitation (MR; murmur intensity increases).

Keep in mind that the murmur of HCM worsens with any drop in left ventricular volume. So, any maneuver that increases ventricular volume decreases the murmur of HCM.

Right-sided murmurs and heart sounds are louder during inspiration and any maneuvers that increase venous return, such as passive leg raises and abdominal compression. Left-sided murmurs and heart sounds are louder during expiration. The only semiexception to this rule is a right-sided ejection click due to pulmonic stenosis; this disappears with inspiration. (On a chest x-ray, pulmonic stenosis can appear as an enlarged pulmonary artery.)

Refer to Table 13-8 on page 13-38 for more on murmurs, and see Figure 13-1 for murmur illustrations.

Heart Sounds

S_1 is caused by the closing of the mitral and tricuspid valves. S_1 intensity is decreased when there is a prolonged PR interval, MR, acute aortic regurgitation (increased LV pressures cause early valve closure), or a severely calcified mitral valve.

S_1 intensity is increased (i.e., the mitral valve slams shut) by a short PR interval, mitral stenosis, or hyperdynamic ventricular function.

S_2 is caused by the closing of the aortic (A_2) and pulmonic (P_2) valves at the end of systole. P_2 usually occurs just after A_2. This physiologic split is increased with inspiration because the increased volume of blood in the right ventricle (RV) prolongs RV systole and delays closure of the pulmonic valve. It generally disappears on expiration.

A persistently (or widely) split S_2 varies with respiration but does not disappear on expiration. A widely split S_2 can be due to pulmonic stenosis, acute pulmonary embolism, ectopic or pacemaker beats originating in the left ventricle, pulmonary hypertension, or right bundle branch block (RBBB)—all of which cause delayed or prolonged contraction of the right ventricle. A widely split S_2 can also be caused by early closure of the aortic valve, as in MR. Pulmonic stenosis is especially likely if the patient has an ejection click that disappears with inspiration.

A fixed split S_2 does not vary with respiration. You hear a fixed split S_2 with atrial septal defect. The patient presents with a fixed split S_2 and a systolic ejection murmur (SEM) and has pulmonary vascular congestion on the chest x-ray. You can also hear a fixed split S_2 with RV failure when the stroke volume is unable to increase with inspiration.

Table 13-1: Maneuvers to Differentiate Murmurs	
Maneuver	**Result**
Passive straight-leg raise (to 45°; listen after 15 seconds)	Increases venous return
Valsalva (hold for 20 sec; listen just before end)	Decreases venous return
Standing (squat for > 30 seconds then quickly stand; listen during first 15 seconds after standing)	Decreases venous return
Transient arterial occlusion (BP cuff on both arms, inflated > 20 mmHg above systolic pressure)	Increases systemic vascular resistance
Handgrip (isomeric; listen at end of 1-minute max grip)	Increases systemic vascular resistance
Squatting	Increases venous return and increases systemic vascular resistance, but preload effect is stronger than afterload effect
Maneuvers for diagnosing systolic murmurs	
To Diagnose HCM	**Result**
Standing (from squat)	Increased murmur intensity
Valsalva (if cannot do squat-to-stand)	Increased murmur intensity
Passive straight-leg raise	Decreased murmur intensity
Handgrip	Decreased murmur intensity
To Diagnose MVP	**Result**
Standing and Valsalva	Click-murmur moves earlier
Transient arterial occlusion	Click-murmur moves later
Handgrip	Click-murmur moves later
To Diagnose VSD	**Result**
Standing and Valsalva	Decreased murmur intensity
Transient arterial occlusion	Increased murmur intensity
Handgrip	Increased murmur intensity
To Diagnose AS	**Result**
Transient arterial occlusion	Decreased murmur intensity
Handgrip	Decreased murmur intensity

AS = aortic stenosis; HCM = hypertrophic cardiomyopathy; MVP = mitral valve prolapse; VSD = ventricular septal defect

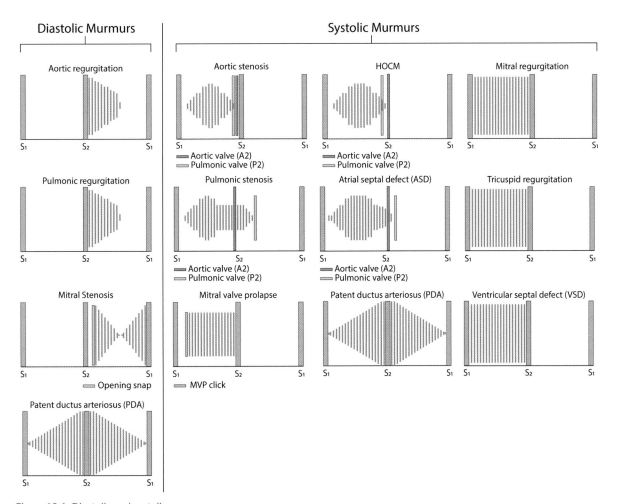

Figure 13-1: Diastolic and systolic murmurs

A delay of aortic closure (A_2) causes a paradoxically split S_2, with P_2 occurring before A_2. In this case, you hear increased splitting with expiration instead of inspiration. This is commonly caused by left bundle branch block (LBBB), advanced HCM, or ectopic or escape beats originating in the right ventricle.

Quick review of split heart sounds:

- Persistently/widely split S_2 (still varies with inspiration but never goes away) occurs with pulmonic stenosis, PE, RBBB, and LV ectopic beats.
- Fixed split S_2 (A_2-P_2 interval remains the same throughout breathing cycle) from ASD.
- Paradoxically split S_2 (P_2 before A_2) is caused by severe HCM, LBBB, RV ectopic beats, AS, and patent ductus arteriosus (PDA).

S_3, when present, follows immediately after S_2 and indicates the end of rapid ventricular filling (sounds like "lub-dub-huh"). This is early diastole, when the first 70% of ventricular filling occurs as the ventricle relaxes. The sound is thought to be due to the tensing of the chordae tendineae. An S_3 is a normal finding in children and in persons with high cardiac output (CO), such as pregnant women. In patients > 40 years of age,

it is usually pathologic. It can be caused by any condition that increases early LV filling rate or volume, such as acute ventricular decompensation or severe aortic or mitral regurgitation. S_3 in a patient with known LV dysfunction is a poor prognostic indicator. Both S_3 and S_4 are best heard in left lateral decubitus position using the bell of the stethoscope.

S_4, when present, is heard just before S_1 at the end of diastole (sounds like "huh-lub-dub"). The S_4 sound is caused by ventricular filling during atrial contraction, and you hear it in patients with decreased ventricular compliance. You may hear an S_4 in ischemic heart disease, AS, HCM, diabetic cardiomyopathy, and hypertensive heart disease with concentric hypertrophy. You do not hear an S_4 in patients with atrial fibrillation (because the sound requires atrial contraction) or mitral stenosis (where there is obstruction of ventricular inflow).

JUGULAR VENOUS WAVEFORMS

Jugular venous pulse (JVP) and jugular venous waveforms are best visualized on the right side of the neck (more direct path to the heart than the left). The JVP is used to assess the right side of the heart (Figure 13-2 on page 13-4 and Table 13-2 on page 13-4). **Know this!**

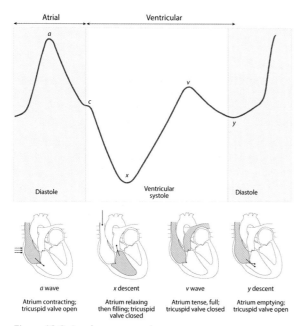

Figure 13-2: Jugular venous pulse

Know the following about jugular waveforms:

- **Large, right-sided *v* waves** are seen in ventricular septal rupture and tricuspid regurgitation.
- **Large *v* waves** are associated with tricuspid regurgitation and heart failure. This may be right heart failure or combined left and right heart failure.
- **Rapid *x* and *y* descents** are seen with constrictive pericarditis, whereas only a rapid *x* descent is seen in tamponade (loss of the *y* descent).
- **Large, right-sided *a* waves** are seen in tricuspid stenosis (TS), severe pulmonic stenosis, and severe noncompliant RVH.

- **Cannon *a* waves** occur in complete heart block, ventricular tachycardia, asynchronous ventricular pacing, and all conditions with AV dissociation (times when the atrium is contracting against a closed tricuspid valve).
- **Slow *y* descent** is from delayed atrial emptying, as in tricuspid stenosis.

The left side of the heart also has "venous" waveforms which are actually left atrial pressures, as seen during PA catheter (Swan-Ganz) monitoring:

- With severe mitral regurgitation, there are tall, **left-sided *v* waves** from the regurgitation during systole.
- **Large, left-sided *a* waves** are seen with mitral stenosis (MS).

Also see Table 13-8 on page 13-38 for a review of the valve defects.

CHEST X-RAYS

PREVIEW | REVIEW

- On a lateral view CXR, extension of the heart border posteriorly and inferiorly indicates enlargement of which ventricle?
- On a lateral view CXR, extension of the cardiac shadow of the lower part of the anterior clear space behind the sternum indicates enlargement of which ventricle?

Know all the following chest x-ray findings!

The chest x-ray (CXR) can tell you about overall heart size and (sometimes) heart chamber sizes.

Table 13-2: Jugular Venous Waveforms		
Condition	**Neck Vein Appearance**	**Other Diagnostic Features**
Pulmonary HTN	Elevated *a* and *v* waves	Other physical exam findings of pulmonary HTN (e.g., accentuated P_2, early systolic click, and midsystolic ejection murmur)
Tricuspid regurgitation	Large *v* waves	TR murmur (see Table 13-8 on page 13-38), pulsatile liver
Constrictive pericarditis	Rapid *x* and *y* descents	Kussmaul sign (paradoxical increase in JVP during inspiration), pericardial knock (an early, sharp S_3)
Tamponade	Rapid *x* descent	Pulsus paradoxus, hypotension
Tricuspid stenosis	Slow *y* descent	TS murmur (see Table 13-8 on page 13-38)
Restrictive cardiomyopathy	Rapid *x* and *y* descents	Low-voltage ECG; diagnose with echo, myocardial biopsy
Tension pneumothorax	Distended neck veins	Dyspnea, unilateral absent breath sounds, deviated trachea; diagnose with chest x-ray
Superior vena cava syndrome	Unilateral distended neck veins	Facial edema and cyanosis, diagnosis of cancer
AV dissociation	Irregular cannon *a* waves	Diagnose with ECG
RV infarction	Elevated *a* and *v* waves	Acute inferior MI, Kussmaul sign
ASD	Large *v* waves and rapid *y* descent	Fixed split S_2; diagnose with echo

On the posteroanterior (PA) view (Figure 13-3), the left ventricle (LV) causes the bulge in the left-lower side of the cardiac shadow. The right atrium (RA) causes the outline on the right. The cardiac "waistline"—between the aortic knob and the LV—is formed by the main pulmonary artery and the left atrial (LA) appendage.

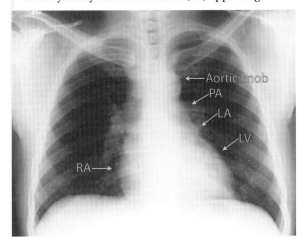

Figure 13-3: Normal posteroanterior chest x-ray

You can also estimate the cardiothoracic ratio from the PA view = the width of the cardiac silhouette divided by the chest diameter (measured from the inside rib margin at the widest point above the costophrenic angles). A cardiothoracic ratio > 0.5 indicates either cardiomegaly or a pericardial effusion. This ratio is valid only for an upright, nonrotated film on full inspiration, with a well-visualized cardiac outline, and when there is no abdominal compression on the diaphragm (e.g., ascites, pregnancy).

On the lateral view (Figure 13-4), if the cardiac shadow extends posteriorly and lower—closer to the diaphragm—this indicates increased LV mass. When the lower part of the anterior clear space behind the sternum is filled in, this indicates increased RV mass.

With **coarctation** of the aorta (COA), the aortic arch is abnormal. Look for the "3" sign (Figure 13-5), which is created by a prominent left subclavian artery, the coarctation, and poststenotic dilation of the descending aorta. The barium swallow can show a "reversed 3" due to the impressions of the arterial structures on the esophagus. CXR in adults can also show intercostal rib notching (Figure 13-6) due to collateral flow through tortuous intercostal arteries.

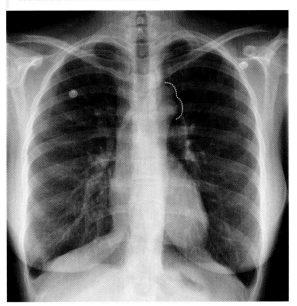

Figure 13-5: "3" sign in COA

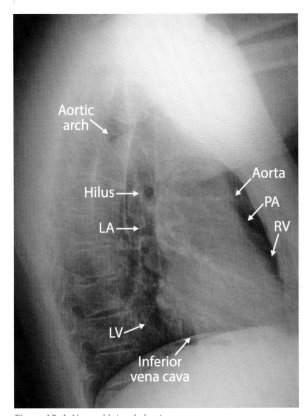

Figure 13-4: Normal lateral chest x-ray
Source: James Heilman, MD

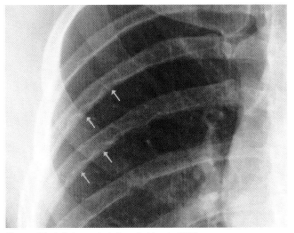

Figure 13-6: Intercostal rib notching in COA

Heart failure (HF; Figure 13-7) is indicated by cardiomegaly, pulmonary vascular redistribution (with visibly thickened upper lobe pulmonary veins), Kerley B (interlobular septal) lines, and pleural effusions (usually right > left), all indicating pulmonary edema.

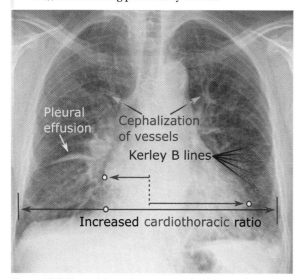

Figure 13-7: Heart failure chest x-ray with edema and Kerley B lines

An **anomalous pulmonary vein** that drains into the inferior vena cava can create a scimitar sign on chest x-ray. This is a curvilinear opacity in the right lower lung field due to associated lung hypoplasia.

Aortic abnormalities seen on CXR include tortuosity, ectasia, and calcification. An aortic aneurysm is sometimes visible on the lateral film. An aortic dissection can show up as mediastinal widening on the posteroanterior projection (Figure 13-8), but remember that the absence of mediastinal widening does not rule out dissection.

Pericardial effusion is suggested by a water bottle or a water balloon shape to the heart, sometimes with significant enlargement of the cardiac silhouette (Figure 13-9).

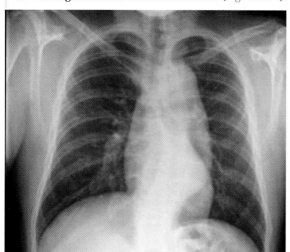

Figure 13-8: Aortic dissection with widened mediastinum and large aortic knob

Shunt vascularity (enlarged, sharply defined pulmonary vasculature) can be visible with ventricular septal defect (VSD), atrial septal defect (ASD), or other left-to-right shunts.

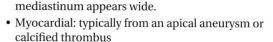

Figure 13-9: Water bottle heart
Source: David Ferry, MD

Areas of calcification on chest x-ray:

- Aortic: Think dissection if you see a separation between calcification and the aortic border, especially if the mediastinum appears wide.
- Myocardial: typically from an apical aneurysm or calcified thrombus
- Valvular: commonly the aortic valve
- Annular (ring-shaped): mitral annular calcification; if it is a perfect ring, then a prosthetic valve is likely (especially if surgical clips are also present).
- Pericardial (Figure 13-10): Think constrictive pericarditis; or think TB if the clinical history suggests exposure.

Know that a single lead in the apex of the RV indicates the presence of an electronic ventricular pacemaker or implanted defibrillator—defibrillator leads are larger and wider than pacemaker leads. 2 leads indicate an atrioventricular (AV) sequential (dual-chamber) pacemaker, and 3 leads indicate a biventricular pacemaker.

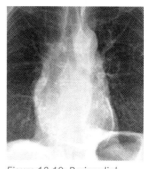

Figure 13-10: Pericardial calcification
Source: David Ferry, MD

See The 12-Lead ECG on page 13-70.

PROCEDURES AND LABS

ECHOCARDIOGRAM

PREVIEW | REVIEW

- Name the anatomic structures and conditions that are evaluated with a TEE.

Echocardiography (echo) is an ultrasound modality used to image the heart. It utilizes M-mode, 2D, and 3D for structural imaging and Doppler for assessing blood flow rate and direction.

Echo is good for assessing:

- Left ventricular systolic or diastolic dysfunction
- Right ventricular systolic dysfunction
- Valvular heart disease
- Congenital heart disease
- Myocardial infarction (including post-MI complications)
- Cardiomyopathy (both decrease in ejection fraction and hypertrophy of myocardium)
- Pericardial disease
- Cardiac masses (tumor, thrombus, and vegetation)
- Diseases of the aorta and pulmonary artery
- Estimation of pulmonary pressure
- Cardiac sources of emboli

Transesophageal echocardiogram (TEE) is an echo performed with an esophageal probe (and is thus an invasive test). It offers higher-resolution images compared to transthoracic imaging and is especially useful for evaluating:

- Valvular structure and function
- Left atrium (including left atrial appendage thrombi)
- Cardiac masses
- Intracardiac shunts
- Endocarditis
- Aortic dissection

A **bubble study** (performed by injecting hand-agitated saline into the venous system) is used to evaluate intracardiac shunts. In technically challenging studies, a contrast agent may be intravenously administered to improve imaging of the chambers.

Doppler echocardiography measures the velocity and direction of the blood flow. Doppler echo determines mean gradients, peak velocities, and valve area. Doppler is useful in determining the severity of valvular stenosis or regurgitation, as well as in evaluating left ventricular diastolic function, left ventricular outflow tract gradients, and intracardiac shunts.

Doppler is also used to estimate pulmonary artery (PA) pressure.

CARDIAC STRESS TESTS

PREVIEW | REVIEW

- What are absolute indications for terminating an ETT?
- When are stress imaging studies done instead of an ETT?
- Which stress imaging tests are used in patients with LBBB? With paced ventricular rhythm?
- When are exercise stress echo and MPI indicated instead of ETT?

Overview

Cardiac stress testing is used in the assessment of patients with coronary artery disease (CAD). Stress testing relies on the increased demand for myocardial oxygen with exercise or pharmacologic agents. Stress tests have an integral role in both the detection of CAD (diagnostic tool) and in stratification of risk (prognostic tool). To appropriately utilize stress tests, you must take into account the pretest probability of CAD. (A positive test in a low-risk patient has a higher likelihood to be a false positive, and a negative test in a high-risk patient has a higher likelihood to be a false negative.) Diagnostic testing is most valuable when pretest probability for CAD is intermediate.

There are 2 general types of cardiac stress tests:

1) Exercise tolerance test (ETT; basic treadmill or stationary bicycle testing without imaging)
2) Stress imaging testing—stress is induced with:
   - exercise (treadmill or bicycle), or
   - pharmacologic stress (either dobutamine or a vasodilator, such as adenosine).

The associated imaging is done with:

- Echocardiography (a.k.a. stress echo)
- Myocardial perfusion imaging (MPI; a.k.a. nuclear stress test)
- Cardiac magnetic resonance imaging (CMR)

Exercise Tolerance Test

Exercise tolerance test (ETT), using either a treadmill or stationary bicycle, is the standard diagnostic testing for ischemia and functional capacity and for determining prognosis (including post-MI).

Despite an overall low sensitivity and specificity (men: sensitivity = 68%, specificity = 77%; women: sensitivity = 61%, specificity = 70%), ETT has a number of advantages, including the ability to test functional capacity, safety, widespread availability, and relatively low cost. Due to the low predictive value, it is most commonly performed in conjunction with nuclear or echocardiographic imaging.

The patient typically exercises on a treadmill using standard exercise protocols, such as the Bruce protocol. The level of maximal exercise achieved on the ETT is measured in metabolic equivalents (METS).

ETT without imaging is not recommended in 2 groups:

1) Patients unable to exercise sufficiently (must achieve 85% of age-predicted maximum heart rate)
2) Patients with baseline ECG abnormalities that can interfere with interpretation of the stress test (e.g., left ventricular hypertrophy [LVH], LBBB, Wolff-Parkinson-White [WPW] syndrome, ventricular pacing, resting ST depression, taking digoxin)

Know the following information related to ETTs.

Definition of a positive ETT: flat or down-sloping ST-segment depression > 1 mm at 80 msec after the J-point in 3 consecutive beats.

Unlike ST elevation, ST depression does not correlate with the anatomic location of myocardial ischemia. Isolated ST depression in inferior leads is far less specific than ST depression in lateral leads (V4–6).

ST elevation during an ETT in 3 contiguous leads without Q waves of prior MI is unusual and suggests marked ischemia (but can also be seen with coronary artery spasm).

Terminate the ETT immediately if you see:

- ST elevation > 1 mm in leads without Q waves from prior MI (excluding aVR, aVL, and V1)
- Decrease in systolic BP > 10 mmHg with other evidence of ischemia or hypoperfusion
- Moderate or severe angina
- CNS symptoms (e.g., ataxia, dizziness, near syncope)
- Signs of poor perfusion (e.g., cyanosis/pallor)
- Sustained 2nd or 3rd degree AV block
- Technical difficulties in monitoring ECG/BP
- Patient requests to stop
- Serious arrhythmia (e.g., sustained ventricular tachycardia)

Achieving target heart rate alone is not a reason to discontinue the ETT; encourage the individual to go as long as tolerated until required to stop for some reason (e.g., dyspnea, fatigue, exhaustion).

Excellent exercise tolerance (> 10 METS) correlates with a good prognosis independent of the degree of coronary artery disease.

Absolute contraindications to ETT:

- Acute MI within 2 days
- Unstable angina not previously stabilized by medical therapy
- Uncontrolled arrhythmias causing symptoms or hemodynamic compromise
- Symptomatic severe aortic stenosis
- Decompensated symptomatic HF
- Acute pulmonary embolus or infarction
- Acute myocarditis or pericarditis
- Acute aortic dissection

Stress Imaging Tests

Overview

The stress imaging studies include the stress echo, MPI, and cardiovascular magnetic resonance (CMR; discussed under Cardiac MRI on page 13-10). The choice of which to use is often based on operator experience at the facility.

Stress imaging studies are used as the initial diagnostic method when a patient is not a candidate for ETT due to inability to exercise adequately or when there are ECG changes at rest that can interfere with interpretation of the test ECG. They are also preferred in patients with prior revascularization.

Stress imaging studies have greater sensitivity and specificity than the regular ETT. They are used when measurement of ejection fraction or myocardial viability is desired in addition to identifying coronary artery disease.

Stressing the Heart for Imaging Studies

The stress portion of imaging study tests can be performed with exercise or pharmacologic agents.

With **exercise**, imaging studies are done with a standard ETT and require the same ability to meet 85% of age-predicted maximum heart rate. Exercise stress is preferred over pharmacologic stress because it provides additional functional and prognostic information. Exercise is not recommended in patients with pacemakers or LBBB because it can cause false-positive left ventricular anteroseptal perfusion defects. The pharmacologic agents used for cardiac imaging studies are dobutamine or vasodilators.

Dobutamine is both inotropic + chronotropic and causes the heart to respond as it would to exercise. As with exercise, a target heart rate must be achieved with dobutamine. Also, as with exercise, dobutamine is usually not used in patients with pacemakers. Dobutamine is used for patients who are unable to exercise and have a contraindication to vasodilators (e.g., bronchospasm, severe carotid artery stenosis).

Vasodilators: Adenosine, dipyridamole, and regadenoson are the main coronary vasodilators used in pharmacologic MPI stress tests. Vasodilators do not stress the heart by increasing heart rate as is done with exercise or dobutamine. These agents increase blood flow in normal coronary vessels while doing little to change the flow in stenotic vessels. The dilated normal vessels steal flow from the stenotic vessels, causing perfusion defects in the region of the left ventricle supplied by the stenotic vessel (and ST segment changes in ECGs). Use vasodilators cautiously in patients with history of bronchospasm.

Regadenoson is a selective adenosine A2A receptor activator that causes less bronchospasm and allows for a faster stress test. Even so, dobutamine remains the pharmacologic agent of choice for patients with a history of bronchospasm.

Stress Echo and Stress MPI Indications

Unlike ETT, exercise stress echo and stress MPI can be used in patients:

- with resting ECG ST changes,
- with WPW syndrome, or
- on digoxin therapy.

Note that it is a common misconception that these patients require pharmacologic stress, but this is definitely not true! If they can exercise, these patients can get a stress echo with exercise or MPI with exercise (i.e., these patients need the imaging, not the pharmacologic stress).

Note: MPI with vasodilators (but not exercise or dobutamine!) is the test of choice for patients with paced ventricular rhythm.

Stress Echo

The stress echo is a widely used test for myocardial ischemia; it detects stress-induced wall motion abnormalities. Stress echo is less sensitive but more specific than MPI for the detection of coronary artery disease.

Use exercise or dobutamine to achieve target heart rate. Abnormal wall motion or failure of the wall to thicken (contract) appropriately suggests ischemia of that region of the myocardium.

In addition to new regional wall motion abnormalities, criteria for abnormal stress echo are left ventricular cavity dilation and decline in global left ventricular systolic function with stress (suggestive of multivessel disease). Stress echo is less expensive than MPI and does not involve radiation exposure.

Vasodilators are not used for stress echo.

Myocardial Perfusion Imaging

Myocardial perfusion imaging (MPI) uses radioisotopes with single-photon emission computed tomography (SPECT). These tracers distribute in heart tissue in proportion to blood flow; this distribution is recorded by a gamma camera. Perfusion is compared visually between the resting and stressed states. With ischemia, myocardial perfusion is normal at rest but decreased during stress (reversible defect). With myocardial infarction, perfusion is reduced both at rest and during stress (fixed defect). Other MPI findings suggestive of multivessel disease include transient ischemic LV dilation (TID), reduced poststress LV ejection fraction, and increased lung or right ventricular uptake.

Again, target heart rate must be achieved with exercise or pharmacologic agents that cause vasodilation, such as adenosine, dipyridamole, or regadenoson. Other imaging modalities that can be used for MPI (as an alternative to SPECT) include cardiac positron emission tomography (PET) and cardiac MRI, both of which can also assess for myocardial ischemia and viability.

MPI is more expensive than stress echo, and it involves radiation exposure.

Picking the Correct Cardiac Stress Test

In review:

- Exercise is the preferred modality for inducing cardiac stress.
- When the ECG is nondiagnostic, or for enhanced diagnostic value, use echocardiographic or nuclear imaging.
- Vasodilators can be used in lieu of exercise for MPI only, while dobutamine can also be used for nonimaged or echocardiographic tests.

- Dobutamine is contraindicated in severe hypertension or ventricular tachycardia.
- Do not use dobutamine in paced ventricular rhythms due to distortion of normal ventricular contraction.
- Many vasodilator agents are contraindicated in bronchospasm or severe carotid artery disease.

CARDIOPULMONARY EXERCISE TESTING

PREVIEW | REVIEW

- Which patients may benefit from CPX?

Cardiopulmonary exercise testing (CPX) is a special exercise test that measures ventilation and concentrations of oxygen and carbon dioxide during progressive exercise (stationary bicycle/treadmill) and is the gold standard aerobic exercise test. CPX provides the most accurate and reproducible measurement of cardiorespiratory fitness, severity of impairment, and response to intervention. CPX is used to evaluate patients with systolic HF, especially those undergoing a pretransplant assessment, and patients with unexplained exertional dyspnea.

CARDIAC CATHETERIZATION AND OTHER CARDIAC IMAGING TESTS

Contrast Cardiac Catheterization

Coronary angiography (a.k.a. left heart catheterization or simply "cath") is the gold standard for the diagnosis of CAD.

Not only can contrast left-heart catheterization assess coronary anatomy, but through contrast ventriculography it can also assess ejection fraction, wall motion abnormalities, ventricular dilatation, degree of mitral regurgitation, and the presence of a ventricular aneurysm. However, cardiac catheterization is an invasive procedure with ~ 1% risk of serious complications (i.e., death, MI, stroke, arrhythmia, renal failure, bleeding).

Left-heart catheterization requires arterial access, radiation, and contrast exposure.

Cardiac CT

Cardiac CT is a noninvasive modality for imaging the heart. Cardiac CT includes:

- Coronary computed tomographic angiography (CCTA)
- Coronary artery calcium (CAC) scoring

CCTA requires IV contrast (check creatinine!); also, the heart rate must be < 60 bpm and regular, and patients must be able to hold their breath.

CCTA is a reasonable diagnostic test for symptomatic patients who are at intermediate risk for CAD or have congenital abnormalities. The negative predictive value of CCTA is very high; that is, a negative CCTA is very helpful in excluding significant coronary artery disease.

Usefulness is reduced in patients with pronounced coronary calcification.

CAC scanning detects atherosclerosis and, unlike CCTA, does not require IV contrast. CAC is used for risk stratification in asymptomatic, intermediate-risk patients. A CAC score of zero is considered low cardiovascular risk, and > 400 indicates an elevated (~ 3-fold) 10-year risk for a cardiovascular event.

Cardiac MRI

Static and dynamic cardiac MRI (CMR) allows high-resolution imaging of ventricular function, valvular motion, and myocardial perfusion.

CMR is useful to assess cardiac structure and function, valvular heart disease, coronary takeoff, the great vessels, pericardial disease, cardiac masses, myocarditis, and infiltrative diseases. CMR also can be used to assess for myocardial ischemia and post-MI tissue viability.

Cardiac MRI involves the use of gadolinium; therefore, avoid use in patients with advanced renal failure due to the risk of nephrogenic systemic fibrosis.

PULMONARY ARTERY CATHETERIZATION

PREVIEW | REVIEW

- When is PCWP increased?
- At which PCWP do you expect to see frank pulmonary edema?
- In which condition is diastolic pressure equal in all 4 chambers?

Pulmonary artery catheterization (PAC) can be used to assess right and left heart filling pressures, CO, RV and PA pressures, and systemic and pulmonary vascular resistance. This is useful to determine a patient's volume status, causes of shock, and existence of pericardial disease. Clinically, it is no longer used as often as in the past, due to no evidence of substantial benefit of outcomes and risk associated with placement (pneumothorax, damage to avascular, infection, and cardiac injury).

The pulmonary capillary wedge pressure (PCWP) is the dampened LA pressure that reflects left ventricular end-diastolic pressure (LVEDP) in most cases. This reflects LVED volume.

Normal pressures:

- RA: < 8 mmHg (JVD in the upright position indicates RA pressure > 5 mmHg)
- RV: 15–30/1–7 mmHg
- PCWP: 4–12 mmHg
- PCWP increases with LV systolic and diastolic failure, mitral stenosis, aortic and mitral insufficiency, tamponade, and constrictive pericarditis. Consider LV failure if the PCWP is > 15–18 mmHg.
- PCWP 15–25 mmHg causes dyspnea on exertion (DOE).
- PCWP 25–35 mmHg causes dyspnea at rest, orthopnea, and interstitial edema.
- PCWP > 35 mmHg (acutely) causes frank pulmonary edema.

Note: Conditions that decrease ventricular compliance, like LVH and right ventricular hypertrophy (RVH), also increase RA and PCWP.

A few PAC scenarios are shown in Table 13-3. Notice that the diastolic PA pressure is typically very close to PCWP (usual difference < 5 mmHg) in all scenarios except pulmonary hypertension (item 6)!

1) Normal

2) Tamponade and constrictive pericarditis: Diastolic pressure in all 4 chambers is equalized. See Pericardial Diseases on page 13-64 for the tests that differentiate between these disorders.

3) RV failure due to RV infarct: The CO and PCWP are decreased and the RA pressure is elevated. It's typically seen with acute inferior MI. The RV has decompensated and is unable to fill the left side of the heart.

4) If the CO is low, PCWP high, and RA pressure high, the patient has biventricular failure with cardiogenic shock.

5) Mitral stenosis (or LV failure) with 2° RV failure

6) Pulmonary hypertension

	RA Press (mmHg)	PA Press (mmHg)	PCWP (mmHg)	BP (mmHg)	Comments
Table 13-3: Pulmonary Artery Catheterization Scenarios					
1) Normal	0–5	(13–28)/(3–13)	3–11	110/70	
2) Tamponade or constrictive pericarditis	18	32/18	19	70/50	Diastolic pressure equal in all 4 chambers!
3) RV failure due to RV infarct	15	21/11	10	70/50	RV unable to fill the L heart: high RA pressure and low PCWP
4) Biventricular failure	18	30/20	20	70/50	Cardiogenic shock is common.
5) Mitral stenosis	18	90/32	30	110/70	
6) Pulmonary HTN	18	90/32	10	110/70	

Also know that septic shock is mainly due to a low systemic vascular resistance. These patients have low BP, systemic vascular resistance (SVR), and PCWP—and a high CO.

CARDIAC BIOPSY

PREVIEW | REVIEW

- Name 1 indication for endomyocardial biopsy.

Consider endomyocardial biopsy in the following situations:

- To diagnose or monitor for rejection after cardiac transplantation
- To determine the etiology of cardiomyopathy or myocarditis when the diagnosis is uncertain and would change management
- In rapidly progressive heart failure or worsening ventricular dysfunction that persists despite appropriate medical therapy
- In suspected myocarditis (particularly giant cell myocarditis) or a myocardial infiltrative process (particularly amyloidosis)

HYPERTENSION

PREVIEW | REVIEW

- In which patients should you suspect secondary hypertension?
- True or false? A systolic abdominal bruit without a diastolic bruit suggests renal vascular hypertension.
- What disorder should you think of if a patient presents with hypertension, hypokalemia, and low renin?

The 2017 ACC/AHA Guidelines for the Prevention, Detection, Evaluation, and Management of High Blood Pressure in Adults define hypertension as SBP > 130 mmHg or DBP > 80 mmHg. This is lower than the > 140/90 definition from previous guidelines.

Here's what you need to know about the 2017 Hypertension Guidelines:

- Everyone with hypertension (> 130/80) should be treated with lifestyle interventions: stop smoking, lose weight, moderate alcohol, exercise, eat a low-sodium healthy diet.
- Low-risk patients (10-year atherosclerotic cardiovascular disease (ASCVD) risk < 10%): Use medications for SBP > 140 mmHg or DBP > 90 mmHg.
- Everyone else: Use medications for SBP > 130 mmHg or DBP > 90 mmHg.

"Everyone else" includes patients with clinical ASCVD (secondary prevention), patients with a 10-year ASCVD risk > 10%, and patients with comorbidities, including diabetes mellitus, chronic kidney disease (including post-kidney transplantation), heart failure, prior stroke, and peripheral arterial disease.

Suspect secondary causes of hypertension (HTN) in patients who develop HTN before 30 years of age, who have drug-resistant HTN, or who develop uncontrolled HTN that was previously well controlled.

Systolic abdominal bruits (without a diastolic bruit) suggest **renal vascular hypertension**. ACE inhibitors and angiotensin receptor blockers (ARBs) are very effective in bringing down the blood pressure in renovascular hypertension but can cause a decline in renal function, especially with bilateral renal artery stenosis (RAS). Large, randomized, controlled trials have shown no benefit of revascularization (angioplasty or stenting) as compared to pharmacologic therapy in atherosclerotic RAS. For this reason, medical therapy is recommended first, and revascularization should be considered if medical therapy fails. If you're considering revascularization, start with noninvasive tests—duplex ultrasonography, CTA (in individuals with normal renal function), and magnetic resonance angiography (MRA). The diagnosis is confirmed by angiography. When clinical suspicion is high and results of noninvasive tests are inconclusive, catheter angiography with intent to revascularize is reasonable.

Think of **primary hyperaldosteronism** in a hypertensive patient with hypokalemia, volume expansion, and low renin.

Think of **pheochromocytoma** in a patient with recurrent and intermittent episodes of severe hypertension frequently accompanied by palpitations, headaches, and severe apprehension.

Much more on hypertension is in Nephrology & Urology, Book 2.

CARDIAC MEDICATIONS

PREVIEW | REVIEW

- True or false? Digoxin prolongs survival.
- Which medication has been shown to prolong survival both post-MI and for patients with heart failure?
- With which medication should a nitrate be paired to improve survival in heart failure patients?

Refer to Table 13-4 on page 13-12 for an overview and comparison of commonly used cardiac medications. Pay particular attention to those that prolong survival! Note the following:

- A **negative inotrope** is a medication that decreases cardiac contractility.
- A **negative chromotrope** is a medication that slows heart rate.

CARDIOLOGY

Table 13-4: Common Cardiac Medications							
Medication	Negative Inotrope	Negative Chrono-trope	Negative Dromo-trope	Vaso-dilator	Anti-anginal	Prolong Survival Post-MI	Prolong Survival in HF	Indications
Digoxin		+	+					Systolic HF, arrhythmias
Metoprolol and bisoprolol	+++	+++	+++		Yes	Yes	Yes	HTN, angina, HF, arrhythmias
Carvedilol	++	+++	+++	Yes	Yes	Yes	Yes	HTN, angina, HF, arrhythmias
Nifedipine	++			Yes	Yes			HTN, angina
Amlodipine	+			Yes	Yes		Yes (in DCM)	HTN, angina, DCM
Diltiazem	++	++	++	Yes	Yes			HTN, angina, arrhythmias
Verapamil	+++	+++	+++	Yes	Yes			HTN, angina, arrhythmias
Nitrates				Yes	Yes		Yes (with hydralazine)	Angina, HF
ACEIs				Yes		Yes	Yes	HTN, HF
ARBs				Yes		Yes	Yes	HTN, HF
Hydralazine				Yes			Yes (with nitrates)	HTN, HF
Spironolactone							Yes	HTN, HF
Eplerenone						Yes (with HF)	Yes (post-MI)	HF (post-MI)

ACEIs = angiotensin-converting enzyme inhibitors; ARBs = angiotensin receptor blockers; DCM = dilated cardiomyopathy; HF = heart failure; MI = myocardial infarction

ANGINA

OVERVIEW

PREVIEW | REVIEW

- What is the most common cause of acute coronary syndrome?
- What is the cause of Prinzmetal angina?
- What does transient ST-segment elevation suggest on an exercise ECG stress test?
- What are causes of resting ST-segment elevation?
- Explain the similarities and differences between hibernating myocardium, reperfusion injury, and stunned myocardium.

Angina is chest pain or discomfort caused by myocardial ischemia. It is typically classified as either stable or unstable:

- **Stable angina**: Chest discomfort occurs predictably and reproducibly—usually with exertion—and remits with rest.
- **Unstable angina**: angina occurring at rest, with new onset, or with increased frequency

Obstructive atherosclerotic coronary artery lesions (supply problem) are the most common cause of stable angina (Figure 13-11). Plaque rupture or erosion with superimposed thrombus is the most common underlying process triggering acute coronary syndrome (ACS).

There are many causes of increased demand (e.g., tachycardia, fever, thyrotoxicosis) and many other causes of a decreased supply (e.g., hypotension, coronary vasospasm, anemia, hypoxia). Coronary blood flow can be impaired in

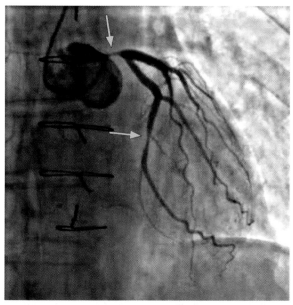

Figure 13-11: Angiogram showing narrowing in coronary artery

severe aortic valve disease with LVH, hypertension, idiopathic dilated cardiomyopathy (DCM), and hypertrophic cardiomyopathy, even in the absence of epicardial CAD.

Note: Only ~ 20% of patients have classic angina at the moment of ischemic ST changes. Silent myocardial ischemia is painless but just as harmful as angina-associated ischemia. Silent ischemia is seen frequently in diabetic patients as well as those with prior ischemic events or prior bypass surgery. Silent ischemia, myocardial infarctions, and thrombotic strokes tend to occur in a circadian pattern, with the highest incidence in the early morning hours.

Distinguishing between stable and unstable angina is key in determining management/diagnostic strategies. Unstable angina is an ACS, along with non-ST-elevation myocardial infarction and ST-elevation myocardial infarction. Long-term risk (death and MI) in patients with ACS is much higher than in patients with stable angina, and therefore patients with ACS warrant emergent medical attention, inpatient management, and, much more commonly, revascularization. (See Acute Coronary Syndrome on page 13-16.) Stable angina, on the other hand, is generally evaluated in the outpatient setting and symptoms are often managed medically.

The most important, easily determinable prognostic factor in patients with CAD is the degree of LV dysfunction. (If severe, it can be a reflection of multivessel or left main/left main–equivalent disease.)

The exercise tolerance test is an excellent, objective way to determine the severity of angina and to determine prognosis. Patients who are able to complete 12 minutes of the Bruce protocol have a nearly 100% 5-year survival, while those who can complete < 3 minutes have only a 50% 5-year survival! Note that coronary angiography is not required for this determination!

> **Coronary spasms** (the cause of **vasospastic** or **Prinzmetal angina**) usually show up as transient ST-segment elevation if they occur during stress testing.
>
> **Cardiac syndrome X** occurs when patients with normal coronary arteries (per cardiac catheterization) have angina and ST depression with cardiac stress testing. This is caused by microvascular dysfunction in the cardiac tissue. It is a diagnosis of exclusion.
>
> What causes resting ST-segment elevation? Acute MI, coronary artery spasm, pericarditis, LV aneurysm, LBBB, ventricular pacing, LVH, and benign early repolarization.
>
> **Hibernating myocardium** is chronically underperfused myocardium. There is no irreversible myocyte injury. When perfusion is restored, contractility may return to normal. Hibernating myocardium can occur with an infarcted region as well, so the degree of viability may determine the extent of myocyte recovery when reperfused.
>
> **Reperfusion injury** occurs when a severely ischemic myocardium is reperfused after ~ 1 hour, causing

further irreversible microvascular damage and damage to the myocardial cells.

Stunned myocardium is the result of acute ischemia. From the time perfusion is restored, it can take 7–10 days for the ventricular function to return to normal.

Treatment of all angina: Modify risk factors and correct aggravating factors such as anemia, hypertension, smoking, drug abuse, and noncompliance. (Good luck!)

ANTIANGINAL DRUGS

PREVIEW | REVIEW

- What are the main drugs used to treat angina?
- Which patients might benefit from ranolazine?
- Which antianginal drugs decrease myocardial oxygen demand?
- Which antianginal drugs decrease afterload?
- Which antianginal drugs decrease preload?
- Which antianginal drug do you avoid in patients with RV infarct? Why?

Beta-blockers and nitrates are the staples of medical treatment of angina, but **calcium channel blockers** can also help. Nifedipine and amlodipine decrease angina by both coronary artery vasodilation and peripheral vasodilation (decreases workload). The main antianginal effect of diltiazem and verapamil is due to their negative chronotropic effect.

ASA (aspirin) decreases mortality and MI occurrence in unstable (and probably stable) angina. Use clopidogrel in patients who cannot tolerate or are allergic to ASA. (Remember to not use ASA in patients with purely vasospastic [a.k.a. Prinzmetal] angina.)

Ranolazine can help patients with persistent angina on maximal standard therapy or as a substitute for beta-blockers. It is thought to work by inhibiting the late Na^+ current in cardiac myocytes, thereby reducing Na^+ and Ca^{2+} overload that follows ischemia. This improves myocardial relaxation and reduces left ventricular diastolic stiffness, which in turn enhances myocardial contractility and perfusion.

More on antianginal drugs:

- Nitrates, beta-blockers, and calcium channel blockers all decrease myocardial O_2 demand, and all decrease afterload.
- Nitrates decrease preload more than afterload and also dilate coronary vessels. Acute preload reduction is why nitrates can cause severe decompensation in patients with an acute right ventricular MI. (Remember, do not give nitrates during acute RV infarct.)
- Nitrates cause sympathetic reflex tachycardia.
- Nitrates are degraded in the liver. Tolerance develops rapidly (tachyphylaxis) but can be avoided by having a

6-hour nitrate-free window once a day (e.g., between midnight and 6 a.m.).

- Beta-blockers decrease myocardial O_2 demand by decreasing HR, BP, and contractility. Beta-blockers complement nitrates well because they decrease the reflex tachycardia.

- Avoid nonselective beta-blockers, such as propranolol, which have been shown to actually prolong the duration of vasospasm in patients with vasospastic angina.

- Calcium antagonists: The combined vasodilatory and antihypertensive effects make them ideal for patients with angina/ischemia and hypertension. See Table 13-4 on page 13-12. Use verapamil and diltiazem cautiously, if at all, in patients with systolic HF due to the negative inotropic effects. Short-acting nifedipine is contraindicated due to steep drops in BP and reflex tachycardia causing an increase in MI.

EVALUATION OF CHRONIC STABLE ANGINA (STABLE ISCHEMIC HEART DISEASE)

PREVIEW | REVIEW

- Why should you determine the probability of CAD in a person with intermittent chest pain?

- What is the most important test for risk stratification in patients with stable ischemic heart disease?

- For which patients with chronic stable angina do you do an echocardiogram? Why?

- A patient undergoing a workup for chronic stable angina is determined to be at high risk for death. What is the next step?

Note

The following is drawn from the 2014 ACC/AHA/AATS/PCNA/SCAI/STS guidelines. First and foremost: Involve and inform your patients. Diagnostic and therapeutic choices should be made through a process of shared decision-making involving the patient and physician, with the physician explaining the risks, benefits, and costs to the patient.

Evaluation of a patient with chest pain is a 3-step process:

1) Determine the probability of CAD.

2) Noninvasive testing for diagnosis and risk stratification

3) Additional workup based on estimated risk

History and Physical Exam — Determine Probability of CAD

First, assess the probability of coronary artery disease. Factors used in the assessment include:

- Type of chest pain (i.e., typical angina, atypical angina, noncardiac chest pain)
- Age
- Gender
- Risk factors (particularly diabetes mellitus [DM], smoking, and HTN)
- ECG abnormalities (Q waves and ST abnormalities)

This step is very important because it determines pretest probability for the rest of the tests, which improves the positive and negative predictive values of these tests.

After other causes of chest pain are ruled out, determine the following:

- Typical vs. atypical vs. noncardiac chest pain. This is determined by assessing quality, location, and duration of the chest pain. Typical angina is provoked by exertion or stress and relieved by rest or nitroglycerin.

- Cardiovascular risk factors: DM, HTN, smoking, hyperlipidemia, family history of CAD, and postmenopausal status in women. Elicit any history of substance abuse: Cocaine accelerates atherosclerosis, enhances platelet aggregation, causes vasospasm, and increases myocardial oxygen demand.

- Comorbid conditions that can precipitate symptoms in the presence of CAD or, when severe, cause angina in the absence of coronary obstruction by:
  - Increasing cardiac demand: hyperthyroidism, cocaine use, severe uncontrolled HTN, significant valvular disease (e.g., aortic stenosis), and HCM
  - Decreasing myocardial oxygen supply: anemia, hypoxemia, and increased blood viscosity

From the above, determine if the patient has high, intermediate, or low probability of CAD. Low probability needs no further testing. Those with intermediate or high probability of CAD should undergo risk stratification with further testing.

Noninvasive Tests for Chronic Stable Angina — Diagnosis and Risk Stratification

ECG: Check first for ST-T wave changes that suggest ischemia, such as T-wave inversions, ST-segment depression, and ST-segment elevation. Also look for signs of prior infarction in the form of Q waves or persistent ST changes. An ECG finding of LVH can alert you to the presence of HTN, which is a strong risk factor for CAD. There are other findings (e.g., RBBB, LBBB, atrial fibrillation, bifascicular block) that can be caused by underlying ischemia, although they are not specific indicators of CAD.

Chest x-ray is recommended if there are signs of HF, valvular disorders, or pericardial disease.

Exercise testing is the most important test in risk stratification. Remember: For those who can exercise, do exercise testing for all with stable angina.

Exercise capacity is one of the stronger indicators of long-term risk. For this reason, it is preferable to perform exercise stress if the patient is able to achieve maximal workload. In addition, exercise can provide a higher physiological stress than pharmacological testing can achieve.

Assess LV systolic function (generally with **echo**) only in patients with prior MI, pathological Q waves, symptoms or signs suggestive of HF, arrhythmias, or heart murmur because it will help guide treatment.

If the test results won't change management (severe comorbid conditions that preclude possibility of revascularization or patient does not want revascularization), further testing is not warranted.

Determination of Further Workup in Chronic Stable Angina

Based on clinical characteristics and stress test results, determine the probability of death or MI and stratify the patient into a high-risk (> 3%/year), intermediate-risk (1–3%/year), or low-risk group (< 1%/year). Refer high-risk patients for coronary angiogram. Patients with low or intermediate risk should be treated with medical therapy to improve symptoms and function, and further workup can be deferred if symptoms can be controlled with medical therapy.

The Duke treadmill score (DTS) uses 3 parameters from the ETT to predict cardiovascular risk: exercise time, magnitude of maximum ST-segment deviation, and occurrence of angina.

TREATMENT OF CHRONIC STABLE ANGINA

PREVIEW | REVIEW

- What is the goal for blood pressure management in a patient with stable ischemic heart disease?

Treatment goals for chronic stable angina include reducing the risk of premature cardiovascular death; preventing complications, including MI and HF; eliminating (or nearly eliminating) symptoms; and improving functional capacity and quality of life.

Medical therapy to prevent MI and death:

- Antiplatelet therapy: aspirin (clopidogrel if ASA is contraindicated)
- High-dose of a high-efficacy statin (e.g., atorvastatin)
- Beta-blockers (if left ventricular ejection fraction [LVEF] < 40% or prior MI)
- ACE inhibitors (if LVEF < 40%, DM, HTN, or CKD)

Medical therapy for relief of symptoms:

- Beta-blockers as initial therapy
- Calcium channel blockers or long-acting nitrates when beta-blockers cannot be used, or in combination with beta-blockers when beta-blockers are not sufficient

- Ranolazine in combination with maximally tolerated beta-blockers

High-risk patients and patients with low or intermediate risk who remain significantly symptomatic despite maximal medical therapy should be referred for coronary angiogram.

Compilation of all recommendations:

- Stepwise strategy smoking cessation (ask, advise, assess, assist, arrange, avoid); avoidance of exposure to environmental tobacco smoke
- Diet: Limit saturated fats to < 7% of total calories, eliminate trans fats, and limit cholesterol intake to < 200 mg/day.
- Physical activity: 30–60 min/day of moderate-intensity aerobic activity for 5–7 days/week
- Weight loss (if BMI > 25 kg/m^2)
- Blood pressure management (goal < 130/80 mmHg per 2017 ACC guidelines): ACEI/ARB first; add thiazide diuretics or calcium channel blockers if needed.
- Influenza vaccine annually
- Statin in all patients (if no contraindications/adverse effects)
- Antiplatelet therapy: aspirin 75–162 mg/day indefinitely; clopidogrel when aspirin is contraindicated
- Beta-blockers: started and continued for 3 years in all patients with normal LV function. Continue indefinitely if LVEF < 40%. Use carvedilol, metoprolol succinate, or bisoprolol in all patients with LVEF < 40%, unless contraindicated.
- ACEIs in all patients who also have hypertension, diabetes mellitus, LVEF < 40%, or CKD, unless contraindicated (use ARB if ACEI intolerant)

CARDIOVASCULAR DISEASE PREVENTION IN WOMEN

PREVIEW | REVIEW

- Would you recommend aspirin in a healthy woman < 65 years of age for primary prevention of MI?

A 2011 update of the AHA guidelines for CVD prevention in women warns that the following should not be used for primary or secondary prevention of cardiovascular disease:

- Hormone therapy
- Antioxidants (e.g., vitamins C and E, beta-carotene)
- Folic acid or vitamin B$_6$
- Garlic, coenzyme Q$_{10}$, selenium, or chromium

Likewise, do not use aspirin in healthy women < 65 years of age for primary prevention of MI. (Aspirin is okay for those ≥ 65 years of age.)

CARDIOLOGY

Other points to remember regarding heart disease in women include:

- Chest pain is the most common angina symptom in both men and women and is described similarly in both.
- Treadmill exercise stress testing has a higher false positive rate in women than in men.
- Women have a lower rate of sudden cardiac death than men at all ages and risk levels.
- Coronary artery disease is more likely to present with chest pain in men than women.

ACUTE CORONARY SYNDROME

CLASSIFICATION OF ACS

PREVIEW | REVIEW

- What are the 2 major categories of ACS?

This is another area from which many exam questions are drawn. Know this well!

Acute coronary syndrome (ACS) is generally caused by atherosclerotic plaque rupture, fissuring, erosion, or a combination with superimposed intracoronary thrombosis. This results in acute ischemia and can lead to myocardial infarction and cardiac death. There are 2 types of acute coronary syndrome:

1) Non-ST-segment elevation ACS

2) ST-segment elevation ACS

Non-ST-elevation ACS includes unstable angina (UA) or non-ST-elevation MI (NSTEMI).

ST-elevation ACS is ST-elevation MI (STEMI).

Rarely, ACS can be due to occlusion by coronary emboli, congenital abnormalities, coronary spasm, and a wide variety of systemic inflammatory diseases.

Patients with NSTEMI have a smaller infarct size and lower risk of early mortality compared to those with STEMI but a higher risk of persistent angina, reinfarction, and death within several months! This is due to the diffuse coronary disease more commonly seen in NSTEMI patients.

So, although patients with NSTEMI have a lower early mortality, they have a higher 6-month mortality compared to patients with STEMI. Also, know that patients with NSTEMI are more likely than those with STEMI to have had a prior MI or angina!

Differential diagnosis of prolonged chest pain includes ACS (MI), aortic dissection, pericarditis, esophageal or biliary tract problems, pneumothorax, pulmonary embolism, pleuritic pain related to pneumonia, musculoskeletal inflammation, and psychogenic causes.

NOTES

PREVIEW | REVIEW

- Name 1 group of patients that is more likely to present with MI without chest pain.

15% of acute myocardial infarctions (AMIs) are asymptomatic.

MI without chest pain or with atypical chest pain is more common in:

- Elderly patients (about 2/3 of silent MI patients are > 75 years of age)
- Diabetics
- Women
- Those with prior CAD

Mitral regurgitation due to papillary muscle dysfunction is seen more commonly with inferior MIs.

Ventricular septal defect (VSD) from septal rupture is seen more commonly with anterior and inferior MIs.

Arrhythmias in the first 48 hours after MI are due to acute ischemia (or are reperfusion-related) and do not imply a need for long-term antiarrhythmic therapy or ICD.

Inferior vs. anterior MI: **Inferior MIs** result in more stable arrhythmias, such as junctional escape and 2nd degree heart block Mobitz 1. **Anterior MIs** result in 2nd degree heart block Mobitz 2, bundle branch blocks (BBBs), and a poorer prognosis. Even when Mobitz 2 or complete heart block is seen in an inferior MI, it is usually temporary. Also, the amount of infarcted myocardium is typically larger with anterior MIs. Unfortunately, septal rupture can occur in either type. (See Complications of Myocardial Infarction on page 13-23.)

MARKERS FOR AMI

PREVIEW | REVIEW

- How are troponin I and T used? How long do they stay elevated after an MI?

Troponins and creatine kinase myocardial bands (CKMBs) are serum markers that increase in response to acute myocardial necrosis. With the better sensitivity of troponin, CKMBs are no longer used for the diagnosis of MI, although they may be used to determine the size of infarction. Since troponin levels will remain elevated for up to 2 weeks, CKMBs may also be useful in estimating timing of the infarction since they will peak at about 1 day and return to baseline in 2–3 days.

Know all of the following!

Assays to detect components of cardiac muscle, troponin I and troponin T (**cTnI** and **cTnT**), are the gold standard for the detection of myocardial necrosis. cTnI and cTnT levels are predictive of both acute MI and cardiac death. The 2 troponin assays are equally useful, and local preferences dictate which is used.

Troponins (**Tns**) first become elevated at 4 hours following an MI and peak at about 44 hours after the event (the "rule of 4s"). They can remain elevated for 10–14 days after an MI. Because they stay elevated so long, troponins are useful even when patients present > 24–48 hours after onset of symptoms.

cTnI or cTnT should be measured at presentation and 3–6 hours after symptom onset in all patients with suspected ACS.

Be aware that troponins can also be elevated in chronic renal failure, myopericarditis, HF, sepsis, pulmonary embolism, and cardiac trauma. In addition, troponins can be elevated with RV strain causing microvascular dysfunction. For this reason, look for the characteristic rise/fall of Tn levels, which is more specific for acute myocardial infarctions (AMIs). Although Tns are sensitive markers for AMI, they are not highly specific; therefore, they are good for excluding AMI but not as good for confirming: sensitive but not specific. In general, the larger the infarct, the higher the troponin level.

Keep in mind that the overall trend is important and gives added information beyond a single elevated value (trending enzymes). An individual whose enzymes continue to rise is a very different patient from someone whose enzymes peaked earlier in the day, even in the absence of symptoms! In the first patient, where the Tn has not yet peaked, you should consider ongoing ischemia or infarction, whereas the second patient has already completed the infarct. This is important for determining the type of further testing and when it should be performed.

TREATMENT OF ACS

PREVIEW | REVIEW

- What are the prehospital guidelines for chest pain?
- What are the major things you should do in early risk stratification of a patient who presents with ACS in the emergency department?

Prehospital Management

Per the 2015 AHA guidelines for emergency cardiovascular care of acute coronary syndromes:

- Call emergency services for transport to hospital by ambulance (rather than friends/relatives).
- Give nonenteric-coated aspirin (ASA; 162–325 mg) as bite and chew × 1.

- Perform ECG.
- If STEMI on ECG, prehospital notification of the receiving hospital (if fibrinolysis is anticipated) or activation of cath lab is appropriate.
- Nitroglycerin (tablets or spray): Administer up to 3 doses at 3–5-minute intervals. Note nitroglycerin is contraindicated in the following situations, due to risk of severe hypotension:
  ◦ Systolic BP < 90 mmHg, or 30 mmHg below baseline
  ◦ RV infarction
  ◦ If the patient has taken a phosphodiesterase-5 inhibitor (e.g., sildenafil, vardenafil) within 24 hours (48 hours for tadalafil)
- Consider morphine in patients with STEMI and chest pain unresponsive to nitrates. (Avoid morphine in unstable angina/NSTEMI—it may increase mortality.)
- Be prepared to recognize and manage ventricular arrhythmias.

Evaluation of Patients with Symptoms Suggestive of ACS

Early evaluation: For patients who present to the emergency department with symptoms suggestive of ACS, immediately (within 10 minutes) get an ECG, draw blood for cardiac markers, give ASA if not contraindicated, and conduct a directed history and physical examination.

High-risk features:

- Ongoing chest pain for > 20 minutes
- Reversible ST-segment changes of ≥ 0.5 mm
- Elevated cardiac enzymes (cTnI or cTnT)
- Signs of LV dysfunction

What happens next depends on the ECG:

- If the ECG is abnormal: Follow guidelines (see below).
- If the ECG is normal or nondiagnostic: Repeat the ECG q 15–30 minutes or do continuous monitoring.

Note: An AMI involving the left circumflex can still present as a nondiagnostic (or normal) 12-lead ECG; consider obtaining V7-9 leads.

Based on this early assessment, assign patients to 1 of the following 3 groups in the ACC/AHA protocol:

1) **Noncardiac** chest pain or chronic stable angina. Treat accordingly. See Treatment of Chronic Stable Angina on page 13-15.

CARDIOLOGY

2) **Possible ACS** with nondiagnostic ECG and normal initial serum markers (Figure 13-12): Observe for ≥ 12 hours following symptom onset. If there is no recurrence of symptoms, a 2nd Tn is negative, and an ECG is unchanged, perform further risk stratification with an appropriate stress test. Patients who have a negative or low-risk stress test can be discharged to home and followed as outpatients (green box in Figure 13-12). If observed patients have recurrent symptoms, subsequent positive Tn, ECG changes, or a positive stress study, admit and manage according to the acute ischemia pathway (Figure 13-13).

3) **Definite ACS**: Immediately determine whether there is ST-segment elevation or new LBBB (Figure 13-14):
- Admit and treat patients without ST-segment elevation or new LBBB according to the acute ischemia protocol (Figure 13-13).
- Consider patients with ST-segment elevation or new LBBB for emergent reperfusion therapy.

We will discuss each of these scenarios shortly, but first let's talk about general measures considered for all patients with ACS.

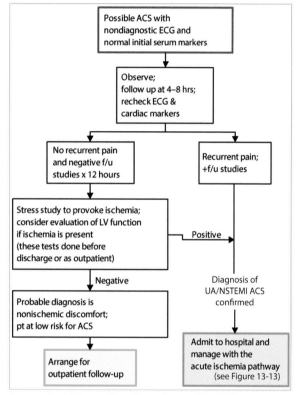

Figure 13-12: Diagnostic pathway for *possible* ACS

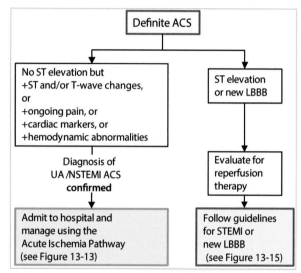

Figure 13-14: Initial Tx pathway for *definite* ACS

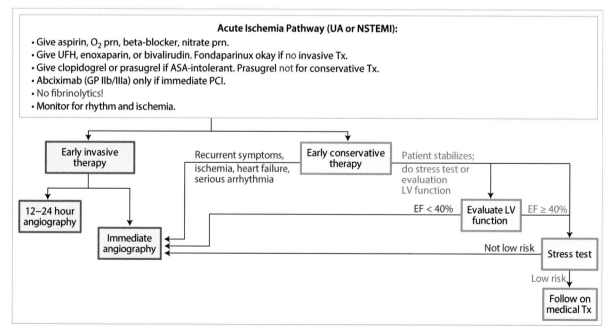

Figure 13-13: Acute ischemia treatment pathway — UA or NSTEMI

ACS — GENERAL MEASURES

PREVIEW | REVIEW

- Which antiischemic measures are done initially for all patients with ACS?

- Which patients should receive a platelet GP IIb/IIIa inhibitor?

- Of those with ACS, which group gets considered for fibrinolytic therapy and which group definitely does not?

ECG, NTG, Morphine, Beta-Blockers, ACEIs, and Atropine

General antiischemic measures for all patients with ACS include:

- Continuous ECG monitoring
- ASA
- Sublingual nitroglycerin (NTG) spray × 3 prn for pain and IV NTG for continued ischemia or hypertension
- Morphine if pain is not relieved by NTG (Note: Never give NSAIDs (except ASA) in ACS; they increase risk of adverse cardiovascular events!)
- Oral beta-blocker and an ACEI if the patient is still hypertensive or has LV dysfunction (EF < 40%)

Administer supplemental **oxygen** to patients with ACS with an arterial saturation < 90%, respiratory distress, or other high-risk features for hypoxemia. (Pulse oximetry is useful for continuous measurement of S_aO_2.)

Note: **Beta-blockers** reduce myocardial O_2 consumption. Also, by blocking the often-excessive sympathetic activity, they reduce the load on the heart and decrease the likelihood of arrhythmias. Oral use is preferred.

Contraindications to beta-blockers include bradycardia, hypotension, 2nd or 3rd degree AV block, pulmonary edema, and asthma. Use caution in giving beta-blockers to patients with signs of acute heart failure. (See Beta-Blockers on page 13-61).

Nondihydropyridine calcium channel blockers (e.g., **verapamil** or **diltiazem**) can be given if beta-blockers are contraindicated and the patient continues to have ischemia and hypertension but no LV dysfunction.

Atropine is indicated for the temporary management of acute sinus bradycardia with signs of low CO while preparing for temporary pacing. Bradycardia seen with (usually inferior) MI can be temporary, and atropine alone may be sufficient.

Anticoagulant / Antiplatelet Therapy in ACS

Overview

Intense antiplatelet and parenteral anticoagulant therapy with multiple agents is a major treatment recommendation for ACS.

There is a high probability of coronary thrombus formation with unstable angina, so always use either IV heparin or subcutaneous low-molecular-weight heparin (LMWH) if there are no contraindications.

According to the 2016 ACC/AHA Guidelines Focused Update on Duration of Dual Antiplatelet Therapy in Patients with Coronary Artery Disease, the following are now recommended concomitantly with heparin and for follow-up medical therapy for unstable angina:

- ASA daily for life
- Clopidogrel or ticagrelor for at least 1 year following MI

Parenteral Anticoagulants

The parenteral anticoagulants are unfractionated heparin (**UFH**), **enoxaparin**, **fondaparinux**, and **bivalirudin**. One of these agents is recommended for most patients with ACS:

- UFH is preferred if coronary artery bypass graft (CABG) is anticipated within 24 hours (or coronary angiography, although this is not as absolute).
- Enoxaparin is commonly used; however, remember to adjust the dose in the patient with renal impairment.
- Fondaparinux can be considered if the patient has increased risk of bleeding, especially if a conservative (noninvasive) strategy is chosen for the patient. It is not used if percutaneous coronary intervention (PCI) is expected (due to increased risk of catheter thrombosis and increased coronary complications).
- Bivalirudin can be used as an alternative to UFH in patients who will undergo catheterization within 4 hours, particularly in patients at high risk of bleeding.

Antiplatelet Therapy

Aspirin

Administer **aspirin** at a dose of 162 or 325 mg immediately to all patients with ACS, and continue daily (indefinitely) unless there are contraindications.

Thienopyridines — Platelet $P2Y_{12}$ Receptor Blockade

Thienopyridines include clopidogrel and prasugrel. Their effect is additive to aspirin. These drugs block the ADP receptor $P2Y_{12}$ on platelets. Ticlopidine is no longer routinely used due to its side effect profile.

The safety of combining proton pump inhibitors (PPIs) and thienopyridines is controversial. Although a 2010 AHA expert consensus statement reported no clear-cut evidence of harm, a 2015 meta-analysis showed an increased risk of cardiovascular events in patients taking PPIs with clopidogrel.

Clopidogrel requires the liver enzyme CYP2C19 to become active. Overall, 16–50% of patients may be clopidogrel-resistant, either due to impaired absorption, drug interactions, or poor CYP enzyme activity. In 2010, clopidogrel received an FDA boxed warning about poor metabolizers and the tests available, but genetic testing is not recommended in any current guidelines.

Prasugrel is a thienopyridine that has a faster onset of action and is effective in clopidogrel-resistant patients. It has significantly more antiplatelet activity and therefore lower cardiovascular events—but also higher rates of significant bleeding and is contraindicated in the elderly, those who weigh < 132 lb (60 kg), and patients with history of previous stroke.

Clopidogrel and prasugrel can be used interchangeably for all proven ACS scenarios except if CABG is imminent (operative bleeding complications).

All patients who undergo PCI with a drug-eluting stent (DES) should be on clopidogrel for 1 year.

Nonthienopyridines — Platelet P2Y$_{12}$ Receptor Blockade

Ticagrelor, a nonthienopyridine, is a reversible oral antagonist of the platelet P2Y$_{12}$ receptor with a rapid onset of action. Like prasugrel, it is more effective than clopidogrel, but without the increased bleeding risk. It can be used as an alternative to clopidogrel/prasugrel. Know that the aspirin maintenance dose in combination with ticagrelor must never exceed 81 mg daily, as higher doses render ticagrelor less effective.

Use dual antiplatelet therapy (aspirin, + agent such as clopidogrel, prasugrel, or ticagrelor) for at least 1 year after receiving a drug-eluting stent (DES) or after MI without revascularization, and ≥ 1 month following a bare-metal stent (BMS), ideally up to a year.

Note: Even if a patient needs surgery, do not stop clopidogrel, prasugrel, or ticagrelor until 6 months after DES placement. Similarly, do not stop these agents until ≥ 30 days after BMS placement. Withholding clopidogrel, prasugrel, or ticagrelor and performing surgery prior to these time frames has an increased risk of death and in-stent thrombosis.

Glycoprotein IIb / IIIa Inhibitors

Glycoprotein (GP) IIb/IIIa inhibitors act on the final common pathway of platelet aggregation—where fibrin binds platelets together by connecting to the GP IIb/IIIa receptor. The most studied drug is **abciximab**. Others are **eptifibatide**, **tirofiban**, and **lamifiban**. Only the IV forms are effective. GP IIb/IIIa inhibitors are considered for high-risk ACS patients (elevated troponin, hemodynamic instability, dynamic ECG changes); however, since introduction of dual oral antiplatelet therapy, they are used less commonly.

Fibrinolytic Therapy in ACS

Do not give fibrinolytic therapy to patients without ST elevation (i.e., those with NSTE-ACS) because it increases mortality. Do give fibrinolytic therapy to those ACS patients with STEMI or new LBBB if immediate PCI is not available and if there are no contraindications (discussed under Fibrinolytic Therapy on page 13-22).

ACS — MANAGEMENT OF NSTE-ACS — THE ACUTE ISCHEMIA PATHWAY

PREVIEW | REVIEW

- Which NSTE-ACS patients should be considered for an early invasive strategy?

Early Invasive vs. Ischemia-Guided Therapy

Note: The 2014 ACC/AHA NSTE-ACS treatment guidelines have 2 areas of focus (Figure 13-13 on page 13-18):

1) Antithrombotic therapy with multiple agents
2) Aggressive use of early percutaneous coronary intervention (cardiac catheterization) in those with moderate-to-high risk

Okay, you have determined the patient is having ACS and have initiated treatment according to the general measures under Treatment of ACS on page 13-17. You've drawn labs and done the ECG, which reveals no acute ST changes. The labs come back, and you determine that the patient has NSTEMI (cTn abnormal) or UA (cTn normal).

You have 2 options:

1) Early invasive therapy (angiography)
2) Ischemia-guided therapy

Early Invasive Therapy in NSTE-ACS

Indications for urgent invasive therapy for NSTE-ACS:

- HF or hemodynamic instability
- Recurrent or refractory angina
- Life-threatening arrhythmias

Indications for invasive therapy for NSTE-ACS within 24–48 hours:

- Elevated cTnI or cTnT
- Dynamic ST changes
- Diabetes
- GFR < 60 mL/min
- EF < 40%
- Recurrent angina
- PCI within the previous 6 months
- Prior MI
- Prior CABG
- Intermediate-/high-risk patients (either by clinical judgment or using a scoring system such as the thrombolysis in myocardial infarction [TIMI] risk score)

Both STEMI and NSTE-ACS patients selected for early invasive therapy get the following medical therapy:

- Parenteral anticoagulant:
  - UFH, enoxaparin, or bivalirudin. Do not give fondaparinux due to increased rate of catheter thrombus formation.
- Antiplatelet therapy:
  - ASA plus either prasugrel, ticagrelor, or clopidogrel (dual therapy). Note: Do not use prasugrel for patients > 75 years of age or those with prior history of stroke/transient ischemic attack (TIA); use clopidogrel in these cases.
  - Ticagrelor or prasugrel are preferred over clopidogrel due to increased efficacy.
  - A GP IIb/IIIa inhibitor can be given if the patient is high risk.

Remember: NSTE-ACS patients do not receive fibrinolytic therapy, as fibrinolytics actually increase mortality in the absence of ST elevation.

Ischemia-Guided Therapy in NSTE-ACS

Patients with NSTE-ACS who respond to intense medical therapy, have none of the indications for invasive therapy above, and do well on post-ACS stress testing are at low risk for immediate and 1-year mortality—and can be followed without invasive evaluation.

Ischemia-guided therapy for NSTE-ACS patients:

- Parenteral anticoagulant:
  - UFH, enoxaparin, or fondaparinux for 48 hours. Fondaparinux is especially useful if there is risk of bleeding.
- Antiplatelet therapy:
  - ASA with either clopidogrel or ticagrelor. Always give dual antiplatelet therapy.
  - Prasugrel or IIb/IIIa inhibitors are not given for conservative therapy.

This is basically the same anticoagulant/antiplatelet treatment as those getting UA/NSTEMI early invasive therapy, except that IIb/IIIa inhibitors and prasugrel are not used and fondaparinux is now a reasonable option.

Long-Term Antiplatelet Therapy after NSTE-ACS

With bare-metal stent:

- ASA 81 mg/day for life
- Clopidogrel or ticagrelor for at least 1 month

With a drug-eluting stent or no stent:

- ASA 81 mg/day for life
- Clopidogrel, prasugrel, or ticagrelor for at least 1 year

ACS — MANAGEMENT WITH STEMI OR NEW LEFT BUNDLE BRANCH BLOCK

PREVIEW | REVIEW

- Which reperfusion therapies are appropriate in patients with STEMI or new LBBB? Who gets what?
- What are the absolute and relative contraindications to fibrinolytic therapy?
- How does management of RV infarction differ from LV infarction?
- Which patients with tachyarrhythmias after an MI get DC cardioversion?
- What are the medical options for hemodynamically stable MI patients with VT?
- What time frame after MI do the major mechanical complications tend to occur? How do they present? What is the best test to diagnose such a complication?
- When should a patient with STEMI be referred for an ICD?

Note

The management of ACS with STEMI is the same as for ACS with a new LBBB; see Figure 13-15. Also know that STEMI includes those with a posterior infarct (ST depression in V1, V2 and tall Rs in V1, V2).

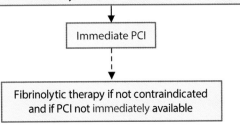

STEMI or new LBBB MI:
- Give aspirin, O_2 prn, beta-blocker, nitrate prn.
- Give UFH, enoxaparin, or bivalirudin.
- Give clopidogrel, prasugrel, or ticagrelor.
- Give abciximab (GP IIb/IIIa) only if immediate PCI.
- Monitor for rhythm and ischemia.

Immediate PCI

Fibrinolytic therapy if not contraindicated and if PCI not immediately available

PCI should be done within 12 hrs of chest pain onset and within 90 min of arrival to emergency department.

Figure 13-15: Acute MI treatment pathway with STEMI or new LBBB

The following are additions to the general measures for all ACS patients discussed above under Treatment of ACS on page 13-17.

STEMI (or new LBBB) patients get the following medical therapy:

- Parenteral anticoagulant:
  - UFH, enoxaparin, or bivalirudin. Give UFH or bivalirudin if going to cath lab.
- Dual antiplatelet therapy:
  - ASA plus clopidogrel, prasugrel, or ticagrelor (in emergency department)
  - IIb/IIIa inhibitors as early as possible when patients are going to the cath lab for PCI

Immediate Reperfusion Therapies

Overview

Consider emergent reperfusion (primary PCI or fibrinolytic therapy) in all patients who present within 12 hours of the onset of symptoms with a STEMI or a new (or presumed-new) LBBB.

Primary PCI

Primary percutaneous coronary intervention (**PCI**) is an urgent reperfusion procedure and usually includes placement of a stent (bare-metal or drug-eluting). BMSs may be used in patients with high bleeding risk, inability to comply with 1 year of dual antiplatelet therapy, or anticipated invasive or surgical procedures in the next year. Remember: no surgery within 1 year of PCI with DES, due to high risk of stent thrombosis.

Primary PCI has been shown to be superior to fibrinolytic therapy when used in patients with STEMI, MI with new LBBB, and new true posterior MI. Outcomes are better than fibrinolytic therapy as long as an experienced practitioner performs the procedure within 12 hours of the onset of symptoms—and within 90 minutes of the arrival of the patient in the emergency department. (Door-to-balloon time is a commonly measured metric for quality of care in STEMI.) Transfer patients with STEMI who present to a hospital without PCI capabilities to a PCI-capable hospital—with a goal of no more than 120 minutes from first medical contact (**FMC**) to stent placement.

Primary PCI is particularly beneficial in patients with highest risk for mortality (e.g., cardiogenic shock) or acute severe heart failure in the setting of a STEMI or new LBBB MI.

In the patient who presents with completed STEMI (beyond 12 hours of the onset of symptoms), coronary angiogram is indicated if the patient continues to have chest pain or is in heart failure, left ventricular ejection fraction (LVEF) is moderately to severely reduced, there is electrical instability (ventricular tachycardia [VT] or ventricular fibrillation [VF]), or post-MI stress test shows significant ischemia.

Fibrinolytic Therapy

When primary PCI cannot be accomplished within 120 minutes of presentation, fibrinolytic therapy should be administered unless otherwise contraindicated.

Many studies show that the sooner the patient receives fibrinolytic therapy, the greater the benefit in reduction of mortality, with the most benefit when treated within the first 4 hours and the greatest when treated within the first hour. Patients with new bundle branch block benefit the most, followed by anterior MI, then inferior MI. Start fibrinolytic therapy within 30 minutes of arrival in the emergency department.

Note: Fibrinolytics are used for patients at facilities that do not have the capabilities for urgent PCI. Following treatment with fibrinolytic therapy, high-risk STEMI patients (recurrent ischemia, cardiogenic shock, severe HF, or other high-risk features) should be transferred to a PCI center to undergo coronary angiography and PCI immediately—without waiting to determine whether reperfusion has occurred.

Fibrinolytic agents include the recombinant, tissue-type plasminogen activators (e.g., rt-PA, TNK), anistreplase, streptokinase, and urokinase.

Contraindications to fibrinolytic therapy can be either absolute or relative.

Absolute contraindications:

- Previous hemorrhagic stroke at any time; other cerebrovascular events within 1 year
- Intracranial neoplasm
- Active internal bleeding
- Suspected aortic dissection

Relative contraindications:

- Persistent BP > 180/110
- Remote nonhemorrhagic CVA (> 1 year)
- Current use of anticoagulants with INR > 2–3; bleeding diathesis
- Recent (2–4 weeks) major trauma or surgical procedure
- Noncompressible vascular puncture
- Previous exposure to streptokinase/anistreplase
- Pregnancy
- Active peptic ulcer

Of the patients with STEMI/new LBBB initially evaluated for fibrinolytic therapy, almost 2/3 do not get fibrinolytic therapy for the reasons listed above. The risk of intracranial hemorrhage increases with age, to as much as 1% in patients > 75 years of age, but age by itself is no longer a contraindication. Many of these patients are still good candidates for primary PCI.

Cocaine and Methamphetamine Users with ST Elevation

Give nitroglycerin, calcium channel blockers, and benzodiazepines (not beta-blockers). Avoid beta-blockers in most of these patients. If ST-segments are elevated and there is no immediate improvement with treatment, proceed with coronary angiogram or fibrinolytics if cath lab is not available. If chest pain resolves with treatment, troponin is not elevated, and there are no ST-segment abnormalities, the patient does not need a stress test.

Additional Treatment Recommendations from the 2013 ACC / AHA STEMI Guidelines

For patients with STEMI:

- Stop all NSAIDs (except ASA), including COX-2s!
- Start an oral beta-blocker within 24 hours for patients who do not have any of the following: signs of HF, evidence of low-output state, increased risk for cardiogenic shock, PR interval > 0.24 seconds, 2nd or 3rd degree heart block, active asthma, or reactive airway disease.
- Do not give fibrinolytic therapy if immediate PCI is anticipated. In addition, there is no role for partial- or low-dose fibrinolytic therapy.
- Give clopidogrel or ticagrelor (no PCI) + ASA (1 year).
- Place patient on a high-dose statin.
- Give ACEIs within 24 hours to all with anterior STEMI, HF, or EF ≤ 40% (unless contraindicated). Use an angiotensin receptor blocker if ACEI intolerant.
- Give an aldosterone antagonist (e.g., spironolactone, eplerenone) to those with no contraindications who are already receiving an ACEI and beta-blocker, have an EF ≤ 40%, and have either symptomatic HF or diabetes mellitus.
- Administer IV nitroglycerin in the first 24 hours for ongoing chest pain or hypertension.
- In patients with diabetes, keep blood sugars < 180 mg/dL using insulin-based regimens while avoiding hypoglycemia.
- Vaccinate for influenza yearly.

Clopidogrel, prasugrel, and/or ticagrelor should be stopped 24 hours before urgent on-pump CABG. Discontinue short-acting intravenous GP IIb/IIIa receptor antagonists (i.e., eptifibatide, tirofiban, abciximab) ≥ 2–4 hours before urgent CABG. Abciximab should be discontinued ≥ 12 hours before urgent CABG.

Complications of Myocardial Infarction

Left Ventricular Dysfunction and Cardiogenic Shock

Left ventricular dysfunction after an MI has a poor prognosis. Historically, patients with cardiogenic shock have had mortality rates of > 85%, but studies from 1999, 2001, and 2008 using PCI or emergent CABG have demonstrated an improvement in these dismal outcomes, with in-hospital mortality rates closer to 50%.

If the CO is low, PCWP high, and RA pressure high, the patient has biventricular failure with cardiogenic shock. Treatment is to give diuretics, preload and afterload reducers, and inotropes. In a typical case, a patient gets nitroprusside, nitroglycerin, milrinone, or dobutamine.

Right Ventricular Infarction Complications

Right ventricular infarction (RVI) frequently accompanies an inferior MI and is almost always due to occlusion of the proximal right coronary artery. Inferior MI complicated by RVI has a significantly worse prognosis than inferior MI alone.

ST-segment elevation in right-sided chest leads (e.g., V3R–V7R) indicates RVI infarction of the right ventricle.

Suspect RVI in all cases of inferior MI, which is typified by the clinical triad of hypotension, clear lung fields, and elevated jugular venous pressure. Kussmaul sign (paradoxical increase in JVP during inspiration) is frequently present.

If you perform right heart catheterization, an elevated RA pressure of ≥ 10 mmHg with low pulmonary capillary wedge pressure (PCWP) and CO are quite specific for right ventricular MI.

Management of RVI is in some ways diametrically opposed to that of LV infarction. Do not give preload-reducing agents such as nitroglycerin and nitrates because CO depends on adequate preload. Treat with IV fluid until the blood pressure returns to normal. This sounds like stressing an already stressed RV—and it is—but there is a net positive effect when BP and, hence, coronary artery blood flow are returned to normal and heart rate is reduced. Inotropic support, typically with dobutamine, may be necessary.

Arrhythmias and Blocks

A variety of tachyarrhythmias can occur with myocardial infarction/ischemia. Remember that any hemodynamically unstable tachyarrhythmia should be cardioverted immediately.

Atrial fibrillation (A-fib) with hemodynamic instability requires emergent treatment with direct current (DC) synchronized cardioversion. If patients do not require cardioversion, control the ventricular rate with beta-blockers, diltiazem, or digoxin.

Treat ventricular fibrillation (VF) and pulseless ventricular tachycardia (VT) with defibrillation (DC unsynchronized cardioversion).

For sustained VT with a pulse accompanied by hemodynamic instability, treat with DC synchronized cardioversion.

CARDIOLOGY

For episodes of sustained VT without hemodynamic instability:

- Amiodarone is the drug of choice. It can be given as a continuous infusion or as boluses every 10–15 minutes. Procainamide is also an option.
- Correct any hypokalemia or hypomagnesemia.
- Routine prophylactic use of lidocaine to prevent VT is no longer recommended.

For patients who develop VT or VF after the first 48 hours, short-term and long-term mortality rates are high. Consider an electrophysiologic study and implantable cardioverter-defibrillator (ICD) placement in these patients.

Note that patients with isolated, premature ventricular contractions or runs of nonsustained (< 30 seconds) VT do not need antiarrhythmic therapy on a routine basis. Beta-blockers are effective for ventricular ectopic activity and preventing arrhythmias.

Bradycardia and AV block are more common with inferior MIs than anterior MIs because of the increased vagal tone and AV nodal ischemia seen with an inferior infarct. Remember: Prognosis is related to the size of the infarct, not the presence of AV block itself. The block is often transient and does not require a permanent pacemaker.

AV block accompanying an anterior MI implies destruction of a large amount of myocardium in the interventricular septum, has a high mortality, and frequently requires permanent pacing if the patient survives.

Indications for temporary pacing at the time of an MI include:

- Symptomatic bradyarrhythmias unresponsive to medical treatment
- Asystole or sinus arrest
- Complete (3rd degree) AV block
- Mobitz Type 2 second-degree AV block

Mechanical Complications after STEMI

Fortunately, the catastrophic complications described below have become much rarer in developed nations due to widespread access to early PCI; however, they do still occur at times, and you must be able to recognize them, as each constitutes a medical emergency. Echocardiography is indicated in any hemodynamically unstable MI patient and is the diagnostic modality of choice for all of these conditions.

- **Papillary muscle rupture**: usually occurs 3–7 days after an inferior MI. The patient rapidly develops shock and acute pulmonary edema. You may (or may not) hear a murmur (classically holosystolic, but sometimes early or midsystolic) at the apex, and it may radiate to the back, sternal border, or axilla. Intensity of this murmur does not correlate with the severity of mitral regurgitation.

Diagnosis is with echo. The treatment is urgent cardiothoracic surgery.

- **Ventricular septal defect** (VSD): Incidence peaks once in the first 24 hours after an anteroseptal MI and again 3–5 days later. Incidence is about 0.3% of MIs (before the reperfusion therapy era, incidence was 1–3%). Again, the patient rapidly develops shock. A holosystolic murmur is heard, loudest at the left sternal border. Confirm the diagnosis by echocardiography. Once again, the mortality rate is very high, and the only treatment is urgent cardiothoracic surgery.
- **Free wall rupture** of the LV: occurs 3–7 days after a large, anterior MI, most frequently in elderly hypertensive women. Sudden syncope is typical. The neck veins are grossly engorged from tamponade; pulsus paradoxus, tachycardia, and hypotension make up the triad. Hemodynamic collapse occurs quickly. There have been a few heroic saves with immediate surgery, but rapid death is the usual outcome.

Diagnose mechanical complications after STEMI with transthoracic echocardiography. Transesophageal echocardiography may be needed in some patients, particularly those suspected to have papillary muscle rupture and/or acute mitral regurgitation. Arterial pressure monitoring with an indwelling arterial line is appropriate in some patients, particularly those requiring mechanical ventilation. Intraaortic balloon counterpulsation is indicated as a bridge to urgent revascularization and/or surgery in patients in cardiogenic shock after STEMI who do not quickly stabilize with pharmacological therapy or in those with a mechanical complication.

Implantable Cardioverter-Defibrillators

Implantable cardioverter-defibrillator (ICD) therapy is indicated before discharge in patients who develop sustained ventricular tachycardia/ventricular fibrillation > 48 hours after STEMI, provided the arrhythmia is not due to transient or reversible ischemia, reinfarction, or metabolic abnormalities.

Studies have shown that ICDs prolong survival in post-MI patients with LVEF < 30–35%, depending on New York Heart Association (NYHA) classification. LVEF is typically reevaluated after 40 days following revascularization to allow stunned or hibernating myocardium to recover. An ICD is particularly indicated if there are baseline episodes of ventricular tachycardia.

CORONARY ARTERY DISEASE

NOTE

The risk factors for coronary artery disease (CAD), recommendations for screening and treatment of hyperlipidemia, and revascularization options will be reviewed here.

RISK FACTORS FOR CAD

PREVIEW | REVIEW

- What are the primary risk factors for CAD?

The primary risk factors for CAD:

- Older age
- Male gender
- Family history of early CAD (i.e., females < 65 years of age, males < 55 years of age)
- Smoking
- Hypertension
- Diabetes mellitus (DM)
- Elevated LDL cholesterol
- Low HDL cholesterol
- Chronic kidney disease

Aerobic exercise and elevated HDL are protective against CAD.

Smoking is an independent risk factor for CAD and multiplies the risk of other CAD risk factors, DM, hyperlipidemia, and hypertension. Smoking cessation should be addressed at every visit for patients with atherosclerosis and those at high risk for atherosclerosis. Benefits of smoking cessation are seen within weeks, and those who abstain for 10 years have returned their risk for CAD to that of nonsmokers. Smokers who quit tobacco use between 25 and 34 years of age add 10 years to their life expectancy. Those who quit smoking between 45 and 54 years of age gain 6 years of life expectancy. Women appear to be more vulnerable to smoking, as the hazard ratio for heart disease in women who smoke is 1.25 compared to men who smoke.

Diabetes is an important independent risk factor for CAD. In fact, diabetes is regarded as an equivalent to having established CAD when performing a risk assessment for ASCVD. All patients with diabetes should be regarded as high risk, meriting high-intensity statin therapy. Diabetes increases the risk of CAD 2.5-fold in both men and women. > 25% of Americans > 65 years of age have diabetes.

In patients with diabetes, as in all individuals at high risk for ASCVD, hypertension should be treated when systolic blood pressure is > 130 mmHg or diastolic blood pressure is > 80 mmHg. Reduction in sodium intake, regular aerobic exercise, and weight loss should be recommended in addition to antihypertensive medications. Patients with congenital heart disease (CHD) and hyperglycemia have worse outcomes than those with normal serum glucose, so patients with CHD and diabetes should be closely monitored for their hyperglycemia.

HYPERLIPIDEMIA SCREENING

PREVIEW | REVIEW

- Which lab tests should general lipid screening include?
- In which situations are LDL receptors down-regulated? Up-regulated?
- Which familial dyslipidemia is the most common? Which lipoproteins are elevated?
- Which lipid test result suggests the need to work up familial hypoalphalipoproteinemia?

Evaluation of Hyperlipidemia

High cholesterol means elevated LDL. High triglycerides mean elevated chylomicrons, elevated VLDL, and/or elevated IDL. Low HDL is a predictor of CAD. Therefore, general cholesterol screening uses the fasting lipid panel (FLP) that includes total cholesterol, LDL, HDL, and triglycerides. LDL is calculated and is the value you care about most (see LDL on page 13-26).

Review of Lipoproteins

Chylomicrons

Lipoprotein review: Follow along in Figure 13-16 on page 13-26.

All **lipoproteins** are particles with a hydrophobic core (triglycerides and/or cholesterol), surrounded by a hydrophilic phospholipid outer layer that facilitates transport through the serum. Apolipoproteins (a.k.a. apos) are embedded and bind enzymes or receptors. **Chylomicrons** (with apos B48, CII, and E) are large globules that consist of mostly triglycerides but some cholesterol and are formed in the intestinal epithelium from dietary fats. The apo B48 on their surface is unique to chylomicrons. Chylomicrons enter the circulation by way of the intestinal lymph ducts. In the circulation, chylomicrons attach to peripheral binding sites in muscles and fat, where the CII apolipoproteins on the surface of the chylomicrons activate lipoprotein lipase (LPL).

The activated LPL removes the triglycerides from the inside of the chylomicrons by breaking down the triglycerides into free fatty acids (FFAs), which are either utilized or stored. The shrunken remnant, now high in cholesterol relative to triglycerides, is called (appropriately enough) a chylomicron remnant. It is taken up by the liver via the liver receptors specific for apo E. The liver degrades the remnants, and the cholesterol goes either into bile or on to further synthesis reactions.

To review: The apo B48 is a chylomicron marker; apo CII activates the LPL to suck out the triglycerides; and the apo E is a marker recognized by the liver. If there is a deficiency of either apo CII or LPL, the patient has hyperchylomicronemia and markedly elevated triglycerides, which can cause acute pancreatitis and eruptive xanthomas.

CARDIOLOGY

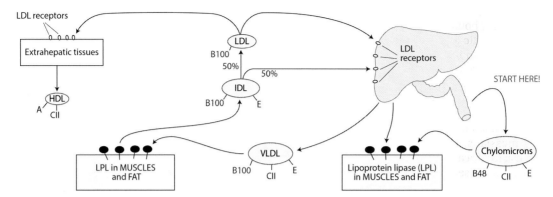

Figure 13-16: Lipoprotein pathways

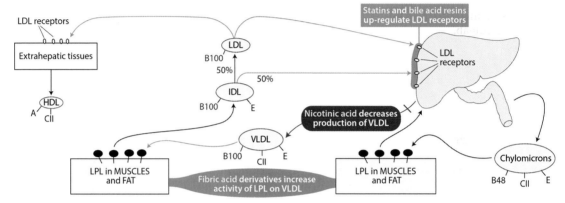

Figure 13-17: Effect of drugs on the lipoprotein pathways

VLDL

Very low-density lipoprotein (**VLDL**; with apos B100, CII, and E) is synthesized by the liver to supply energy to the body. All subsequent lipoproteins except HDL have apo B100. VLDL is similar to chylomicrons, except that it is smaller and contains less triglyceride and more cholesterol. VLDL function is analogous to chylomicrons in that VLDL transports triglycerides to the capillaries of the muscle and fat and is metabolized by the peripheral LPL (activated by CII).

IDL

Following its excretion from the liver and catalyzation by LPL, VLDL forms a remnant called **intermediate-density lipoproteins** (**IDLs**). These still have the triglycerides and some cholesterol. 50% of IDLs are identified and consumed by the liver via the LDL receptor, which recognizes apo E and apo B100. The other 50% remain in the plasma, where they lose the rest of the triglycerides and all of the apolipoproteins, except B100, and thereby are converted to low-density lipoprotein (LDL). If there is a deficiency of apo E, patients have a high IDL.

LDL

LDL is formed from IDL. LDL (cholesterol only; apo B100 only) provides cholesterol for the synthesis of hormones, cell membranes, and bile acids. The only apolipoprotein on LDL you need to remember is apo B100!

LDL is either taken up by a specific LDL receptor (2/3) or scavenged (1/3)—usually by monocytes or smooth muscle cells. The LDL receptor is present on all cells, but it is much denser in the liver (80%). This receptor binds lipoproteins with apos E and B100. Affinity is greater for those with both apo E and apo B100, which is why there is no accumulation of IDL in a healthy person.

LDL receptors are down-regulated or decreased:

• When dietary cholesterol or saturated fats are high
• With age (increasing cholesterol with age)
• In patients with familial hypercholesterolemia (heterozygotes = 50%, homozygotes = 0)

LDL receptors are up-regulated or increased by:

• Dietary cholesterol or saturated fats
• Estrogen
• Thyroxine
• Statins (HMG-CoA reductase inhibitors)
• Decreased bile acid uptake from the intestines (as with bile acid resins)

Lipoprotein(a) [**Lp(a)**] contains apolipoprotein(a) [apo(a)], which is covalently bound by a disulfide bond to the apo B100 of LDL. Genetic and epidemiologic studies have identified Lp(a) as an independent risk factor for coronary heart disease and stroke. Its exact mechanism is still unknown; however, because of the high homology of apo(a) and plasminogen, it has been hypothesized that Lp(a) is prothrombotic. Lp(a) levels are genetically inherited and are 2× higher in African Americans than in Caucasians, although they may not cause increased risk in African Americans. Nicotinic acid and mipomersen, an antisense oligonucleotide to apo B100, can decrease Lp(a). Nicotinic acid decreases Lp(a) only in those patients with concomitant hypertriglyceridemia. Mipomersen, however, decreases Lp(a) levels by 21–27% in patients with familial hypercholesterolemia and severe hypercholesterolemia. The new PCSK9 inhibitors (i.e., alirocumab, evolocumab, both FDA approved in 2015) also reduce Lp(a).

Small LDL particle size carries an increased risk of CAD and endothelial dysfunction. The smaller particles are more easily oxidized, bind arterial wall proteoglycans with more affinity, and bind the LDL receptor with less affinity, thereby reducing their clearance from the blood stream. These mechanisms contribute to their proatherogenic nature. Also, the presence of small, dense LDL particles seems to parallel a state of decreased high-density lipoprotein (HDL).

HDL

HDL is mainly composed of protein and phospholipids, with very little cholesterol or triglycerides. It scavenges the unesterified cholesterol from cell breakdown. HDL contains mainly apo AI and AII but also apo C.

Apo AI (expressed by the *apo AI* gene) helps esterify the scavenged cholesterol. Then, it is transferred to IDL or LDL and removed via the liver. In this way, the HDL is a sort of reverse transport system. Do not confuse apo AI in HDL with apo(a) in Lp(a)—they are completely different lipoproteins.

ABCA1 is a transmembrane protein expressed by the *ABCA1* gene that helps to move cholesterol from inside the cell to the cell membrane. ABCA1 is expressed when cholesterol loads onto the cell surface and is removed when the apolipoproteins pick up the cholesterol.

Problems arise in HDL levels when something goes wrong with apo AI or *ABCA1* (protein or gene). Low HDL is common in cases of premature CAD and is usually either isolated or occurs in combination with elevated triglycerides (TGs). Low HDL occurs because of low levels of apo AI (termed hypoalphalipoproteinemia) and happens because the synthesis of apo A is reduced or its breakdown is increased. (There are diseases associated with these, but you do not need to know them.)

When the HDL level is low, the apo CII level lowers because HDL also acts as a reservoir for apo CII. Because CII activates LPL, there is decreased processing of VLDL and chylomicrons by LPL in the muscle and fat. The end result can be hypertriglyceridemia—as in familial hypertriglyceridemia.

Hereditary Dyslipidemias

Overview

Dyslipidemias can be classified as familial/primary or acquired/secondary (due to DM2, hypothyroidism, and nephrotic syndrome). Of the familial dyslipidemias, known monogenic causes include mutations in the LDL receptor, the PCSK9 enzyme, and the microsomal triglyceride transfer protein (MTTP). It is important to know that the majority of cases of dyslipidemia seen in an internist's clinic are polygenic in origin, which may contribute to the variable response rates to different lipid-lowering therapies. However, regardless of the genetic etiology of a particular dyslipidemia, clinical management is primarily determined based on clinical history, family history, CV risk assessment, and, most importantly, serum LDL-C.

Many cases of premature CAD are related to a familial dyslipidemia. Start screening for lipid disorders at 20 years of age using the basic fasting lipid panel (FLP). Some experts look for the less common familial dyslipidemias by measuring apo B100, apo AI, and Lp(a) when they observe CAD in a patient with a normal lipid profile or if there is a strong family history of CAD and/or ischemic events.

LDL-Associated Dyslipidemias

Familial combined hyperlipidemia (FCHL) is the most common dyslipidemia. 1% of the population is autosomal dominant for FCHL, and up to 10% of those with premature CAD have FCHL. It is the most common cause of lactescent (milky) plasma. FCHL has an extremely variable presentation, with varying elevations of LDL and VLDL. In FCHL, there is increased production of both apo B100 and VLDL, and the increased VLDL stresses the pathways toward increased LDL production. The LDL levels in FCHL are usually less than those in familial hypercholesterolemia (< 230 mg/dL [5.96 mmol/L]).

Familial hypercholesterolemia (FH) presents as premature atherosclerosis and tendon xanthomas on physical exam. Homozygous FH (1:1,000,000 incidence) is uncommon, and patients present with an extremely high LDL (usually > 400 mg/dL [10.36 mmol/L]). Homozygous FH patients have no functional LDL receptors, so they are typically unresponsive to statins. Heterozygous FH is more common, with an incidence of 1:500. Heterozygous FH patients have baseline LDL-C levels > 200 mg/dL (5.18 mmol/L) and have variable response to statins.

Diagnosis is suggested by family history of premature CAD, tendon xanthomas, elevated LDL levels, and an LDL:apo B ratio < 1.2 (vs. > 1.4 normally).

Familial defective apolipoprotein B100 is an autosomal dominant genetic disorder that causes a problem on the LDL particle at the apo B100 ligand. Like heterozygous

CARDIOLOGY

FH, LDL levels are 2–2.5× higher than normal. Distinguish these 2 disorders using genetic testing.

Hyperapobetalipoproteinemia is also caused by excess production of apo B, but LDL levels are normal. Suspect this in patients with premature CAD, especially if they have prominent xanthelasma (yellowish deposits under the skin, often around the eyelids). Labs show a normal LDL but increased apo B with LDL:apo B < 1.2.

Polygenic hypercholesterolemia is another cause of premature CAD that clusters in families. LDL is increased, but the genetic specifics are unclear.

Other Dyslipidemias

Familial hypertriglyceridemia contrasts with FCHL in that the apo B and VLDL numbers are normal but VLDL size is larger and less dense. Like FCHL, it is an autosomal dominant inheritance!

Dysbetalipoproteinemia is autosomal recessive and presents with a high IDL, meaning elevated TGs and cholesterol. The IDL has an abnormal apo E, which interferes with the attachment of IDL on the LDL receptor in the liver. The patient must be homozygous (E2/E2) for the defect—plus have DM, be obese, or have an alcohol problem to have significantly elevated IDL levels.

HDL-Associated Dyslipidemias

Familial hypoalphalipoproteinemia is autosomal dominant and results from a mutation in the gene for apo AI (*APOA1*) or for the genes *ABCA1* or *LCAT*. It results in an isolated low HDL. Data shows that the condition is seen in 6% of Japanese patients who have low HDL.

Familial HDL deficiency is also autosomal dominant and is caused by mutations in the gene encoding *ABCA1*. Theoretically, the altered intracellular transport of cholesterol that occurs with an *ABCA1* mutation increases catabolism of apo AI. It results in an isolated low HDL with premature CAD.

Tangier disease is also due to an *ABCA1* mutation leading to increased catabolism of apo AI. Patients heterozygous for the mutation have low HDL (50% of normal), and homozygous patients have no HDL. This leads to very defective cholesterol handling and diffuse deposition of foam cells, causing hepatosplenomegaly, neuropathy, and premature CAD.

TREATMENT OF HYPERLIPIDEMIA

PREVIEW | REVIEW

- What is the primary endpoint of lipid screening done for primary prevention of ASCVD?
- Per ACC/AHA ASCVD guidelines, name the 4 statin benefit groups.
- How is a high-intensity statin defined? A moderate-intensity statin?
- Which fats are the "good" fats? The "bad" fats?
- Which class of drugs is recommended 1st line to reduce LDL?
- What are the major side effects of statins?
- What are side effects of bile resins?
- What is the main action of the fibrate drugs?
- What are relative contraindications to niacin?
- Which lifestyle activities increase HDL? Lower HDL?

Overview

The treatment goal for hyperlipidemia can be:

- **Primary** prevention of atherosclerotic cardiovascular disease (ASCVD; e.g., MI, ischemic stroke) in patients without known clinical ASCVD
- **Secondary** prevention of recurrent cardiovascular events in patients with known ASCVD

Dozens of randomized trials, summarized in a 2016 meta-analysis, have confirmed the benefit of treating dyslipidemia for primary prevention of ASCVD.

Our discussion of lipids is based on the 2013 ACC/AHA guidelines, 2015 National Lipid Association recommendations, 2016 ACC guidelines on nonstatin therapy, and the current body of literature.

General Concepts of Primary Prevention

Start screening with a fasting lipid panel at 20 years of age, with follow-up in 5 years if normal or yearly if borderline and < 2 CAD risk factors. If abnormal, start treatment and follow up in 4–6 weeks.

The primary screening endpoint is LDL. LDL is usually a derived value:

$$LDL = \text{total cholesterol} - HDL - VLDL$$

$$= \text{total cholesterol} - HDL - \text{triglycerides}/5$$

Note: This calculation is valid only if triglycerides < 400 mg/dL [4.52 mmol/L]. If triglycerides are > 400 mg/dL [4.52 mmol/L], measure LDL directly.

LDL is the most important measure for determining if there is a need for treatment and assessing response to therapy. Non-HDL cholesterol is a secondary target in patients with hypertriglyceridemia > 200 mg/dL (2.26 mmol/L):

$$\text{Non-HDL} = \text{Total cholesterol} - HDL$$

The non-HDL result is theoretically equivalent to the sum of the remaining atherogenic lipoproteins: LDL + Lp(a) + IDL + VLDL, and may do a better job of predicting plaque formation than LDL alone in those patients with elevated LDL and triglycerides.

After obtaining the FLP, identify the patient's risk category using the ASCVD risk estimator (see next topic).

2013 ACC / AHA Clinical Practice Guidelines on Blood Cholesterol to Reduce ASCVD Risk in Adults

Recommendations from these guidelines:

* Encourage therapeutic lifestyle changes in all patients.
* Estimate 10-year risk using the ASCVD Risk Estimator (available at tools.acc.org/ascvd-risk-estimator-plus) to guide decisions on use of statins for primary prevention.
* There are 4 groups for whom there is strong evidence a statin should be initiated or continued:

  1) Clinical ASCVD—treat with a high-intensity statin (see below).
  2) LDL > 190 mg/dL (4.92 mmol/L), including those with familial hypercholesterolemia—treat with a high-intensity statin.
  3) Patients with diabetes 40–75 years of age with LDL of 70–189 mg/dL (1.81–4.90 mmol/L)—treat with a moderate- or high-intensity statin.
  4) Those with LDL of 70–189 mg/dL (1.81–4.90 mmol/L) and a 10-year risk of cardiovascular disease > 7.5%—treat with a moderate- or high-intensity statin.
* Statin intensity is defined as:

  ◦ High-intensity statin therapy (e.g., atorvastatin 40–80 mg/day, rosuvastatin 20 mg/day) lowers LDL-C by approximately 50%.
  ◦ Moderate-intensity statin therapy (e.g., atorvastatin 10–20 mg/day, simvastatin 20–40 mg/day) lowers LDL-C by 30–50%.
  ◦ Low-intensity statin therapy (e.g., simvastatin 10 mg/day, pravastatin 10–20 mg/day) lowers LDL-C by < 30%.
* No recommendation was made for the initiation or continuation of statin therapy in patients with NYHA Class II–IV heart failure and patients receiving maintenance hemodialysis (insufficient data).
* Groups at high risk for adverse effects include age > 75, renal/hepatic dysfunction, unexplained ALT elevation (> 3× the upper limit of normal), and previous statin intolerance or muscle disorders.

Note: For those with LDL of 70–189 mg/dL (1.81–4.90 mmol/L) and a 10-year ASCVD risk of 5–7.5%, the guideline gives a weaker recommendation: It is reasonable to consider moderate-intensity statin.

Dietary Therapy

Diet is always the 1st line of treatment for the hyperlipidemias. Total fat consumption should be < 30% of daily calories. More specifically, saturated fat should be < 7% of daily calories and cholesterol < 200 mg a day for patients with ASCVD and < 300 mg daily for others.

Regarding types of fats:

* Hydrogenated (trans fat) vegetable oils (e.g., margarines) not only raise LDL but also lower HDL—doubly bad!
* Decreasing dietary saturated fats increases LDL receptors and so decreases LDL, but HDL also decreases—not good!
* Similarly, changing to a diet high in polyunsaturated fats decreases LDL and VLDL as well as HDL. In all of these cases, the LDL:HDL ratio is the same or increased—not good!
* On the other hand, monounsaturated fats (e.g., olive/peanut/canola oils) decrease LDL but not HDL—good!
* Omega-3 fatty acids decrease only VLDL (triglycerides)—pretty good.
* Table 13-5 summarizes this information.

Drugs for Dyslipidemias

Statins are 1st line drugs for LDL reduction and decrease both cardiovascular events and cardiovascular mortality by about 25% and overall mortality by 15%. Niacin decreases cardiac events but has inconsistent effects on mortality. Gemfibrozil and cholestyramine decrease cardiac endpoints but not overall mortality. See Figure 13-17 on page 13-26 and Table 13-6 on page 13-31.

HMG-CoA reductase inhibitors are the **statins**: lovastatin, pravastatin, simvastatin, fluvastatin, atorvastatin, pitavastatin, and rosuvastatin. These are the primary cholesterol-lowering drugs. HMG-CoA reductase is the enzyme in the rate-limiting step of lipid metabolism. Statins inhibit this enzyme and, thereby, up-regulate the LDL receptors—as do the bile acids.

Statins decrease LDL and may decrease VLDL. There are only modest gains in HDL with statins. As mentioned, put all persons with established ASCVD on a statin long-term, if they can tolerate it.

Statins may cause myalgias, an elevated CPK, and, rarely, rhabdomyolysis. Check liver transaminases if the patient develops nausea, abdominal pain, or other signs/

Table 13-5: Dietary Therapy and Cholesterol				
Diet Modification	LDL	HDL	LDL:HDL	Verdict
Change to hydrogenated vegetable oils (trans)	Increase	Decrease	Increase	Doubly bad!
Decrease saturated fats	Decrease	Decrease	Same or increase	Neutral to bad
Change to polyunsaturated fats	Decrease	Decrease	Same or increase	Bad
Change to monounsaturated fats	Decrease	May increase	Decrease	Good!

symptoms of hepatotoxicity. There is no indication for checking liver function tests as a baseline test.

The risk of myopathy with statins increases significantly when used in combination with cyclosporine, gemfibrozil (but not as much with fenofibrate!), erythromycin, and ketoconazole.

Statins can cause mild hyperglycemia. Statins may cause memory loss and confusion in some people. The FDA added blood sugar and cognitive changes to the warnings in 2012. Both are generally reversible after stopping the drug.

Inhibitor of intestinal cholesterol absorption (ezetimibe): 2nd line LDL-lowering drug (after statins). Ezetimibe is used as adjuvant therapy in combination with statins or as monotherapy in patients who cannot take statins. It is approved for use alone or in combination with a statin or fenofibrate to reduce LDL and apo B in patients with primary or mixed hyperlipidemias. It is also approved for use with atorvastatin or simvastatin to reduce LDL in patients with familial homozygous hypercholesterolemia. Alone, ezetimibe can reduce LDL by up to 17%; in combination with a statin, it provides a further 14% reduction in LDL over the effect of the statin. Avoid using ezetimibe with gemfibrozil. Moderate or severe hepatic impairment is a contraindication.

The IMPROVE-IT trial, published in 2015, is the first study done to directly assess clinical outcomes in ezetimibe + simvastatin vs. simvastatin alone. After 7 years, the combination of ezetimibe and simvastatin had a very small decrease in the primary outcome of cardiovascular disease (2% absolute risk reduction) compared to simvastatin alone.

Bile acid resins (cholestyramine, colestipol, and colesevelam) are also 2nd line LDL-lowering drugs. Similar to ezetimibe, bile acid resins are used primarily as adjuvant therapy in combination with statins or monotherapy in patients who cannot take statins. Resins decrease LDL, slightly increase HDL, and may increase triglycerides. By binding bile acids in the intestine, and thereby preventing their reabsorption, they cause up-regulation of the LDL receptors in the liver, which increases the processing of serum LDL needed to synthesize replacement bile acids. Although the HDL level remains the same, the LDL:HDL ratio decreases.

Bile acid resins may also increase the synthesis of VLDL, potentially increasing triglycerides. Side effects of these resins are nausea, vomiting, constipation, and bloating. The resins impair absorption of other oral drugs, so patients should take other medicines at least 1 hour before or 4 hours after the resins.

Fibric acid derivatives (mainly gemfibrozil and fenofibrate) are used primarily to treat hypertriglyceridemia. These drugs decrease VLDL and raise HDL. Their main mechanism of action is increasing the activity of LPL on VLDL—thus increasing its rate of conversion to IDL. Some of this IDL is then converted to LDL, occasionally causing an increase in LDL. They also increase production of apo

AI and AII, which increases HDL and increases excretion of cholesterol into the bile.

Fenofibrate appears to have more efficacy than gemfibrozil in lowering LDL. Unlike gemfibrozil, it does not inhibit statin breakdown (thus does not increase risk for statin myopathy). Fenofibrate is the drug of choice when combining a fibrate with a statin.

The 2010 ACCORD trial included diabetic patients who were treated with a statin vs. statin + fibrate to determine if the addition of the fibric acid derivative reduced rates of nonfatal MI, stroke, or cardiovascular death. The end result: The addition did not change these endpoints. So, high-risk patients should generally be treated using a statin only.

Nicotinic acid (a.k.a. niacin) is great if the patient can tolerate it. It is by far the least expensive agent of those listed. It lowers triglycerides and cholesterol (LDL) and increases HDL. It is the most effective drug available for raising HDL (up to 30%). It lowers triglycerides by blocking the production of VLDL (and therefore LDL). Initially, give nicotinic acid 100 mg tid, then raise it 100 mg tid each week to the full dose of 1–2 gm tid. Important metabolic side effects include hyperuricemia and insulin resistance; gout and diabetes mellitus are relative contraindications. Annoying side effects include flushing (especially), dry skin, and nausea/abdominal pain. Give 325 mg ASA 30 minutes before the dose to block the flushing reaction. This reaction usually disappears after 1–2 weeks. Niacin has been shown to reduce cardiovascular events, but the data is not as strong as the data for statins. The AIM-HIGH trial, which concluded in 2011, failed to show a clinical benefit of adding niacin to statin therapy even though lipid levels improved.

The omega-3 fatty acids (eicosapentaenoic acid and docosahexaenoic acid) in moderate doses appear to decrease mortality and sudden cardiac death in patients with known ASCVD. High doses decrease platelet and neutrophil aggregation, decrease BP, and decrease triglycerides (VLDL) but increase LDL. Very high doses may decrease restenosis rate after coronary angioplasty. Generally, if a patient has ASCVD, adding fatty fish (e.g., salmon, mackerel, herring, sardines, albacore tuna) to the diet 2×/week or a daily fish oil supplement is recommended.

Proprotein convertase subtilisin/kexin Type 9 (PCSK9) inhibitors (alirocumab and evolocumab) are monoclonal antibodies approved by the FDA in 2015 for the treatment of elevated LDL. PCSK9 is a serine protease produced predominantly in the liver that leads to the degradation of hepatocyte LDL receptors and increased LDL-C levels. Early studies support huge efficacy in LDL-lowering, safety, and possible cardiovascular mortality and morbidity benefits. A large clinical trial (FOURIER) combining a PCSK9 inhibitor and optimal statin therapy was stopped early when the addition of the PCSK9 therapy showed significant benefit. The 2016 ACC Expert Consensus document suggests that patients with ASCVD who do not achieve > 50% reduction in LDL on high-intensity statin may consider a PCSK9 drug.

Summary (see Table 13-6):

- Statins block HMG-CoA reductase. Ezetimibe inhibits intestinal cholesterol absorption. Nicotinic acid decreases triglycerides by blocking synthesis of VLDL. Fibrates increase LPL action on VLDL.
- Statins and nicotinic acid are the only drugs that both decrease LDL and increase HDL.
- Ezetimibe is used in conjunction with either a statin or fenofibrate to reduce LDL and/or apo B.
- Both fibric acid derivatives (e.g., gemfibrozil, fenofibrate) and nicotinic acid decrease triglycerides; but, whereas nicotinic acid also decreases LDL (good), gemfibrozil may increase the levels of LDL (bad). Fenofibrate increases LDL less than gemfibrozil.
- Combining gemfibrozil with statins significantly increases the risk of myositis. Use fenofibrate if you need to combine with a statin.
- What increases HDL? Nicotinic acid, fibrates, statins, omega-3 fatty acids, moderate alcohol intake, exercise, smoking cessation, losing weight if obese, and reducing intake of trans fats.
- What lowers HDL? Beta-blockers (except labetalol), smoking, weight gain, and eating a diet high in hydrogenated (trans) fats or polyunsaturated fats.
- What has no effect on HDL? Bile resins. Monounsaturated fats (peanut, olive, and canola oils) have no effect or may raise HDL only slightly.

LIPIDS IN ACUTE CORONARY SYNDROME

PREVIEW | REVIEW

- What happens to the lipid panel in ACS?

Statins do more to reduce CAD mortality than just reducing LDL. They stabilize plaques, reduce inflammation and thrombogenicity, and reverse endothelial dysfunction.

Give all patients with acute coronary syndrome (ACS) a high-dose statin no matter what the LDL measures. (You can also consider adding ezetimibe to the statin based on the IMPROVE-IT trial, but statins are always indicated). If the patient is already taking a statin, increase the dose for the acute event. Continuing the statin during an ACS hospitalization results in an improved outcome. Some experts specifically recommend atorvastatin based on data that high-dose atorvastatin decreases mortality during ACS, but other experts believe the benefit is a drug-class effect. High-dose statin regimens have more side effects (especially myalgias) than low-/moderate-dose regimens.

Remember: A recent MI or any serious illness may affect the lipid panel. These effects include decreasing LDL and HDL levels and raising or lowering triglyceride levels. So do not use the FLP drawn at admission for ACS to determine how to treat the patient. Start the statin at a high dose. Redraw the FLP 8 weeks later for a better idea of the patient's true lipid profile.

GOAL LEVELS OF LDL IN PATIENTS WITH CAD

Know all of the following:

Give all patients with CAD long-term statin therapy for secondary prevention, even if their LDL is in the normal range. Prescribe high-intensity statin for these patients, atorvastatin 40 or 80 mg, or rosuvastatin 20 or 40 mg. High-intensity statin is expected to reduce serum LDL by 50%.

The target LDL is not well-defined, but the trend is to treat to an LDL < 70 mg/dL (1.81 mmol/L) for CAD patients with comorbidities or < 100 mg/dL (2.59 mmol/L) for those without comorbidities per 2016 ACC Consensus.

Experts caution, however, that if a patient with CAD is unable to achieve an LDL < 70 mg/dL (1.81 mmol/L) with statin therapy, there is no evidence to support adding a 2nd drug. As always, you must weigh the risk vs. the benefit of an additional medication. Intensively treated patients can experience side effects that outweigh the benefit of further LDL reduction.

Reevaluate the lipids after initiating treatment to reduce LDL, and then consider interventions to reduce non-HDL and/or raise HDL.

Table 13-6: Uses of Currently Available Lipid Drugs			
Drug Class	**Most Common Drugs**	**Use**	**Side Effects**
HMG-CoA reductase inhibitors (statins)	Atorvastatin, rosuvastatin	Drug of choice for LDL reduction	Myalgias, myositis, elevated transaminases
Cholesterol uptake inhibitors	Ezetimibe	Alternative drug for LDL reduction	Elevated transaminases
Bile resins	Cholestyramine, colesevelam, colestipol	Alternative drug for LDL reduction	N/V, constipation, bloating
PCSK9 inhibitors	Evolocumab	Alternative drug for LDL reduction	Injection site irritation
Fibric acid derivatives	Gemfibrozil, fenofibrate	Drug of choice for triglyceride reduction	Possible: abdominal pain, gall bladder disease, malignancy
Nicotinic acid		Alternative drug for LDL and triglyceride reduction	Flushing, dry skin, N/V/abdominal pain

CARDIOLOGY

REVASCULARIZATION

PREVIEW | REVIEW

- Which patient groups definitely should get CABG?

- Which patient groups could get either PCI or CABG?

- In 3-vessel disease, what is the benefit of CABG—survival, symptoms, or both?

- Why is dual antiplatelet therapy so important after stent placement?

Overview

The revascularization options for coronary artery disease are:

- Coronary artery bypass graft (CABG)
- Percutaneous coronary intervention (PCI) with either stents or angioplasty

CABG vs. PCI

The following recommendations are based on the 2012 ACC/AHA Guidelines for the Diagnosis and Management of Patients with Stable Ischemic Heart Disease and the 2014 ACC/AHA Focused Update. For patients with stable ischemic heart disease, revascularization (PCI or CABG) should be performed when there are unacceptable angina symptoms despite maximal medical therapy, or when there is a survival benefit based on anatomy of coronary disease (location, severity, and number of diseased vessels), or presence of LV dysfunction:

- CABG is recommended to improve survival for all patients with significant left main CAD (> 50% diameter stenosis) and in patients with significant (> 70% diameter) stenoses in 3 major coronary arteries or in the proximal LAD artery plus 1 other major coronary artery (e.g., proximal circumflex).
- CABG is reasonable to improve survival in patients with significant (> 70% diameter) stenoses in 2 major coronary arteries with severe or extensive myocardial ischemia (i.e., high-risk criteria on stress testing, abnormal intracoronary hemodynamic evaluation, or > 20% perfusion defect by myocardial perfusion stress imaging) or target vessels supplying a large area of viable myocardium.
- CABG is reasonable to improve survival in patients with mild-to-moderate left ventricle systolic dysfunction (LVEF 35–50%) and significant (> 70% diameter stenosis) multivessel CAD or proximal LAD coronary artery stenosis, when viable myocardium is present in the region of intended revascularization.
- CABG is recommended in patients with multivessel CAD and diabetes mellitus for which revascularization is likely to improve survival (3-vessel CAD or complex 2-vessel CAD involving the proximal LAD), particularly if a left internal mammary artery graft can be anastomosed to the LAD artery.
- PCI or CABG to improve symptoms is beneficial in patients with ≥ 1 significant (> 70% diameter) coronary artery stenoses amenable to revascularization and unacceptable angina despite optimal medical therapy.
- PCI or CABG is recommended to improve survival for survivors of sudden cardiac arrest with presumed ischemia-mediated ventricular tachycardia caused by significant (> 70% diameter) stenosis in a major coronary artery.
- PCI is reasonable as an alternative to CABG in select stable patients with significant (> 50% diameter stenosis) unprotected left main CAD with anatomy compatible with a low risk of PCI complications and clinical characteristics predicting a significantly increased surgical morbidity/mortality.

So, CABG improves symptoms and survival in:

- Left main, left main–equivalent (2-vessel disease with 1 vessel being proximal LAD), or 3-vessel CAD
- Multivessel CAD or proximal LAD disease with LV dysfunction and viable myocardium
- Complex 3-vessel CAD
- Multivessel CAD with DM

CABG vs. PCI: In most of the recent trials (SYNTAX 2011 and 2014; BEST 2015; Everolimus-Eluting Stents or Bypass Surgery for Multivessel Coronary Disease), patients have the same survival results, but the need for revascularization is greater in the PCI group. For patients with diabetes, the 2012 FREEDOM trial and other studies have shown a survival benefit with CABG as compared with PCI.

Again: When compared with PCI, CABG does not improve survival after bypass unless the patient has:

- 3-vessel disease with significant LV dysfunction, or
- left main or left main–equivalent disease, or
- diabetes.

Stents

Stents are the mainstay of PCI. These are placed in the area of blockage and then expanded, thereby opening the lumen to normal size. Stents stabilize the dissection of the plaque produced by angioplasty and are not susceptible to elastic recoil—both of which can occur with angioplasty alone. Stents also have a lower restenosis rate than plain angioplasty. In-stent restenosis is almost always due to neointimal hyperplasia, but stents also carry a risk of in-stent thrombosis, particularly during the early period after placement. This is why dual antiplatelet therapy is so important after stent placement.

Drug-eluting stents (DESs) are made with a metallic stent backbone supporting a polymer covering that contains a slow-release drug. These drugs have properties that decrease the neointimal hyperplasia that is the cause of most restenoses. Commonly used DESs contain medications such as zotarolimus and everolimus. With these agents, the restenosis rate drops dramatically (to 5%) compared to bare-metal stents ([BMSs]; 25%), although there is a slight increase in late stent thrombosis (0.4%). As opposed to BMSs, DESs require prolonged obligatory dual-antiplatelet therapy (i.e., clopidogrel + ASA) due to the delay in neointimal-ization: a minimum of 1 year as opposed to 30 days with a BMS. For patients who are not at increased risk of bleeding, prolonged dual antiplatelet therapy up to 30 months is recommended. Elective, noncardiac surgery should be delayed 1 year after DES for acute MI to avoid stent thrombosis.

Other PCI Techniques

Balloon angioplasty stretches the plaque and vessel wall to enlarge the lumen. There is a 30–50% chance of restenosis within 6 months. Balloon angioplasty is currently used for vessels too small to allow coronary stenting. It is also used to predilate vessels before stent placement.

Rotational ablation atherectomy (catheter with diamond grinding chips in it) has a role for heavily calcified lesions.

PERIPHERAL ARTERIAL DISEASE

PREVIEW | REVIEW

- What are the causes of arteriosclerotic PAD?
- What is Buerger disease?
- What is the difference between claudication and pseudoclaudication?
- What is the first test to establish the diagnosis of lower extremity PAD? What result is considered abnormal?
- Which antiplatelet therapy is recommended for patients with PAD?

CAUSES OF PAD AND INTERMITTENT CLAUDICATION

Peripheral arterial disease (PAD), previously called peripheral vascular disease (PVD), has many causes, including the following:

- Arteriosclerosis (e.g., arteriosclerosis obliterans; most common cause in middle-aged and older). 2 major risk factors for arteriosclerotic PAD are diabetes (5× greater chance) and smoking. Other modifiable risk factors include hyperhomocysteinemia, hyperlipidemia, and hypertension. Note: Patients with arteriosclerotic PAD are at increased risk of MI and stroke.
- Arteritis (e.g., connective tissue disease, Takayasu arteritis). Vasculitides are discussed in Rheumatology, Book 3.
- Trauma (e.g., jackhammer hands)
- Thromboangiitis obliterans (a.k.a. Buerger disease). Classically seen in young, male smokers. It involves medium and small arteries and often affects arteries of the wrists (positive Allen test) and hands. Due to the diffuse, distal nature of this vascular disease, there is rarely a revascularization option. Calcium channel blockers can reduce symptoms of painful or cold fingers. However, no therapy will be effective without smoking cessation.
- Entrapment—think especially of thoracic outlet syndrome and popliteal artery entrapment. Thoracic outlet syndrome results in upper extremity claudication due to compression of nerves or blood vessels at the thoracic outlet. Muscle enlargement from weight lifting, trauma, rare tumors, and the rare cervical rib can all cause thoracic outlet syndrome. Popliteal artery entrapment occurs primarily in young men. Symptoms are intermittent claudication of the calf or foot arch with walking.

It is important to differentiate vascular claudication from lumbar spinal stenosis (or other neurogenic causes; Table 13-7) and know that the latter causes a pseudoclaudication. Lumbar spinal stenosis is relieved by sitting down (flexing the spine), but not by standing still. It is exacerbated by anything that extends the spine, such as standing or walking (especially downhill). Vascular claudication is

CARDIOLOGY

Table 13-7: Causes of Lower Extremity Pain					
	Description of Pain	Location	Precipitant	Onset of Symptoms	Relief
Claudication	Achy, cramping, fatigue	Calf first, then thigh	Exercise	Reliable relationship to exertion	Stop walking
Spinal stenosis	Similar to claudication; may have tingling or weakness	Buttock, thigh, and hip	Walking or standing	Variable	Sitting or other change in position
Arthritis	Aching pain	Joints of knees and hips	Exercise (use of affected joints)	Variable	Rest, nonweightbearing
Venous insufficiency	Fatigue, heavy sensation to legs	Feet and lower legs	Prolonged standing	Variable	Leg elevation, compression therapy, exercise

relieved by sitting down or standing still. Neither disease causes nocturnal leg cramps. When the distance to onset of claudication or severity abruptly changes, consider thrombosis *in situ* or an embolic event.

DIAGNOSIS OF PAD

On physical examination, the degree of diminishment of peripheral pulses (including popliteal, posterior tibial, dorsalis pedis, and even radial and ulnar) correlates with the severity of PAD in that extremity.

Use the resting ankle brachial index (ABI; ankle/arm BP ratio) to establish the diagnosis of lower extremity PAD in those with ≥ 2 of the following: exertional leg symptoms, diminished or absent pulses, nonhealing lower extremity wounds, or age ≥ 65 years (age ≥ 50 years if history of smoking/diabetes).

ABI classification: noncompressible > 1.40, normal 1.00–1.40, borderline 0.91–0.99, and abnormal (i.e., PAD) < 0.90. Therefore, an ABI measurement < 0.90 indicates definite PAD. ABI < 0.50 indicates severe stenosis.

Continuous-wave Doppler ultrasound is useful to diagnose anatomic location and degree of stenosis of PAD.

Exercise tolerance tests (ETTs) are recommended to objectively measure functional limitation of claudication and response to therapy. ETTs with preexercise and postexercise ABI values can differentiate arterial claudication from nonarterial claudication (pseudoclaudication).

Magnetic resonance angiography (MRA) of the extremities (with gadolinium enhancement) is useful to diagnose anatomic location and degree of stenosis of PAD. Computed tomographic angiography (CTA) can be considered as a substitute if there are contraindications to MRA.

Contrast angiography provides detailed information about arterial anatomy and is recommended for evaluation of patients with lower extremity PAD when revascularization is contemplated.

Aneurysms of limb arteries can lead to thromboembolism. Aneurysm of the popliteal artery is often diagnosed by U/S or CT scan. In patients with femoral or popliteal aneurysms, U/S (or CTA or magnetic resonance) imaging is recommended to exclude contralateral femoral or popliteal aneurysms and abdominal aortic aneurysms (AAAs).

Cholesterol emboli may also be seen in patients with extensive atherosclerosis of the aorta and extremities as well as in patients with aneurysmal disease. Look for signs of painful feet with intact distal pulses and livedo reticularis. Cholesterol crystals may be seen on kidney biopsy when there is renal involvement.

TREATMENT OF PAD

Recommendations:

- **Statin** in all patients
- Keep BP < 130/80 mmHg; beta-blockers are effective and not contraindicated.

- Proper foot care
- Smoking: Counsel to stop smoking, offer behavioral and pharmacologic Rx (varenicline, bupropion, and nicotine replacement therapy); ask smokers/former smokers about tobacco use at every visit.
- **Antiplatelet therapy** with aspirin 75–325 mg/day or clopidogrel 75 mg/day to decrease cardiovascular events (warfarin is of no benefit!)
- Exercise 30–45 minutes at least 3 days/week.
- **Cilostazol**, a phosphodiesterase inhibitor, increases cAMP in platelets and blood vessels and reversibly inhibits platelet aggregation. This agent was previously used to increase walking distance and was used only if LV function was normal because phosphodiesterase inhibitors increase mortality in patients with Class III or IV heart failure. This agent is no longer available.
- The benefit of pentoxifylline is marginal and not well established.

If PAD is due to Buerger disease, stop tobacco use. If Takayasu arteritis is present, treat the disease with steroids. (Please refer to Rheumatology, Book 3, for additional information.)

Other treatment: Many forms of PAD can be effectively treated with percutaneous intervention (angioplasty and stents)—with low restenosis rates. Surgical bypass can also effectively relieve symptoms and ischemia.

ACUTE LIMB ISCHEMIA

With acute peripheral arterial occlusion, rapid evaluation and intervention are necessary to avoid limb loss. Patients present with sudden onset of unremitting limb pain. The onset of pain is abrupt and severe enough that they are specific about the time and circumstances of onset. Acute limb ischemia is identified by the 6 **P**s: **p**ain, **p**allor, **p**ulselessness, **p**aresthesia, **p**oikilothermia (coolness), and **p**aralysis.

Urgent evaluation can include imaging with ultrasound, CTA, or catheter-based angiography. Consultation should be obtained from vascular surgery and/or interventional cardiology to establish a revascularization strategy. If the limb is immediately threatened (i.e., sensory loss, rest pain, absent pulses), urgent surgical intervention may be appropriate. Heparin protects the collateral circulation during evaluation by preventing thrombus formation around the new clot. Embolectomy/thrombectomy is the treatment of choice. After revascularization, ongoing pain with evidence of myonecrosis (often in conjunction with renal failure) suggests compartment syndrome. Perform manometry to exclude compartment syndrome.

Many arterial emboli to the lower extremities come from the heart, but atheromatous emboli from a diseased aorta can also occur, which can cause renal failure and ischemia of the toes (Figure 13-18). Perform echocardiography to identify cardiac sources of emboli.

Ultrasound of the aorta can exclude AAA as another possible source. ECG and possibly Holter monitoring should also be performed to exclude atrial fibrillation.

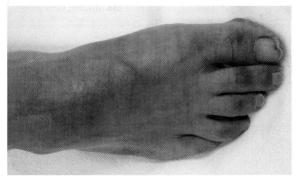

Figure 13-18: Thromboangiitis obliterans (a.k.a. Buerger disease) symptoms on toes
Source: James Heilman, MD

RENAL ARTERY STENOSIS

Atherosclerotic disease of the aorta may encroach upon the ostium of the renal arteries. Renal artery stenosis (RAS; see Nephrology and Urology, Book 2) is an important cause of hypertension in people with early or late onset of hypertension and for those with sudden worsening of chronic hypertension. Randomized data on angioplasty with stenting vs. medical therapy for resistant hypertension in patients with RAS, including the National Heart, Lung, and Blood Institute's 2013 CORAL trial, failed to show benefit for routine treatment with angioplasty. 2013 ACC/AHA guidelines recommend percutaneous revascularization of renal artery stenosis only in patients with 1 of the following:

1) Recurrent heart failure
2) Unstable angina
3) Accelerated, resistant, or malignant hypertension

Bulky aortic disease may also compromise flow to the mesenteric arteries. Ischemic bowel disease (ischemic colitis) is discussed in full in Gastroenterology, Book 5.

CAROTID ARTERY DISEASE

PREVIEW | REVIEW

- Which of these adverse cardiovascular events is most likely to occur in a patient with atherosclerotic disease of the carotid artery: MI, stroke, or TIA?
- When is carotid endarterectomy indicated?
- How might spontaneous dissection of the internal carotid artery present clinically? What is its prognosis?

CAROTID ARTERY ATHEROSCLEROSIS

Atherosclerosis within the carotid artery occurs most frequently within the common carotid bifurcation and proximal internal carotid artery. Patients with atherosclerotic carotid artery disease are at a higher risk of having an MI than of having a transient ischemic attack (TIA) or stroke!

Carotid artery atherosclerosis (a.k.a. carotid stenosis) can be symptomatic or asymptomatic. Focal neurologic symptoms in the internal carotid artery territories can include weakness or numbness in the face or an extremity (contralateral to the stenotic vessel), dysarthria, and vision loss. Carotid duplex ultrasound is the best initial diagnostic test to detect hemodynamically significant carotid stenosis in both symptomatic and asymptomatic patients. Use MRA or CTA when ultrasound cannot be obtained or yields equivocal/nondiagnostic results.

Symptomatic patients who have experienced nondisabling ischemic stroke or TIA symptoms within 6 months should undergo carotid endarterectomy (**CEA**) if:

1) the diameter of the lumen of the ipsilateral internal carotid artery is reduced (> 70% by noninvasive imaging or > 50% by catheter angiography) and
2) the anticipated rate of perioperative stroke/mortality is < 6%.

Carotid artery stenting is an alternative to CEA for these same patients. The choice between these 2 methods of revascularization is based on patient and anatomic characteristics.

Medical therapy for atherosclerotic carotid disease includes:

- Aspirin, clopidogrel, or low-dose aspirin + extended-release dipyridamole
- Treat blood pressure to goal < 130/80 mmHg.
- Statins for all
- Smokers should quit!

INTERNAL CAROTID ARTERY DISSECTION

Suspect spontaneous dissection of the internal carotid artery (cervical area) in a patient with unilateral headache along with either TIAs or a constricted pupil. It can also present as unilateral neck pain in a hypertensive patient. Look for cholesterol emboli on the funduscopic exam. Spontaneous dissection of the internal carotid artery typically resolves with no treatment and with excellent recovery. Occasionally, anticoagulation or a stent is needed.

CEREBRAL EMBOLIC DISEASE

PREVIEW | REVIEW

- What is the most common cause of cerebral embolic events?

CARDIOLOGY

OVERVIEW

The causes of cerebral embolic events of cardiac origin (and the approximate percentage of events they cause):

- Atrial fibrillation (45%)
- Acute MI (15%)
- Ventricular aneurysm (10%)
- Mechanical valve prosthesis (10%)
- Valvular heart diseases, including endocarditis (10%)
- Other cardiac abnormalities (10%)

Other cardiac abnormalities include patent foramen ovale or persistent ASD (which allows an intermittent right-to-left shunt and paradoxical emboli) and dilated cardiomyopathy (which allows formation of a mural thrombus).

The noncardiac causes of embolic cerebral events are aortic and carotid atherosclerosis.

Nonembolic causes of cerebral ischemic attacks or strokes are thrombosis, systemic hypoperfusion, and blood disorders (especially clotting disorders).

Patients with ischemic cerebral vascular accidents (CVAs) should be evaluated for the source of ischemia. A minority of CVAs are due to obstructive disease of intracranial cerebral vessels. A CT angiogram of the vessels of the neck and brain will identify intracranial lesions. An electrocardiogram should be performed to exclude atrial fibrillation, but telemetry or a Holter monitor should be considered since paroxysmal AF may be the source for emboli. The majority of patients with CVA will have an embolic source for their stroke. Carotid artery U/S should be performed in patients with CVA. A transthoracic echocardiogram should be performed in all patients with CVA to exclude cardiac abnormalities discussed above as sources of emboli. In young patients without a source for carotid or cardiac embolus on initial evaluation, a transesophageal echocardiogram with bubble study may be considered to exclude patent foramen ovale.

TRANSIENT ISCHEMIC ATTACK

The definition of transient ischemic attack (TIA) has changed and is no longer related to duration of symptoms. TIA is defined as any period of CNS ischemia without infarction. Ischemic stroke is defined as ischemia with infarction. The CNS includes the brain, spinal cord, and retina. (More on TIAs is in Neurology, Book 4.)

Medical treatment of TIA: If there is a history of TIA but no history of cardioembolic stroke, no significant lesion is found, and the patient does not have atrial fibrillation, the cause is likely atherosclerosis; therefore, place the patient on antiplatelet therapy: ASA + dipyridamole, ASA alone, clopidogrel alone or aspirin + clopidogrel short-term followed by monotherapy.

AORTIC DISEASE

PREVIEW | REVIEW

- What are the procedures of choice for diagnosing a dissecting aortic aneurysm?
- At what size is surgery indicated for a thoracic aortic aneurysm?
- At what size is surgery indicated for an abdominal aortic aneurysm?

AORTIC ANEURYSMS

Overview

The causes of aortic aneurysms can be broadly categorized as degenerative diseases, inherited or developmental diseases, infections, vasculitis, and trauma. With aortic aneurysms, rupture is the biggest threat. Atheroembolism is another complication of abdominal aortic aneurysm. Signs of atheroembolism are livedo reticularis, then blue toes, then ischemic ulceration. (Remember, though, that most emboli to the lower extremities originate in the heart!) Hypertension from renovascular disease can occur if abdominal aneurysms are not treated.

Thoracic Aortic Aneurysms

Thoracic aortic aneurysms tend to dissect as well as rupture. Aortic dissection is an intimal tear in the aorta, resulting in a dissecting hematoma that can cause severe pain and occlusion of the aorta and involved vessels. Systemic hypertension, cystic medial necrosis, bicuspid aortic valve, coarctation of the aorta, and the 3rd trimester of pregnancy are predisposing factors. Aortic dissection is a major cause of death in those with Marfan syndrome.

Cystic medial necrosis is the most common pathology in **ascending aortic** aneurysms, whereas atherosclerosis results most frequently in aneurysms of the **aortic arch** and **descending thoracic** aorta. The average growth rate of thoracic aneurysms is 0.1–0.2 cm per year.

The traditional **DeBakey** classification of aortic dissection lists 3 types:

- **Type I**: Involves the ascending aorta, aortic arch, and descending aorta
- **Type II**: Proximal in the ascending aorta alone
- **Type III**: Involves the descending aorta alone, commonly just after the subclavian artery

The **Stanford** classification is now more commonly used to categorize aortic dissections and lists 2 types:

- **Type A**: Any dissection involving the ascending aorta
- **Type B**: Limited to the descending aorta only

Proximal dissection (Type A) can cause aortic regurgitation, hemopericardium with tamponade, and MI due to involvement of a coronary artery (usually the right coronary artery). Dissections typically present with severe anterior chest pain and/or severe interscapular pain. Patients often describe the pain of aortic dissection as a ripping or tearing sensation down the back.

On physical exam, look for pulse differentials (e.g., between upper extremities, or between upper and lower extremities), blood pressure differentials, a new diastolic murmur indicating acute aortic regurgitation, or signs of cardiac tamponade (indicating hemopericardium).

Diagnosis: Low clinical suspicion and a negative D-dimer score rules out dissection! Negative D-dimer is ≤ 500 µg/mL (2.74 nmol/L) up to 50 years of age; for > 50 years of age, use age × 0.01 µg/mL (0.05 nmol/L).

Transesophageal echo is the diagnostic procedure of choice for suspected proximal thoracic aortic dissection (Type A). For all others, chest or cardiac CT and MRI are the diagnostic procedures of choice. If the initial diagnostic test is unrevealing and you still suspect dissection, get a 2nd test using a different imaging modality. You cannot afford to miss this diagnosis!

Treatment of aortic dissection: Lower elevated blood pressure immediately with beta-blockers and nitroprusside. (Start beta-blockade 1st before giving nitroprusside in order to minimize reflex tachycardia.)

Ascending (Type A) aortic dissections are at greater risk for complications, so they always require surgery. Descending aortic dissections are mainly treated medically unless evidence of end-organ damage develops (e.g., renal insufficiency, GI ischemia, limb compromise), which suggests continuing dissection and the need for emergent surgery.

For chronic, stable thoracic aortic aneurysm: Surgery is indicated at a width of 5.5 cm in the ascending aorta (5 cm if Marfan's) and 6 cm in the descending aorta.

Also, surgery is indicated if the aneurysm is small but enlarging rapidly (> 10 mm in a year), causing symptoms, compressing surrounding structures, or is of traumatic origin.

For nonruptured aneurysms, there is preliminary evidence that aneurysms related to Marfan's should be treated with an ACEI or ARB to block transforming growth factor (TGF) signaling, in addition to beta-blockers.

Abdominal Aortic Aneurysm

Screening is covered in General Internal Medicine, Book 5.

Abdominal aortic aneurysms (AAAs) are more common in men with a history of smoking. They tend to rupture rather than dissect. Treat BP and lipids as for patients with CAD and advise to stop smoking (and recommend smoking cessation interventions).

If asymptomatic, aneurysms 4–5.4 cm should be monitored with ultrasound or CT every 6–12 months. Aneurysms that are ≥ 5.5 cm or symptomatic (abdominal/back pain + pulsatile mass + hypotension) should undergo surgical repair. AAAs that expand > 0.5 cm in 6 months should undergo surgical repair as well. Put the patient on beta-blockers during the observation period.

Know that acute MI and other CAD-related problems are the cause of 70% of perioperative mortality for AAA repair. Surgical risk is lower if the patient does not have CAD, so perform CAD screening with a nuclear stress test if the patient has ≥ 2 CAD risk factors (listed under Risk Factors for CAD on page 13-25). Use perioperative beta-blockers in patients with CAD undergoing surgical repair of AAA.

Open and endovascular repair are both options for infrarenal AAAs and/or common iliac aneurysms in good surgical candidates; however, endovascular repair requires periodic long-term surveillance imaging to monitor for endoleak (persistent arterial perfusion of the aneurysmal sac after endovascular repair) and for shrinkage/stability of the excluded aneurysm sac and to determine need for further intervention.

COARCTATION OF THE AORTA

Coarctation of the aorta (COA) is a congenital anomaly that causes persistent hypertension, sometimes even after surgical correction. CO responds normally to exercise. Blood pressure is higher in the upper extremities than in the lower. Brachiofemoral delay, the femoral pulse occurring after the brachial pulse, is present in COA. People with COA have a high risk of developing subsequent aortic disease, including aneurysms and dissection, even after correction of the lesion. A bicuspid aortic valve is often seen (~ 50%) in COA patients. Patients with COA have a higher incidence of intracerebral aneurysms. See more on COA under Coarctation of the Aorta on page 13-67.

VALVULAR HEART DISEASE

SPECIFIC VALVE LESIONS

PREVIEW | REVIEW

- With which common clinical symptoms do patients with aortic valve stenosis present?
- When should valve replacement occur for aortic valve stenosis?
- Name 2 conditions that cause chronic aortic regurgitation.
- What is the usual treatment for acute aortic regurgitation with associated heart failure?
- When the mitral stenosis is more severe, is the S_2-OS interval smaller or larger?
- Which type of murmur occurs in mitral stenosis?

- Hemoptysis is seen with which mitral lesion?

- Describe the murmur sometimes heard with MVP. Does that murmur's intensity decrease or increase with standing? With Valsalva maneuver?

- Carcinoid usually results in which type of tricuspid murmur?

- On physical exam, in patients with tricuspid regurgitation, what large waves are noted on the jugular waveform?

- True or false? Pulmonic stenosis is virtually always acquired.

- Ebstein anomaly is occasionally seen with which structural and electrical abnormalities?

Note

The 2014 AHA/ACC Valvular Heart Disease Guidelines stage all valvular heart disease (VHD) as:

- Stage **A**: At risk
- Stage **B**: Progressive
- Stage **C**: Asymptomatic severe
- Stage **D**: Symptomatic severe

Stages C and D usually require valve repair/replacement.

Table 13-8: Heart Defects and Associated Sounds

Valve Defect	Murmurs	Clicks	Change in Heart Sounds	Pulse Waveforms; a/v Waves
AS	S: SEM at RUSB, mid-to-late peaking, diamond-shaped	S: Ejection click if congenital or bicuspid	Absent S_2 (occ); S_4; paradoxically split S_2	Slowed carotid upstroke
Acute AR	D: Short diastolic murmur		S_3 if severe	Thready
Chronic AR	S: Occasional early systole SEM D: 1) High pitched, decrescendo early to holodiastolic (regurgitation through the valve); 2) Austin Flint: low, rumbling diastolic (regurgitant stream striking the anterior mitral leaflets)		S_3 if severe	Corrigan or water-hammer pulse (rapidly increasing and falling)
MS	D: Diastolic rumble	D: Opening snap (the only click that occurs in diastole!)	S_1 is enhanced, sometimes "snapping." May be silent if severely calcified.	Large left a waves and y descent
MVP with murmur; chronic MR	S: MVP—late SEM follows click. Chronic mitral regurgitation—pansystolic constant murmur	S: MVP—midsystolic click (click-murmur syndrome)	S_3 if severe; S_4	
Acute MR	S: Pansystolic decrescendo at apex		S_3 if severe	Large left v waves
TS	D: Diastolic at LSB			Giant right a wave
TR	S + D: Systolic at LLSB			Large right v waves
PS	SEM, maximal at LUSB with radiation to the back	S: Ejection click	Persistently/widely split S_2	Large right (jugular) a wave
VSD	S: Holosystolic at LLSB			
ASD—ostium secundum	S: SEM at LSB (increased flow across pulmonic valve)		Fixed split S_2	
ASD—ostium primum	S: SEM at LSB (increased flow across pulmonic valve); +/− TR or MR murmur		Fixed split S_2	
COA	Midsystolic to continuous murmur (depending on severity) in the upper back			
HCM	S: Harsh midsystolic murmur		S_4	Brisk carotid upstroke that is bifid in 2/3
PDA	S + D: Continuous machinery-like murmur at LUSB		Paradoxically split S_2	

Note that S_4 is also heard in ischemic heart disease, diabetic cardiomyopathy, and hypertensive heart disease with concentric hypertrophy.
Note: Right-sided murmurs sound louder on Inspiration, lEft on Expiration; all right-sided valve problems can rarely be caused by carcinoid.
Cannon a waves occur in complete heart block and with ventricular pacing.

Refer to Table 13-8 as you study these valve lesions. It is important for both hospitalists and clinicians to be able to identify a specific valvular defect based on physical exam findings.

Aortic Stenosis

Aortic stenosis (AS) is generally due to age-related, calcific valve degeneration. Congenital bicuspid aortic valves usually start getting calcified and stenotic between 40 and 70 years of age, while the normal trileaflet aortic valves

Murmur Louder with:	CXR	Other	Valve Defect
Table 13-8: Heart Defects and Associated Sounds (Continued)			
Squatting*; expiration after PVCs	LVH	Sustained apical impulse Etiology: bicuspid valve SSx: Classic triad is LVF, angina, and syncope with exercise.	Aortic stenosis
Squatting*; expiration	Normal	Cardiogenic shock and pulmonary edema Consider aortic dissection.	Acute aortic regurgitation
Squatting*; expiration	LVH	Etiology: congenital, endocarditis, or dilated aortic root from Marfan's, VSD, arteritis, polychondritis, syphilis	Chronic aortic regurgitation
Squatting*; expiration	LAE	Etiology: virtually always rheumatic fever SSx: hemoptysis, secondary pulmonary HTN	Mitral stenosis
Standing or Valsalva: longer—moves earlier into systole; sustained handgrip; expiration	LAE	Etio of MVP: congenital; ischemia	MVP with murmur; Chronic mitral regurgitation
Squatting*; expiration	Normal	Etiology: endocarditis, MI with papillary muscle ischemia or rupture, chordae tendineae rupture SSx: pulm edema	Acute mitral regurgitation
Squatting*; inspiration	RAE	TS is rare. Etiology: usually rheumatic fever but also congenital and carcinoid synd. with carcinoid; pt. typically also has TR. SSx: venous congestion	Tricuspid stenosis
Squatting*; inspiration	RVE	Etiology: usually dilation from pulmonary HTN; other—rheumatic fever, endocarditis (IVDA), carcinoid SSx: Liver pulsations, JVD	Tricuspid regurgitation
Inspiration	RVH; enlarged pulmonary artery	Etiology: virtually always congenital—rarely caused by rheumatic fever and carcinoid; congenital type typically does not progress.	Pulmonic stenosis
Handgrip	RVE + LVE	Consider in new MI with new systolic murmur	VSD
	RVE; shunt vascularity	ECG: RAD, RBBB	ASD—ostium secundum
	RVE	ECG: LAD, RBBB	ASD—ostium primum
	Rib notching, loss of aortic notch		COA
Standing, Valsalva; note—Sustained handgrip decreases murmur.	LVE	Apical impulse may have double- or triple-taps.	HCM
	Calcification of ductus arteriosus		PDA

* Squatting or lying down or raising legs if already supine

AR = aortic regurgitation
AS = aortic stenosis
ASD = atrial septal defect
COA = coarctation of the aorta
D = diastolic
HCM = hypertrophic cardiomyopathy
HTN = hypertension
IVDA = IV drug abuse
JVD = jugular venous distension
LAD = left axis deviation

LAE = left atrial enlargement
LBBB = left bundle branch block
LSB = left sternal border
LUSB = left upper sternal border
LV = left ventricle
LVE = left ventricular enlargement
LVF = left ventricular failure
LVH = left ventricular hypertrophy
MI = myocardial infarction

MR = mitral regurgitation
MS = mitral stenosis
MVP = mitral valve prolapse
PDA = patent ductus arteriosus
PE = pulmonary embolus
PS = pulmonic stenosis
RAD = right axis deviation
RAE = right atrial enlargement
RBBB = right bundle branch block

RUSB = right upper sternal border
RV = right ventricle
RVE = right ventricular enlargement
RVH = right ventricular hypertrophy
S = systolic
SEM = systolic ejection murmur
TR = tricuspid regurgitation
TS = tricuspid stenosis
VSD = ventricular septal defect

CARDIOLOGY

become stenotic at > 75 years of age. A bicuspid aortic valve is the most common congenital valve disorder (1–2%). Less frequently, rheumatic heart disease can also cause AS, usually together with mitral valve disease.

Presenting signs and symptoms include the classic triad of heart failure, angina, and syncope with exercise.

Physical exam with significant AS: The carotid pulse has a decreased amplitude and slowed upstroke (parvus et tardus), and the heart has a sustained apical impulse. Associated heart sounds include:

- A mid-to-late-peaking, diamond-shaped systolic ejection murmur at the right upper sternal border (RUSB) or suprasternal notch that radiates to the neck
- An S_4 gallop
- Often a decreased or absent aortic component of the 2nd heart sound due to decreased mobility of the aortic valve leaflets
- A paradoxical S_2 split with severe AS

Occasionally, an AS murmur is transmitted to the apex, where it can be confused with the systolic murmur of mitral regurgitation (the Gallavardin effect).

The systolic ejection murmur of AS is louder with squatting, whereas the murmur of hypertrophic cardio-myopathy (HCM) decreases.

An ejection click sounds like a guitar string being plucked immediately after S_1. This ejection click is classic and common in bicuspid aortic valve patients but is not heard with age-related calcific AS. Ejection clicks can also be heard in patients with pulmonic stenosis but will show respiratory variation.

With aortic stenosis, a systolic thrill can sometimes be felt over the upper precordium and the suprasternal notch. This thrill is a palpable sensation similar to feeling the purring of a cat.

Doppler echo is very accurate in detecting severe AS.

A left heart cath is typically used to diagnose AS if there is a discrepancy between clinical and echo findings—or to detect concomitant coronary artery disease (CAD).

Patients with AS have a high rate of CAD: 1/3 of those 40–60 years of age and 2/3 of those > 60 years of age.

AS severity is usually assessed by mean valve pressure gradient (in mmHg) or maximum velocity across the valve (in m/s):

- Mild: < 25 mmHg
- Moderate: 25–40 mmHg
- Severe: > 40 mmHg (~ > 4.0 m/s)

Low flow states (e.g., heart failure) give artificially low pressure and velocity readings. In this case, determine valve area:

- Mild: 1.9–1.6 cm²
- Moderate: 1.5–1.1 cm²
- Severe: ≤ 1 cm²

Patients with symptomatic, severe AS have at least a 10% risk of sudden death. Without surgical intervention, clinical symptoms predict median survival, given by the mnemonic S:ASH.

Survival in AS:

- **A**ngina: 5 years
- **S**yncope: 3 years
- **H**eart failure: 2 years

Do aortic valve replacement (AVR) for all symptomatic (Stage D) patients and all with asymptomatic severe AS (Stage C)—i.e., with a gradient > 40 mmHg, velocity > 4.0 m/s, or valve area ≤ 1 cm². It is also indicated for patients with severe asymptomatic AS who have an EF < 50% or those who need CABG.

Transcatheter aortic valve replacement (TAVR) is recommended for patients with prohibitive risk for surgical AVR and a predicted post-TAVR survival > 12 months.

Use caution when treating ventricular failure due to AS with vasodilators. Aortic stenosis has the worst prognosis of all valvular lesions, and medical therapy alone is not effective.

Chronic Aortic Regurgitation

Chronic aortic regurgitation (AR) occurs as a result of valve deformity (e.g., bicuspid valve, rheumatic fever, endocarditis, or degenerative valve disease) or an abnormal aortic root (e.g., dilation seen in Marfan syndrome, senile aortic disease, giant cell arteritis, relapsing polychondritis, or syphilis).

Patients with AR may be asymptomatic and typically have good exercise tolerance. Exercise induces peripheral vasodilation, reducing afterload and augmenting forward flow. Exercise also causes tachycardia, which reduces regurgitation by shortening the time for regurgitation during diastole.

Chronic AR causes LV volume overload, which eventually causes LV dilation and a drop in LV systolic function. Once this happens, symptoms of heart failure occur, with exertional dyspnea and angina.

Physical exam with chronic AR has several classic physical findings:

- A decrescendo, diastolic, high-pitched blowing murmur caused by the regurgitation through the valve. It is loudest at the **left** sternal border (3rd space) if due to the aortic **l**eaflet and at the **right** sternal border (RSB) if due to aortic **r**oot disease (because the root is closer to the RSB). The high-pitched blowing sound of this murmur indicates a high flow, whereas mitral stenosis, which also causes a diastolic murmur, causes a low-flow, diastolic rumble.
- Occasionally, you hear an Austin Flint murmur, which does sound similar to the low-flow rumble of mitral stenosis. It is thought to be due to the high-pressure regurgitant jet striking the anterior mitral leaflet and impeding mitral valve inflow by causing early closure.

This murmur does not have an associated presystolic accentuation as seen in MS.

- A wide and bounding carotid Corrigan pulse and water-hammer in the limbs 2° to elevated systolic and low diastolic components of BP
- There are many other exam findings seen with chronic AR that have eponyms and are all related to pulsations; e.g., Becker sign = visible pulsations of the retinal arteries; de Musset sign = bobbing of the head with the pulse; Müller sign = bobbing of uvula during systole.

Chest x-ray shows an enlarged left ventricle and may show dilation of the ascending aorta. Aortic angiography can be performed at the time of cardiac cath to diagnose AR—although it is more frequently diagnosed with echo.

Monitor patients with chronic AR using echocardiograms to follow LV size and function.

Medical therapy for severe AR is vasodilators. Routine use of vasodilator therapy is no longer recommended for nonsevere AR. ACEIs/ARBs are typically used, along with diuretics, to treat symptoms.

Aortic valve replacement (AVR) surgery is indicated if the patient is symptomatic (Stage D) or if asymptomatic and AR is severe or EF is < 50% (Stage C). Intraaortic balloon pump placement is contraindicated in patients with aortic regurgitation.

Acute Aortic Regurgitation

Native acute AR is normally caused by a flail leaflet due to:

- Endocarditis
- Type A aortic dissection
- Trauma

Prosthetic valve acute AR can be caused by:

- Tissue valve leaflet rupture
- Mechanical valve closure problem (e.g., thrombosis)
- Paravalvular regurgitation due to infection

Patients with acute AR present with severe pulmonary edema and low CO. Because the CO and BP are low, there is no bounding arterial pulse. The diastolic murmur is short because it ends when the ventricular pressure rises to the level of the low aortic pressure. The LV in these patients does not have time to compensate for the LV volume overload. Patients with significant acute AR and heart failure (HF) need immediate AVR.

Mitral Stenosis

Mitral stenosis (MS) is relatively rare in the U.S. It is almost always due to rheumatic fever. Other causes are SLE, rheumatoid arthritis, and severe valve calcification. Atrial fibrillation is common. MS can cause HF, but sometimes 2° pulmonary hypertension is the main complication.

Physical exam with MS: Patients have a diastolic murmur with a diastolic opening snap (OS) caused by the tensing of the chordae tendineae and stenotic leaflets (best heard at the apex as opposed to a split S_2 heard best at the upper sternal border). The time interval between the 2nd heart sound (S_2) and the OS (the S_2-OS interval) is inversely related to the severity of the MS: The more severe the MS, the higher the left atrial (LA) pressure, and thus the earlier the mitral valve is forced open in diastole, the smaller the S_2-OS interval.

As mentioned in the section on heart sounds, the S_1 is accentuated and can also have a snapping quality. The diastolic murmur is often described as a rumble, which suggests low flow, in contrast to the high-pitched, high-flow diastolic murmur heard in aortic regurgitation.

The chest x-ray shows the following triad:

1) Prominent pulmonary artery vascularity
2) An enlarged left atrium
3) Normal-sized LV

A biphasic P wave in V1 on the ECG is seen with an enlarged left atrium (Figure 13-24 on page 13-72). Do an echo to confirm the diagnosis. Hemoptysis can occur with MS; it is due to rupture of the pulmonary bronchial vessels distended by pulmonary venous hypertension.

All nonpregnant patients with atrial fibrillation due to MS should be anticoagulated with warfarin.

Percutaneous mitral balloon valvotomy (PMV) is recommended for patients with symptomatic MS (Stage D) or asymptomatic severe MS (Stage C; mitral valve area ≤ 1.5 cm^2 or pulmonary hypertension).

Surgical mitral valve replacement or repair is less desirable but is an alternative for patients who are not PMV candidates or fail PMV. Mitral valve surgery is also considered for patients with moderate stenosis (1.6–2.0 cm^2) who are undergoing other cardiac surgery.

Chronic Mitral Regurgitation

Chronic mitral regurgitation (chronic MR) can be due to rheumatic heart disease, mitral valve prolapse (discussed below), annulus dilatation from left ventricular dilatation, prior episode of endocarditis, and/or ischemic effects on the papillary muscle (from coronary artery disease or MI).

Chronic MR presents differently from acute MR. Because the heart has an enlarged left atrium in the chronic form, there is less back pressure to the flow across the incompetent mitral valve, resulting in a constant intensity, holosystolic murmur instead of decrescendo (as in acute MR). Atrial fibrillation is common. In both severe chronic and acute MR, the S_1 is soft or absent and S_2 is widely split. (The aortic valves close early because of decreased volume ejected from the left ventricle.) An S_3 is common in severe MR.

The left ventricular ejection fraction (LVEF) in chronic MR is frequently normal or above normal because LV outflow now has 2 routes of exit during systole (forward through the aorta and backward through the regurgitant mitral valve).

Treat significant chronic MR with diuretics and afterload reducing agents (ACEIs/ARBs). Beta-blockade can help to prolong diastole. Do surgery if the patient is symptomatic (Stage D) or if asymptomatic (Stage C) with:

- LVEF < 60%, and/or
- LV enlargement with left ventricular end-systolic diameter ≥ 40 mm, or
- PAH with pulmonary arterial pressure > 50 mmHg, or
- new onset atrial fibrillation.

Repair (if possible) is preferable to replacement in patients with Stage C and D disease. A percutaneous valve repair device (mitral clip) was approved by the FDA in 2013 and may be a good option in patients with severely symptomatic chronic MR who are poor surgical candidates.

Mitral Valve Prolapse

Mitral valve prolapse (MVP) is the most common valvular problem seen in practice (up to 2.4%) and is more common in women. There are different causes of MVP. Most MVPs are considered a normal variant; in these, the chordae tendineae are weakened, causing a billowing of the otherwise normal mitral valve leaflets. On the other hand, myxomatous changes in the mitral valve leaflets (determined by echo) invariably progress to mitral regurgitation. Many symptoms (e.g., dyspnea, panic attacks, chest pain) previously attributed to MVP have been shown to occur with no greater frequency than in individuals without MVP. Patients with MVP should receive reassurance of its generally benign course and be advised to follow a healthy lifestyle. Beta blocker agents may help with symptom management.

Physical exam with MVP: These patients have a midsystolic click. If there is also MR, this is followed by a mid-to-late systolic murmur (click-murmur syndrome).

The murmur of MVP is like the murmur in hypertrophic cardiomyopathy (HCM) in that decreased preload increases the intensity of the murmur. The click and murmur become louder and move earlier into systole with standing or Valsalva, both of which decrease preload and, hence, LV volume. (An earlier click means a longer murmur.) This gives the clue for how you can tell the difference between an ejection click (aortic or pulmonary stenosis) and the midsystolic click—an ejection click is fixed, whereas the midsystolic click varies in timing with changes in the patient's position. Stand the patient up, and the midsystolic click sounds just like an ejection click. Squatting or supine position increases LV size and causes the click to occur later, thereby shortening the murmur. Dynamic auscultation is required to diagnose MVP clinically.

Acute Mitral Regurgitation

Acute mitral regurgitation (acute MR) commonly presents with acute-onset pulmonary edema.

Causes of native valve acute MR include:

- Flail leaflet (due to endocarditis, MVP, or trauma)
- Papillary muscle ischemia or rupture (MI, trauma)
- Chordae tendineae rupture (endocarditis, acute rheumatic fever, trauma, spontaneous)

Causes of prosthetic valve acute MR include:

- Tissue valve leaflet rupture
- Mechanical valve closure problem (e.g., thrombosis)
- Paravalvular regurgitation due to infection

Physical exam with acute MR: decrescendo systolic murmur at the apex. Echocardiogram shows a hyperactive LV with normal-to-high ejection fraction and a normal-sized left atrium. There are large, left-sided v waves on wedge pressure tracing.

Treat with afterload reduction and diurese. Unlike severe AR, intraaortic balloon pump can be helpful for patients in heart failure from acute MR. Urgent surgery is often required.

Tricuspid Stenosis

Tricuspid stenosis (TS) is rare. Causes are rheumatic fever (usual), congenital, carcinoid syndrome, and endocarditis. With TS caused by carcinoid, tricuspid regurgitation is usually present also. Note: Carcinoid can affect either right-sided heart valve and typically implies a hepatic tumor if valvular involvement is present. (The pulmonary vascular bed is generally quite effective in removing the active 5-HIAA products that lead to valve damage.) Patients have systemic venous congestion without pulmonary venous congestion or pulmonary hypertension.

Physical exam with TS: a diastolic murmur along the left sternal border that increases with inspiration (as do all right-sided murmurs). They have a giant a wave caused by backflow during atrial contraction against a stenotic tricuspid valve. There may be ascites and lower extremity edema.

The ECG shows the tall, peaked P waves in II and V1 (evidence of the right atrial hypertrophy) but no indications of right ventricular hypertrophy (RVH). Chest x-ray shows an enlarged right atrium.

Treat the underlying disease, and consider tricuspid valve surgery for patients with Stage C or D disease.

Tricuspid Regurgitation

Tricuspid regurgitation (TR) is often a functional result of RV dilation, which can be caused by end-stage left ventricular failure, pulmonary embolism, or other causes of pulmonary hypertension. TR can also be caused by rheumatic heart disease, endocarditis, carcinoid, and congenital disease (Ebstein anomaly). Endocarditis affecting the tricuspid valve is typically seen in IV drug abusers, and it is often caused by *Staphylococcus*; also consider *Candida*.

Physical exam with TR: Patients have a holosystolic murmur along the lower left sternal border (increases with inspiration) that does not radiate to the axilla. Severe TR can cause a parasternal heave, liver pulsations, venous distention, ascites, and lower extremity edema (signs of RV failure). There are large, jugular *v* waves, reflecting the backflow through the tricuspid valve during ventricular contraction.

Diagnose with echo. Treat the underlying disease. Antibiotic treatment is usually sufficient for endocarditis; the valve rarely needs to be removed, unless the cause is *Candida*. Surgery also can be indicated in circumstances of severe destruction of the valve (Stage D). Tricuspid surgery is considered in patients with Stage C TR who are undergoing other right-sided valve surgery.

Pulmonic Stenosis

Pulmonic stenosis is virtually always congenital, and it typically does not progress! It is a fairly common congenital valve anomaly in adults. Rarely is it caused by rheumatic heart disease or carcinoid. It can cause RV hypertrophy. Although it generally is not seen along with other abnormalities, it does occur in Noonan syndrome, in which the patient also has low-set ears and hairline.

Physical exam with severe pulmonic stenosis: an ejection click and a crescendo-decrescendo systolic murmur that changes in intensity with respiration. A prominent jugular *a* wave may be present, which is caused by backflow during atrial contraction against an inadequately emptied right ventricle.

If needed, open the stenotic pulmonic valve with percutaneous balloon valvuloplasty.

Pulmonic Regurgitation

Pulmonic regurgitation is typically secondary to pulmonary hypertension (e.g., primary, cor pulmonale, mitral stenosis), but it may be due to a primary valve lesion (e.g., congenital, rheumatic heart disease, endocarditis, carcinoid). Pulmonary artery pressure is > 60 mmHg in patients with secondary pulmonic regurgitation. The murmur of pulmonic regurgitation is diastolic, high pitched, and best heard over the 2nd and 3rd intercostal spaces. It classically is louder during inspiration.

Ebstein Anomaly

With Ebstein anomaly, the tricuspid septal leaflet is positioned lower in the ventricle than normal (apically displaced)—so the RA appears huge and the RV small. TR murmur is common. A sound like a flapping sail may be heard due to the abnormally displaced septal leaflet. It is occasionally seen with atrial septal defect (ASD) and

with WPW syndrome. (See ASD on page 13-66 and WPW on page 13-50.)

INFECTIVE ENDOCARDITIS

PREVIEW | REVIEW

- Are blood cultures more frequently positive with right-sided or left-sided endocarditis?
- Which type of ASD requires antibiotic prophylaxis before a dental procedure?
- Which of these require antibiotic prophylaxis: previous CABG? VSD? Mitral valve prolapse without murmur? Mitral valve prolapse with murmur? Prosthetic valve? Are your answers based on the ACC/AHA 2014 guidelines update?

Overview

Know this topic well.

More information on the causes, diagnosis, and prophylactic treatment of infective endocarditis (IE) is in Infectious Disease, Book 1.

Occasionally, endocarditis presents only with signs of embolic events, such as black toes or septic emboli to other organs. It can also present as an illness of smoldering, nonspecific symptoms (e.g., weight loss, fevers, chills, night sweats) or heart failure due to valvular insufficiency.

Classic physical exam findings include new regurgitant heart murmurs, Osler nodes (tender nodules on the pads of the digits), Janeway lesions (nontender erythematous/ hemorrhagic macular/ nodular lesions on the palms or soles), splinter hemorrhages (Figure 13-19), and Roth spots.

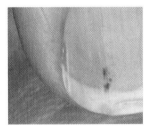
Figure 13-19: Splinter hemorrhage on fingernail in endocarditis

Blood cultures are positive in right- and left-sided endocarditis with equal frequency (95%). This is because there is a constant level of bacteremia in endocarditis, whereas with most other bacterial causes of fever, the bacteremia precedes the temperature spike.

Diagnosis of endocarditis is by the Duke criteria; echo, including TEE, is frequently used to help make the diagnosis.

Endocarditis occurring within 2 months of prosthetic valve placement means the valve was seeded when the valve was implanted. It is harder to treat (especially if *S. epidermidis*); if there is no response to 1 round of adequate antibiotics, replace the valve.

CARDIOLOGY

If it has been > 2 months since the prosthetic valve placement, antibiotic treatment is generally sufficient. The valve must also be replaced if there is evidence of valve ring infection, myocardial penetration, or unstable prosthesis. These can appear as a new heart block or a new BBB.

Surgery is indicated in endocarditis for refractory heart failure, usually from acute valve regurgitation, extension of the infection to the myocardium (or perivalvular abscess), failure of medical therapy, or large vegetations with systemic emboli or recurrent emboli on adequate therapy.

Antibiotic Prophylaxis

Overview

Know the following from the ACC/AHA 2008 Focused Update on Infective Endocarditis.

Significant changes to the bacterial endocarditis prophylaxis prevention guidelines were made because it has become clear that infective endocarditis is more likely to occur from bacteremia caused by brushing teeth than from medical procedures. It appears that medical procedures cause little if any infective endocarditis.

Indications for Prophylaxis

Prophylaxis is no longer indicated for GI/GU surgeries. Prophylaxis prior to dental procedures is now indicated only for patients with specific highest-risk-for-IE cardiac conditions:

- Prosthetic valves
- Previous episode of endocarditis
- Congenital heart disease (CHD)
  - Unrepaired cyanotic CHD
  - Repaired CHD within 6 months of procedure
  - Repaired CHD with residual defects
- Cardiac transplant patients with valve lesions

Prophylaxis is no longer indicated for bicuspid aortic valve, any ASD or VSD (unless unrepaired and cyanotic, or repaired with residual defect), native valvular stenosis or regurgitation, mitral valve prolapse (with or without murmur), coronary artery bypass graft (CABG), or HCM (unless repair occurs within 6 months of procedure).

Antibiotic Selection for Prophylaxis

Know the following:

Dental procedures: All dental procedures that involve manipulation of gingival tissue or the periapical region of teeth or perforation of the oral mucosa require prophylaxis in high-risk patients. See Table 13-9.

Table 13-9: Endocarditis Prophylaxis — Dental Procedures

Situation	Antibiotic	Regimen
Oral prophylaxis	Amoxicillin	2 g orally
Unable to take oral medications	Ampicillin or Cefazolin* or ceftriaxone	2 g IM/IV 1 g IM/IV
Allergic to penicillin	Clindamycin or Cephalexin* or Azithromycin or clarithromycin	600 mg orally 2 g orally 500 mg orally
Both allergic to penicillin and unable to take oral meds	Clindamycin or Cefazolin* or ceftriaxone	600 mg IM 1 g IM/IV

Note: Antibiotics (PO or parenteral) are given 30–60 minutes before the procedure.
* Cephalosporins should not be used if the PCN allergy is an immediate-type hypersensitivity reaction.

GU/GI procedures: Prophylaxis is not indicated in these high-risk patients for any GI or GU procedures.

Respiratory tract procedures, or **skin** or **musculoskeletal** tissue infection: The high-risk patient should receive prophylaxis that covers staphylococci and beta-hemolytic streptococci.

RHEUMATIC FEVER

PREVIEW | REVIEW

- Following acute rheumatic fever, how many years on average does it take for valvular dysfunction to occur, if it does?

Acute rheumatic fever is a syndrome that occurs 2–4 weeks after acute group A streptococcal pharyngitis. In patients with pharyngitis, always swab throats for a strep screen.

Acute rheumatic fever is rare in the U.S. and developed countries (< 2 cases/100,000), but rheumatic fever remains common outside of the U.S. (> 470,000 cases/year worldwide). It occurs more frequently in overcrowded areas and is the most common cause of mitral stenosis and tricuspid stenosis.

Table 13-10 lists the diagnostic criteria for rheumatic fever. Joint affliction in rheumatic fever is distinguished from rheumatoid arthritis by the lack of typical joint deformities and a negative rheumatoid factor. The associated carditis typically has no symptoms referable to the heart!

Table 13-10: Modified Jones Criteria for the Diagnosis of Rheumatic Fever	
Major	**Minor**
Carditis	Previous rheumatic fever
Polyarthritis	Arthralgias
Chorea	Fever
Erythema marginatum	Acute phase reactants (high sed rate or WBC)
Subcutaneous nodules	ECG changes: prolonged PR interval

Diagnosis requires 2 major criteria or 1 major and 2 minor criteria and evidence of a preceding group A strep infection (positive strep test or rising or elevated [> 250 Todd units] ASO titers).

Treat group A *Streptococcus* with IM or oral penicillin and consider ongoing prophylactic parenteral penicillin. In adults, administer 1.2 million units benzathine penicillin intramuscularly on diagnosis. For patients with evidence of carditis, this should be repeated monthly for 10 years or up to 21 years of age, whichever is longer. If there is residual heart disease, it should continue until 40 years of age. For patients with rheumatic fever without carditis, therapy is recommended to continue for 5 years or to 21 years of age, whichever is longer.

Up to 72% of children with acute rheumatic fever develop chronic valvular disease. Symptoms of valvular dysfunction occur, on average, 20 years following acute rheumatic fever infection. See Rheumatology, Book 3, for more on acute rheumatic fever.

VALVE SURGERY

PREVIEW | REVIEW

• What are the major prognostic factors after valve surgery?

In general, valve surgery is indicated for any valve problem if the patient is symptomatic at rest (Stage D) or asymptomatic with severe disease (Stage C). Even though there is high mortality, valve surgery is better than no surgery in patients with severe valve disease and ventricular failure (since the natural history in these cases is 100% early mortality).

Bioprosthetic valves are less durable (especially in young patients and those on hemodialysis) but do not require anticoagulation. These are indicated for patients > 70 years of age and those with contraindications to anticoagulation (e.g., chronic bleeding problems, ulcers). They also are often given to women of childbearing age to avoid having to use anticoagulants during pregnancy.

Mechanical valves are used for younger patients and do require anticoagulation, but they are very durable—typically lifelong in most cases. Either a bioprosthetic or mechanical valve is reasonable in patients between 60 and 70 years of age.

Percutaneous balloon valvuloplasty is the procedure of choice in pulmonic valve stenosis and rheumatic mitral stenosis—but not aortic stenosis due to a very high short-term restenosis rate (6–12 months).

For mitral regurgitation (MR), if surgery is required, do valve reconstruction whenever possible because it has better outcomes and about 50% the morbidity of MV replacement. Reconstruction is valve repair and/or annuloplasty with an annuloplasty ring; it is especially useful for MVP, ruptured chordae, flail leaflets, endocarditis, and annular dilation. Valve replacement is usually necessary in MR due to rheumatic fever.

Since 2013, percutaneous transcatheter MV repair has been available. This procedure is ordinarily reserved for patients who are high risk for traditional repair. Similarly, percutaneous aortic valve replacement is now available for patients who are at high risk for surgery.

The major prognostic factors after valve surgery are ejection fraction, severity of symptoms, and type of valve surgery (valve repair is better than replacement). Echocardiography is best for checking for prosthetic valvular function. A transesophageal echocardiogram (TEE) is especially useful for checking mitral valve prosthesis. Fluoroscopy is also a useful tool for documenting leaflet motion with mechanical valves if valve dysfunction is suspected.

When anticoagulating for mechanical aortic valves, keep an INR of 2.5 (if no additional risk factors for emboli) or 3.0 (if additional risk for emboli) and an INR of 3.0 for the mitral valve. Additional risk factors for thromboemboli that should be considered in the INR target include atrial fibrillation, hypercoagulable state, LV dysfunction, and prior thromboembolic event. A mechanical mitral valve has a higher risk for a thrombus formation compared to a mechanical aortic valve (hence the 3.0 INR for all). Use unfractionated heparin for all mitral valve patients having warfarin withheld for surgery. ASA (75–100 mg) is additionally given to all mechanical prosthesis patients.

FINAL PEARLS ABOUT MURMURS

PREVIEW | REVIEW

• Describe the abnormal heart sounds found in AS, chronic AR, and MS.

Know:

• Aortic stenosis (AS): suprasternal notch thrill with systolic murmur; paradoxically split S_2
• Chronic aortic regurgitation: early diastolic, blowing, decrescendo murmur heard best at left sternal border, 3rd intercostal space, with patient leaning forward and exhaling; also, low-pitched late-diastolic rumble (Austin Flint)
• Mitral stenosis: hemoptysis; opening snap; low-pitched, diastolic murmur at the apex

Valsalva (one last time): decreases the murmur of AS, increases the murmur of hypertrophic cardiomyopathy, and increases the murmur of mitral valve prolapse.

ARRHYTHMIAS

MECHANISMS OF ARRHYTHMIAS

The 3 usual mechanisms of abnormal rhythms are reentry, triggered activity, and automaticity. Reentry is the most common mechanism of arrhythmias, especially AV node reentrant tachycardia (AVNRT), atrial flutter, and most ventricular tachycardias. AVNRT is the most common type of reentrant tachycardia—hence it is also the most common supraventricular tachycardia (SVT). Be able to diagnose all rhythms at a glance; some case studies are provided in ECG — Analysis Summary on page 13-78.

BRADYARRHYTHMIAS

Although bradycardia is normal in athletes, exclude a secondary cause when present in others. A 12-lead ECG should be obtained to identify heart block (see ECG — Analysis Summary on page 13-78). Hypothyroidism is an important cause of bradycardia: Think of this in patients with weight gain, cold intolerance, and delayed reflexes. Digoxin toxicity causes bradycardia; think of this in a patient on digoxin with worsening renal function. Excessive administration of any AV nodal agent may cause bradycardia.

Patients with severe symptomatic bradycardia should be admitted and placed on telemetry. Admit the patient to a coronary care unit (CCU) if the ECG suggests increased risk for complete heart block (e.g., 2:1 AV block, long PR interval and wide QRS, high-grade Mobitz 2 block, alternating right and left bundle branch block). Atropine should be at the bedside and administered if hypotension develops or the patient becomes symptomatic. If permanent pacing is delayed for patients with heart block, employ a temporary pacing wire or transcutaneous pacing.

SICK SINUS SYNDROME

Sick sinus syndrome causes any 1 (or combination) of several sinoatrial node problems, including sinus bradycardia, sinus pauses/sinus arrest, and tachy-brady syndrome (typically baseline sinus bradycardia or sinus pauses with intermittent episodes of rapidly conducting atrial fibrillation/atrial flutter). These patients generally do not need electrophysiologic testing. Because prognosis is good, there are only 2 indications for treatment with a pacemaker:

1) Symptomatic patient
2) Patient with tachy-brady syndrome where treatment of tachyarrhythmias might precipitate or worsen bradycardia

HEART BLOCK

1st degree heart block: PR interval > 200 msec. Can be caused by medications and generally requires no treatment.

2nd degree heart block (**Mobitz 1**, **Wenckebach**): gradual prolongation of PR interval until QRS drops; return PR interval shorter than last conducted PR interval.

Results in grouped beating on ECG. It can occur during periods of high vagal tone during sleep (obstructive sleep apnea) or in endurance athletes. It generally does not require treatment unless it is causing symptoms.

2nd degree heart block (**Mobitz 2**): abrupt loss of P-wave conduction to the ventricle with no evidence of gradual prolongation of the PR interval. Thus, there is no warning prior to the dropped beat. Generally, it indicates higher-grade AV block, and associated symptoms can necessitate pacemaker placement.

3rd degree heart block (**complete** heart block): None of the P waves are conducted to the ventricles, and there is often a regular, narrow junctional (40–60 bpm) or wide ventricular (20–40 bpm) escape rhythm.

Permanent pacing is indicated if there is a Mobitz 2 or complete heart block—especially if symptomatic. See Arrhythmias and Blocks on page 13-23 for more detailed pacing criteria post-MI.

To differentiate between AV node block vs. infranodal block: AV node block typically has narrow QRS complexes, has escape focus rate > 40 bpm (usually 40–60 bpm), and is responsive to atropine. Infranodal block (involving the His-Purkinje system) usually has widening of the QRS complex.

TACHYARRHYTHMIAS

PREVIEW | REVIEW

- What is the treatment sequence for atrial flutter?
- What procedure can cure the most common types of atrial flutter with 85–95% success rate?
- In which circumstance is immediate DC cardioversion indicated for A-fib?
- What can happen after DC cardioversion to the patient who has A-fib with a slow rate? What intervention prevents this complication?
- According to the 2013 update to the ACC/AHA Practice Guidelines: Management of Patients with Atrial Fibrillation, what HR is an acceptable target for patients with A-fib and stable ventricular function? For others, how is strict control of heart rate defined?
- Which medication should you use to prevent postoperative A-fib in patients undergoing cardiac surgery?

- How is the CHA_2DS_2-VASc score calculated? At what score should you treat with warfarin/DOACs (unless contraindicated)?
- In which patient group is MAT found?
- What is the treatment for acute A-fib in WPW?

Note

Patients with sinus tachycardia typically have an underlying pathology as an instigator. Fever, infection, pain, hypoxia, anemia, ongoing bleeding, and pulmonary embolism are possible causes. Exclude hyperthyroidism causing tachycardia by checking a TSH. Perform an ECG and draw blood work for patients with tachycardia.

Atrial Flutter

Typical (Type I) atrial flutter, the common form, has a characteristic atrial rate of 300 bpm (240–340 bpm), commonly with a 2:1 AV block. Look for atrial flutter in any ECG with a heart rate of 150 bpm; atrial flutter waves at 300 bpm with 2:1 AV block gives a heart rate of 150 bpm.

Atrial flutter can be:

- counterclockwise rotation around the right atrium (most common), characterized by negative sawtooth flutter waves in ECG leads II, III, and aVF (with positive deflection in V1); or
- clockwise, characterized by positive flutter waves in ECG leads II, III, and aVF (with prominent negative deflection in V1).

These 2 atrial flutter types share the same right atrial reentrant circuit around the cavo-tricuspid isthmus (circuit running between the inferior vena cava and the tricuspid valve).

Atrial flutter is generally an indication of disease, most often either organic heart disease or pulmonary disease. Flutter is a relatively unstable rhythm and often spontaneously converts to either atrial fibrillation or a normal sinus rhythm.

AV block is usually 2:1 with a ventricular rate 50% of the atrial rate. If it is ≥ 3:1, the cause is either medications or advanced AV conduction system disease. Atrial flutter (as well as atrial fibrillation) can cause systemic embolization (most notably TIA/stroke); thus, anticoagulation needs to be considered in both disorders. Indeed, up to 60% of patients with atrial flutter had atrial fibrillation in the preceding year.

Vagal maneuvers or adenosine cannot terminate atrial flutter; however, they can slow the ventricular rate and assist diagnosis. Rule out pulmonary emboli (often multiple) and thyroid disease—especially if there is no heart or lung history.

The most effective treatment for atrial flutter is synchronized direct current (DC) cardioversion. Always shock if the patient is hemodynamically compromised.

Do not continue DC cardioversion if the patient repeatedly reverts back to atrial flutter.

Antiarrhythmic drugs can be used for nonemergent cardioversion. IV ibutilide is most effective and can be considered a 1st line pharmacologic cardioversion for atrial flutter; however, be aware that it can cause QT prolongation (8%) and *torsades de pointes*. Make sure K^+ and Mg^{2+} levels are normal prior to administering ibutilide to minimize risks of *torsades*.

Procainamide, flecainide, and propafenone can be used as well. See Antiarrhythmic Therapy on page 13-53.

In patients with atrial flutter and preexcitation syndrome (Wolff-Parkinson-White syndrome [WPW]), avoid digoxin, calcium channel blockers, and beta-blockers. See WPW on page 13-50.

Radiofrequency ablation is a treatment modality that can cure the most common types of atrial flutter (success rate 85–95%). It is usually reserved for persistent or recurrent atrial flutter, although studies have suggested it is a reasonable 1st line approach in some circumstances.

Atrial Fibrillation

Overview

Atrial fibrillation (A-fib) is the most common sustained arrhythmia. Ventricular rhythm is irregularly irregular, with ventricular rate generally in the range of 120–180 bpm in the absence of drug therapy. Many patients with atrial fibrillation have structural heart disease. It is commonly seen with hypertension, heart failure, valvular heart disease, coronary artery disease, chronic lung disease, and obstructive sleep apnea.

A-fib can be classified as **first detected** (only 1 diagnosed episode), **paroxysmal** (≥ 2 episodes, self-terminating; each lasts ≤ 7 days, most < 24 hours), **persistent** (≥ 2 episodes; each lasts > 7 days), or **permanent** (> 6–12 months).

The symptoms of A-fib vary widely between patients.

Some patients are asymptomatic, and others have severe, functionally disabling symptoms. Complications are embolic events—mainly stroke—and tachycardia-induced cardiomyopathy.

With new-onset A-fib or in A-fib not responsive to the usual treatment, consider hyperthyroidism, untreated or undertreated obstructive sleep apnea, hypomagnesemia, alcoholism/cocaine abuse, excessive caffeine (including energy beverages), and nicotine as possible causes.

Always work up new-onset A-fib with an echocardiogram, TSH, and complete metabolic panel to check electrolytes. These initial results will guide further testing.

CARDIOLOGY

Treatment of Atrial Fibrillation

Rhythm Control vs. Rate Control

Remember that any hemodynamically unstable tachycardia, including atrial fibrillation, should be cardioverted emergently! This includes patients with severe ongoing myocardial ischemia, symptomatic hypotension, angina, or heart failure.

For stable A-fib, you have 2 choices for treatment:

1) Rhythm control (restoration and maintenance of sinus rhythm)

2) Rate control (control of ventricular response)

There are no significant differences in mortality or morbidity between the 2 treatments. Rate control is the common strategy for asymptomatic or minimally symptomatic patients, while rhythm control is often selected for significantly symptomatic and younger patients.

A-Fib Rhythm Control — DC Cardioversion

DC cardioversion is the most effective method to restore sinus rhythm. Rates of successful pharmacologic cardioversion are lower and depend on the antiarrhythmic drug used and clinical scenario. If possible, DC cardioversion should be carried out under sedation with appropriate cardiac and hemodynamic monitoring.

Again, emergent/urgent DC cardioversion is recommended for patients with hemodynamic instability (angina pectoris, MI, shock, or pulmonary edema), ongoing myocardial ischemia, symptomatic hypotension, angina or heart failure, and WPW syndrome with rapid ventricular rate.

Important points regarding DC cardioversion:

- With slow A-fib, consider inserting a temporary pacemaker before DC cardioversion because the patient could have sinus node disease and may have asystole after cardioversion.
- If time of A-fib onset is unknown or A-fib is known to be present > 48 hours, you must do TEE (to rule out left atrial thrombus) or at least 3 weeks of anticoagulation prior to cardioversion, due to the risk of thromboembolism.
- TEE-guided cardioversion allows you to rule out thrombus at the time of cardioversion. It is especially useful when the time of onset of the A-fib is unclear. It is fast and cost effective.
- Just as with atrial flutter, do not continue DC cardioversion if the patient repeatedly goes right back into A-fib shortly after being shocked.

Note: In what other scenarios do you not shock a patient with an abnormal tachycardic atrial rhythm (but who is stable hemodynamically)? Digitalis intoxication and hypokalemia.

A-Fib Rhythm Control — Pharmacologic Cardioversion

When attempting pharmacologic cardioversion, use these guidelines. Again, use is based on duration of symptoms.

- For A-fib > 7 days:
  - 1st line: dofetilide
  - 2nd line: amiodarone or ibutilide
- For A-fib < 7 days:
  - 1st line: dofetilide, flecainide, ibutilide, or propafenone (previously, dronedarone; see caution below)
  - 2nd line: amiodarone (Exception: If < 48 hours and poor cardiac function, amiodarone is 1st line.)

As with DC cardioversion, when A-fib has been present for more than 48 hours or duration is unknown, you must first rule out atrial thrombus with TEE or do anticoagulation for 3 weeks prior to pharmacologic cardioversion.

Caution: Do not prescribe dronedarone to patients with Class IV heart failure or those who have had decompensated heart failure in the past month, especially if LVEF < 35%, because it increases mortality in these patients. In addition, do not use dronedarone in patients who have had pulmonary toxicity on amiodarone or elevated LFTs.

Maintenance Drugs for Rhythm Control

Pharmacological therapy can be useful in patients with recurrent paroxysmal or permanent A-fib to maintain sinus rhythm. Before initiating antiarrhythmic drug therapy, treat precipitating or reversible causes of A-fib (e.g., thyroid disorders, electrolyte abnormalities). Drug selection is based on the presence of structural heart disease (safety) and, to a lesser degree, on efficacy:

- No or minimal heart disease: flecainide, propafenone, sotalol, and dronedarone; if ineffective, then amiodarone, dofetilide, or catheter ablation (see below)
- Heart failure (EF < 35%): amiodarone or dofetilide (definitely not dronedarone!); if ineffective, use catheter ablation
- Coronary artery disease: dofetilide or sotalol; if ineffective, then amiodarone or catheter ablation
- Hypertension:
  - Left ventricular hypertrophy (LVH) present: Use amiodarone; if ineffective, then catheter ablation.
  - LVH not present: Use flecainide, propafenone, or sotalol. If these fail, then go to amiodarone, dofetilide, or catheter ablation.

Use of Class IC agents (e.g., flecainide, propafenone) for atrial fibrillation:

The unopposed use of Class IC agents (i.e., without concomitant AV nodal blocking agents) can organize atrial fibrillation into atrial flutter conducting to the ventricles much more rapidly. This rapid conduction could degenerate into ventricular tachycardia (VT) or ventricular fibrillation (VF). To avoid this potentially fatal event, always use Class IC agents with AV nodal agents such as beta-blockers, nondihydropyridine calcium channel blockers, or digoxin.

Dofetilide and sotalol require hospital monitoring to initiate therapy.

Catheter ablation (which includes radiofrequency ablation and cryothermal ablation) can help maintain sinus rhythm for selected patients with symptomatic, paroxysmal A-fib who have failed treatment with an antiarrhythmic drug, have a normal or mildly dilated left atrium, normal or mildly reduced LV systolic function, and no severe pulmonary disease. Catheter ablation is less useful (yet can be considered) in treatment of patients with symptomatic persistent A-fib.

A-Fib Rate Control

The 2014 ACC/AHA Guidelines for the Management of Patients with Atrial Fibrillation state that a strict rate-control strategy (resting heart rate < 80 bpm) is reasonable for management of symptomatic A-fib. However, a lenient rate-control strategy (resting heart rate < 110 bpm) may also be okay if symptoms are controlled and LV function is normal. Uncontrolled tachycardia may, over time, result in a reversible decline in ventricular performance.

Use beta-blockers (e.g., atenolol, metoprolol) or nondihydropyridine calcium channel blockers (e.g., verapamil, diltiazem) for rate control at rest and with exercise. Digoxin can have a synergistic effect for rate control when combined with these medications.

A-fib with HF: acute setting and no preexcitation (i.e., WPW)—IV beta-blockers (esmolol, metoprolol, or propranolol) to slow ventricular rate or amiodarone to slow ventricular rate and possibly restore sinus rhythm. Use nondihydropyridine calcium channel blockers (e.g., verapamil, diltiazem) with caution to slow the ventricular response in patients with hypotension or HF because of negative inotropic effects.

IV digoxin or amiodarone is used to control the heart rate acutely in patients with A-fib and HF who do not have an accessory pathway. Remember: An accessory pathway, a.k.a. preexcitation, is usually indicated by a short PR interval and a delta wave (see WPW on page 13-50).

If exertional symptoms related to A-fib are present, assess heart rate control during exercise, adjusting pharmacological treatment to keep the rate in physiological range.

Digoxin is useful to control the heart rate at rest in patients with A-fib with HF, patients with LV dysfunction, or sedentary individuals.

Radiofrequency ablation of the AV node with subsequent permanent pacing is a treatment for patients with refractory A-fib and for those who cannot tolerate the medications needed for rate or rhythm control. This strategy provides definitive rate control but does not cure the underlying atrial fibrillation—hence, patients still require anticoagulation.

In many patients, A-fib originates as abnormal impulses arising in the pulmonary veins. Radiofrequency ablation, or isolation of the pulmonary veins, is becoming increasingly popular in treating recurrent, drug-refractory, symptomatic A-fib, although it is not yet established as 1st line therapy.

Postoperative A-Fib

For patients undergoing cardiac surgery, give an oral beta-blocker to prevent postoperative A-fib (unless contraindicated). For those who develop postoperative A-fib, achieve rate control with AV nodal blocking drugs (beta-blockers, calcium channel blockers, or digoxin). Routine postoperative amiodarone is not indicated for the prevention of atrial fibrillation.

Anticoagulation for Atrial Fibrillation

Before and After Cardioversion

If it has been < 48 hours since the onset of A-fib, most patients can be safely cardioverted without any preceding anticoagulation.

As noted earlier, if it has been > 48 hours since the onset of A-fib (or duration of A-fib is unknown) and the patient is stable, you must achieve adequate anticoagulation × 3 weeks before you attempt cardioversion. As an alternative to preceding anticoagulation, it is reasonable to perform TEE, and if there is no identifiable thrombus, perform a cardioversion.

After cardioversion: Treat with low-molecular-weight or unfractionated heparin until INR = 2–3 on warfarin. As an alternative to heparin/warfarin, one of the direct oral anticoagulants (DOACs) can be considered.

Anticoagulation

Antithrombotic therapy to prevent thromboembolism is recommended for all patients with A-fib (irrespective of rate or rhythm control strategy), except for those with lone A-fib (< 60 years of age without heart disease and without risk factors), those with end-stage kidney disease on dialysis, or those with contraindications to anticoagulation. The selection of the antithrombotic agent should be based upon the absolute risk of stroke. Patients with rheumatic mitral stenosis and prior thromboembolism are at highest risk. For patients with nonvalvular A-fib (without rheumatic mitral stenosis or prosthetic valves), the **CHA$_2$DS$_2$-VASc** scoring system is often used for risk stratification:

- (**C**ongestive) HF during last year or EF < 35% (any history): 1 point
- **H**TN (prior history): 1 point
- **A**ge ≥ 75 years: **2 points**

- **D**M: 1 point
- Prior **s**troke, TIA, or embolic event: **2** points
- **V**ascular disease, known (e.g., CAD, PAD, aortic aneurysm): 1 point
- **A**ge 65–74: 1 point
- **S**ex category = female: 1 point

Medications based on CHA_2DS_2-VASc:

- 0 points = ASA alone
- 1 point = oral anticoagulation or ASA
- ≥ 2 points = oral anticoagulation

Oral anticoagulation can be achieved with vitamin K antagonists such as warfarin or with direct oral anticoagulants (DOACs)—e.g., dabigatran, rivaroxaban, apixaban, edoxaban. DOACs do not require monitoring INR; however, they cannot be used in patients with prosthetic valves, rheumatic mitral stenosis, severe renal insufficiency (with the exception of apixaban and edoxaban), and advanced liver disease.

MAT

Multifocal atrial tachycardia (MAT) is mainly diagnosed by ECG criteria of an irregular atrial rate > 100 bpm with P waves of at least 3 distinct morphologies.

MAT is usually seen in patients with pulmonary disease and can be a result of theophylline use. MAT can also be caused by very low K^+ or Mg^{2+}.

Therapy is directed at underlying illness. If medications are deemed necessary, calcium channel blockers or amiodarone might be useful. Digoxin is of no use in MAT! It can actually worsen it, in addition to causing digoxin-toxic arrhythmias.

SVT

Supraventricular tachycardia (SVT) refers to narrow QRS complex tachycardias originating above the ventricles. It is key to recognize the presence and position of P waves in comparison to QRS:

If no P wave is seen (buried in QRS) or is seen at the end of the QRS (very short R-P interval), the patient has AV node reentrant tachycardia (AVNRT). Representing 60–70% of regular SVT, AVNRT is the most common reentrant tachycardia.

If a P wave is somewhere in the ST segment (short R-P interval), AV reentrant tachycardia ([AVRT]; 20–30% of regular SVT) should be considered.

If a P wave is seen after a T wave (long R-P interval), atrial tachycardia (10% of regular SVT) is most likely the diagnosis.

In acute management of SVT, treatment options include vagal maneuvers, beta-blockers, adenosine, or calcium channel blockers.

Most SVTs are due to a reentrant mechanism. Again, the most common SVT is AVNRT. Rate is typically 150–250 bpm (although it can be slower or faster). Radiofrequency ablation is highly successful and can be considered equally with medical therapy as 1st line long-term therapy. Situations where ablation is preferred include hemodynamic instability, severe symptoms, failed medical therapy, public safety (e.g., pilots and bus drivers), and clear patient preference. If medical therapy is chosen, beta-blockers, calcium channel blockers, or digoxin are 1st line options, followed by antiarrhythmic drugs (typically flecainide or propafenone if there is no structural heart disease).

WPW

In Wolff-Parkinson-White (WPW; a.k.a. preexcitation syndrome), the PR interval is < 0.12 seconds due to a delta wave and symptoms of tachycardia. Total QRS is > 0.12 seconds because of the fusion between the impulse that uses the normal conduction system and that which uses the abnormal (accessory) pathway, which bypasses the AV node. This bypass tract (accessory pathway) conducts faster than the AV node; therefore, a portion of the electrical current reaches the ventricle sooner (the delta wave on the ECG) and preexcites the ventricle—hence the alternative name preexcitation syndrome. Occasionally, the accessory pathway is concealed and the delta wave is not visible. An unusual cause of WPW can involve Ebstein anomaly of the tricuspid valve (more under Ebstein Anomaly on page 13-43).

The spectrum of arrhythmias related to WPW includes orthodromic AVRT (narrow QRS complex regular tachycardia, which uses the AV node antegrade and accessory pathway node retrograde), antidromic AVRT (wide QRS complex regular tachycardia, which uses the accessory pathway node antegrade and AV node retrograde), and atrial fibrillation (irregularly irregular wide QRS complex tachycardia using antegrade accessory pathway conduction).

Treatment of accessory pathways: Many patients have a completely asymptomatic accessory pathway and no dysrhythmias. Patients with an accessory pathway and symptoms of tachycardia (a.k.a. WPW syndrome) can be treated with vagal maneuvers, adenosine, or calcium channel blockers—same as any SVT! In these cases, the impulses are moving down the normal conduction system and returning via the accessory pathway to complete the circuit. Never treat acute A-fib in WPW with digoxin, verapamil, or beta-blockers. Although verapamil and digoxin increase the refractory period in the AV node, they can preferentially enhance conduction down the accessory pathway and precipitate ventricular fibrillation (V-fib).

Instead, treat acute A-fib in WPW with IV procainamide, ibutilide, or amiodarone. Shock if there are any signs of hemodynamic deterioration in any WPW tachyarrhythmia; especially watch those with ventricular rate > 285 bpm because they are at greatest risk of V-fib.

Definitive treatment is by electrophysiology-guided radiofrequency ablation of the accessory pathway. Without treatment, WPW syndrome carries a low but definitive risk of sudden death.

VENTRICULAR ARRHYTHMIAS

PREVIEW | REVIEW

- On an ECG, PVCs are often followed by what type of pause?
- VT is defined as ≥ 3 sequential PVCs occurring at what bpm?
- List the ECG criteria consistent with VT.
- With which type of tachycardia should you never use verapamil?
- ICDs are recommended for primary prevention in which situations with ischemic and nonischemic cardiomyopathy?
- Which antiarrhythmic drugs can cause TdP by prolonging the QT interval?
- What is the treatment for *torsades de pointes*?

PVCs

Premature ventricular contractions (PVCs) often have a compensatory pause; that is, they do not reset the sinoatrial node, and the time between the sinus beats that are on either side of the PVC = 2 basic RR intervals.

Asymptomatic, simple PVCs do not need to be treated if LV function is normal and there is no structural heart disease. Without treatment, most patients have spontaneous resolution or improvement. If you do attempt treatment (beta-blockers are 1st line), the PVCs should decrease by 80% for the treatment to be considered successful—otherwise, stop treatment. Simple PVCs occur beyond the T wave, are uniform, and have constant coupling (reentrant).

Complex PVCs (pairs, triplets) also do not need to be treated if the patient is asymptomatic and has no heart disease!

If a patient has had an MI and has an ejection fraction of < 40%, frequent PVCs (> 10/hour) indicate a high risk of sudden cardiac death—especially if they are sequential.

Ventricular Tachycardia

ECG Findings

Study tip: Now is a good time to review ventricular tachycardias vs. aberrant conduction. Refer to Arrhythmias on page 13-76.

Ventricular tachycardia (VT) is defined as ≥ 3 sequential QRS complexes of ventricular origin at a rate of ≥ 100 bpm. Based on duration and symptoms, VT can be defined as nonsustained (duration of < 30 seconds) or sustained (duration of > 30 seconds, or causes hemodynamic collapse in < 30 seconds). VT can be monomorphic or polymorphic.

Monomorphic VT is generally regular in rate and appearance. It needs to be differentiated from SVT with aberrant conduction, bundle branch block, pacing, and QRS changes due to severe hyperkalemia. The majority of patients with monomorphic VT have structural heart disease (particularly ischemic heart disease). Idiopathic VT occurs in otherwise structurally normal hearts and has much better prognosis. The most common idiopathic VT is right ventricular outflow tract (RVOT) VT.

Know the ECG criteria indicative of VT:

- AV dissociation
- Fusion and capture beats
- Northwest axis (between –90° and +/–180°; see Figure 13-22 on page 13-70)
- Positive or negative concordance in precordial leads (Recall concordance is when QRS complexes in all 6 precordial leads are monophasic with the same polarity.)
- Absence of rS complex in all precordial leads
- If rS is present, r to S time > 100 msec
- QRS width of > 140 msec with a RBBB
- QRS width > 160 msec with a LBBB

If a patient with a history of structural heart disease develops a wide QRS complex regular tachycardia, VT is significantly more likely than SVT.

VT can also be bidirectional, with the complexes alternating in direction; this is usually due to digitalis intoxication but also can be seen post-MI and in a relatively rare genetic condition called catecholaminergic polymorphic ventricular tachycardia.

Polymorphic VT generally has an irregular ventricular rate and polymorphic QRS morphology. QRS complexes appear to twist around an isoelectric axis. Duration of polymorphic VT is typically brief; however, it can be sustained and can degenerate into V-fib. It can occur in patients with prolonged QT interval (*torsades de pointes*) or in patients with normal QT interval (usually in the setting of ischemia/MI).

Treatment

For sustained monomorphic VT, do the following:

- Stable: Give IV amiodarone.
- Hemodynamically compromised: shock (electrical cardioversion)
- Unstable and refractory to electrical cardioversion: Give IV amiodarone/procainamide.
- VT with acute MI: Most use amiodarone 1st. IV lidocaine can be useful.

For sustained polymorphic VT, do the same as monomorphic, except:

- IV beta-blockers if ischemia is suspected or cannot be excluded
- IV amiodarone, as long as there is no prolonged QT
- Urgent cath if ischemia is suspected

CARDIOLOGY

• Assess for *torsades de pointes* (See *Torsades de Pointes.*)

Never use verapamil with any wide-complex tachycardias in the emergency setting. 30% of those with ventricular tachycardia will rapidly deteriorate!

RVOT VT can be terminated acutely with adenosine. Beta-blockers or calcium channel blockers (CCBs) can be used for long-term management. Remember, you generally do not want to use CCBs for wide-complex tachycardias.

Implantable Cardioverter-Defibrillators

Implantable cardioverter-defibrillators (ICDs) can be used for secondary (after event occurs) or primary prevention.

The following are Class I indications for ICDs from the 2008 ACC/AHA Device Therapy Guidelines and 2012 Focused Update:

• Patients who are survivors of cardiac arrest due to VF or who have hemodynamically unstable sustained VT, after evaluation has excluded any completely reversible causes
• Patients with structural heart disease and spontaneous sustained VT (> 30 seconds), whether hemodynamically stable or unstable
• Patients with syncope of undetermined origin with clinically relevant, hemodynamically significant sustained VT or VF induced at electrophysiologic study
• Patients with LVEF ≤ 35% due to prior MI who are at least 40 days post-MI and are in the NYHA functional Class II or III; also, LVEF < 30% and in the NYHA functional Class I
• Patients with nonischemic dilated cardiomyopathy (DCM) who have an LVEF ≤ 35% and who are in the NYHA functional Class II or III
• Patients with nonsustained VT due to prior MI, LVEF ≤ 40%, and inducible VF or sustained VT at electrophysiologic study

Torsades de Pointes

Know this topic! *Torsades de pointes* is a common type of polymorphic VT. It occurs in patients with prolonged QT interval (congenital or acquired). Acquired forms are most often drug induced.

Drugs that can cause *torsades de pointes* are:

• Class Ia antiarrhythmic drugs (e.g., quinidine, procainamide, disopyramide)
• Class III antiarrhythmics (e.g., sotalol, dofetilide, amiodarone)
• Haloperidol and tricyclic antidepressants
• Antibiotics (e.g., macrolides)
• Antihistamines (e.g., astemizole, terfenadine)
• Antifungal agents (e.g., ketoconazole)

Torsades de pointes can occur in association with very low K^+ or Mg^{2+}, and bradycardia can promote it in patients with prolonged QT.

Treat *torsades de pointes* with:

• DC cardioversion for sustained episodes
• Mg^{2+} sulfate 2–4 grams IV over 10–15 minutes
• Correction of hypokalemia
• Correction of bradycardia (isoproterenol or pacing)
• Never treat with Class Ia or Class III antiarrhythmic drugs.

To prevent recurrence of TdP: 1) discontinue any offending medications, 2) prevent bradycardia with isoproterenol or overdrive pacing, and 3) supplement K^+ and Mg^{2+}.

Nonsustained Ventricular Tachycardia

Nonsustained ventricular tachycardia (NSVT) is defined as asymptomatic VT (> 3 sequential PVCs with HR > 100 bpm) lasting for < 30 seconds.

NSVT increases risk for death in patients with heart disease, particularly ischemic cardiomyopathy. NSVT patients are at risk of sustained VT and sudden death when:

• they have ischemic cardiomyopathy (LVEF < 40%), or
• sustained VT can be induced at electrophysiologic testing.

These patients benefit from ICD implantation.

Patients with NSVT without structural heart disease have good prognosis, and they do not require further management.

PACEMAKERS

Permanent pacing is indicated for patients with:

• symptomatic bradycardia,
• sinus node dysfunction (sick sinus syndrome), and/or
• AV conduction problems.

In the absence of symptoms, permanent pacing should be strongly considered for patients with complete heart block and advanced (i.e., not Wenckebach) Type 2 second-degree AV block (particularly with wide QRS).

The most common pacemaker (Table 13-11) is **DDD**, which stands for **d**ual-chamber paced, **d**ual-chamber sensed, and **d**ual response to sensing: triggered and inhibited. Most clinicians use DDD unless the patient is in chronic, slow atrial fibrillation. The DDD is the most physiologic and provides better exercise tolerance.

Pacemaker syndrome (associated lightheadedness and/or syncope) can occur with single-chamber ventricular pacing and is commonly cured by dual-chamber (DDD) pacers, which restore the atrial kick.

Pacemaker-mediated tachycardia can occur when paced ventricular complexes are sensed by the atrial lead and then trigger subsequent ventricular paced beats; this cycle can continue indefinitely.

ANTIARRHYTHMIC THERAPY

PREVIEW | REVIEW

- How long do you have to wait for an antiarrhythmic to reach steady-state therapeutic levels?

- When is it not okay to use verapamil? When is it okay?

- Which antiarrhythmic drug can cause lupus?

- Name the side effects seen with amiodarone.

- Which test is the best indicator of digoxin toxicity?

- For which condition is the treatment of choice radiofrequency ablation?

Drugs

Overview

Class I: Sodium channel blockers that slow electrical conduction in the heart

Ia: quinidine, procainamide, disopyramide—slow conduction velocity, prolong action potential duration, and can prolong QT interval

Ib: lidocaine, tocainide, mexiletine, phenytoin—shorten action potential duration slightly with no significant QT prolongation

Ic: flecainide and propafenone—slow conduction velocity without effect on potential duration or QT interval

Class II: beta-blockers—decrease heart rate and blood pressure by blocking impulses that can cause irregular heart rhythm and decreasing hormonal effects (e.g., adrenaline) on the heart

Class III: amiodarone, sotalol, and the relatively new agents dofetilide and dronedarone—prolong the action potential by potassium channel blockade. These agents can cause QT prolongation. Note: See side effects of dronedarone under Major Side Effects of AADs on page 13-54.

Class IV: calcium channel blockers, especially verapamil and diltiazem—slow inward current. They decrease heart rate and blood pressure like Class II.

Notes:

- With antiarrhythmic drugs (AADs), always wait 4–5 half-lives before determining whether a drug is effective.

- All AADs have a proarrhythmic potential.

- Per the 1989 and 1992 CAST studies, there is evidence that Ic AADs decrease survival in patients with ventricular arrhythmias that occur post-MI.

- The only AAD that has a proven mortality benefit after an ST-elevation MI is a beta-blocker.

- Mexiletine is effective in most patients who respond to lidocaine.

- Quinidine increases digoxin levels.

Digoxin and Adenosine

Digoxin is not in the above classes of antiarrhythmics, but it has antiarrhythmic effects and occasionally is used for this. Digoxin works by inhibiting membrane ATPase. It increases contractility and slows AV conduction and HR. Remember that digoxin is usually reserved for treating severe heart failure.

Adenosine is also not in the above groups. Adenosine slows conduction in the AV node and is used for conversion of SVT (AV node reentry) to normal sinus rhythm. It also induces coronary artery vasodilation and is used in cardiac perfusion imaging. It depresses LV function, but it has such a short half-life, it can be used even in patients with decreased LV function.

Notes on Verapamil

Avoid verapamil with:

- A-fib or atrial flutter occurring in WPW

- Wide-complex tachycardias

- Beta-blockers—relative contraindication because they are both negative chronotropes and negative inotropes

- Patients with asymptomatic hypertrophic cardiomyopathy (HCM)

- Patients with obstructive HCM in the setting of systemic hypotension or severe dyspnea at rest

Table 13-11: Permanent Pacemakers — The North American Society of Pacing and Electrophysiology / British Pacing and Electrophysiology Group Generic (NBG Code) Pacemaker
1st letter = chamber(s) paced—**V/A/D** (**v**entricle, **a**trium, or **d**ual [V + A])
2nd letter = chamber(s) sensed—**V/A/D/O** (**v**entricle, **a**trium, **d**ual [V + A], or **n**one)
3rd letter = mode(s) of response—**T/I/D/O** (**t**riggered, **i**nhibited, **d**ual [T + I], or **n**one)
4th letter = programmability—**P/M/C/R/O** (**p**rogrammable rate and output, **m**ultiprogrammable, **c**ommunicating, **r**ate-modulated, or **n**one)
5th letter = arrhythmia control—**P/S/D/O** (**p**acing, **s**hock, **d**ual [P + S], or **n**one)

Okay to use verapamil in these cases:

- To control the ventricular response to A-fib or atrial flutter in an otherwise healthy heart
- MAT
- SVT (2nd choice after adenosine)
- Symptomatic treatment in HCM (but look above regarding avoiding verapamil in HCM)
- Severe, concentric LVH
- Hypertension

Major Side Effects of AADs

Know! All AADs are, by their nature, arrhythmogenic. Especially remember the following:

Class Ia:

- Quinidine: prolongs the QRS complex and the QT interval—occasionally leading to *torsades de pointes*, diarrhea, and (rarely) autoimmune thrombocytopenic purpura. Cinchonism (hearing loss, tinnitus, and psychosis) may occur.
- Procainamide: prolongs QT and QRS but also causes blood dyscrasias, such as agranulocytosis, neutropenia, and thrombocytopenia, in ~ 0.5%. It also causes drug-induced lupus and must be used with caution in HF patients because it has a mild myocardial depressive effect.
- Disopyramide: prolongs QT and QRS and can cause *torsades de pointes*. It is anticholinergic and vagolytic, so it causes urinary retention, constipation, and dry mouth. Disopyramide has a negative inotropic effect, so avoid in patients with HF. This drug is occasionally used in patients with hypertrophic obstructive cardiomyopathy (HOCM).
- Because quinidine and disopyramide prolong both the QRS and QT intervals, avoid them in patients with 2nd or 3rd degree heart block.

Class Ib: lidocaine—seizures

Class II: Beta-blockers can cause decreased libido and impotence. They must be tapered slowly; stopping a beta-blocker abruptly can precipitate angina.

Class III: All of them can cause prolonged QT, QRS, and *torsades de pointes*:

- Amiodarone is the most effective, but also, due to the extremely high iodine content, it is the most toxic antiarrhythmic drug. It causes corneal deposits in 98% of patients(!) as well as hyper/ hypothyroidism, pulmonary fibrosis, gray skin, and sun sensitivity, but not hematologic changes. Mild transaminitis occurs in 25% of patients; LFTs should be monitored and amiodarone stopped if LFTs increase more than 2-fold. Pulmonary fibrosis from amiodarone can be severe and is fatal 10% of the time. It ordinarily occurs in the 1st year of treatment. It tends to occur only in older patients (> 40 years old) and in those with low carbon monoxide diffusing capacity. Pulmonary fibrosis is unlikely to develop on a maintenance dosage of < 200 mg/day. Amiodarone also causes a less common acute form of pulmonary toxicity. Again, amiodarone: hepatic toxicity, extremely long half-life (40–55 days), hyper/ hypothyroidism, gray skin, pulmonary fibrosis.
- Dronedarone: recommended by the 2014 ACC/ AHA/HRS Guidelines and the 2016 ESC Guidelines as a 1st line agent for recurrent paroxysmal or persistent A-fib without LVH or HF. Contraindicated in patients with Class IV HF or decompensated HF within 4 weeks, especially if EF is < 35% (2× increase in HF mortality in these patients, per a 2008 study).
- Dofetilide: works by blocking the cardiac ion channel carrying the delayed rectifier K+ current (I_{Kr}). It is used to treat highly symptomatic A-fib and can be used in patients with CAD and HF. Dofetilide must be started as an inpatient by approved prescribers and is renally dosed. It can cause significant QT prolongation requiring dose reduction or discontinuation. Do not use dofetilide with the following medications: cimetidine, verapamil, ketoconazole, trimethoprim, prochlorperazine, megestrol, or any form of hydrochlorothiazide; these agents can increase the activity of the CYP3A4 liver enzyme and increase dofetilide levels.

Digitalis toxicity is more likely to occur in elderly patients and in those with low K+, low Mg^{2+}, or low pO_2 (low, low, low) and impaired renal function. Symptoms of digoxin toxicity are nonspecific and can include confusion, nausea, vomiting, vague abdominal pain, or visual changes. The toxicity of digoxin is best determined by changes in the ECG, not by blood levels. The most common ECG changes are bradycardia and prolonged PR interval. Note: In patients with chronic atrial fibrillation, the development of a regular pulse could be a manifestation of digoxin toxicity.

Patients with digoxin toxicity should receive digoxin-binding antibodies to remove it from the circulation. They should be monitored in an intensive care setting.

Electrophysiologic Testing

Electrophysiologic (EP) studies are used to identify and characterize SVTs and VTs, often as a precursor to radiofrequency ablation.

Radiofrequency Ablation

Radiofrequency ablation is the treatment of choice for WPW syndrome.

It is also used for the following if the patient prefers it over drug therapy or the condition is not responsive to meds:

- AVNRT
- Atrial tachycardia
- Atrial flutter
- Idiopathic VT

Radiofrequency ablation is also used to treat atrial fibrillation by ablating a focal source of A-fib or by destroying the AV node and placing a ventricular pacemaker.

SYNCOPE

PREVIEW | REVIEW

- What is the most common cause of syncope?

- Explain how you approach the diagnostic workup in a patient with probable neurocardiogenic (vasovagal) syncope.

- What are the tests used to work up high-risk patients with syncope?

Syncope is sudden transient loss of consciousness with associated loss of postural tone and spontaneous recovery. It is important to differentiate syncope from other types of loss of consciousness, such as seizures or narcolepsy. Classifications of syncope:

Neurally mediated (reflex) syncope symptoms include dizziness, lightheadedness, and fatigue, with prodromal features such as diaphoresis, pallor, palpitations, nausea, hyperventilation, and yawning. Myoclonic jerks can occur when the patient is unconscious, sometimes causing confusion with seizure.

Subtypes of neurally mediated syncope:

- Vasovagal syncope, as in the common faint, is the most common cause of syncope. It is triggered by intense emotion, pain, prolonged standing, alcohol, or heat exposure. Vasovagal episodes are typically preceded by a prodrome that includes nausea, vomiting, flushing, hot flashes, and diaphoresis. Extremely elderly patients may not have a classic prodrome.

- Situational reflex syncope is brought on by specific scenarios such as cough, micturition, straining, or squatting. These triggers provoke reflex vasodilation and bradycardia leading to syncope.

- Carotid sinus hypersensitivity may be responsible for up to 40% of falls in the elderly and is diagnosed with a pause > 3 seconds during carotid sinus massage (CSM). Absolute contraindications to CSM include MI within 3 months and TIA/CVA within 3 months. Relative contraindications to CSM include previous VT/VF or carotid bruit.

Arrhythmia: bradycardia, SVT, or VT

Orthostatic hypotension: Syncope from orthostatic hypotension can be caused by volume depletion or autonomic dysfunction. With volume depletion, the blood pressure drops and the HR rises with standing. Syncope and orthostatic hypotension 2° autonomic dysfunction causes symptoms with no increase in the patient's heart rate with standing or during the vertical phase of tilt-table testing.

To treat autonomic dysfunction, try nonpharmacologic therapy 1st (e.g., support hose and increased dietary salt). Medications include midodrine and fludrocortisone. Midodrine is a prodrug for desglymidodrine, an alpha-agonist that stimulates the alpha-adrenergic receptors of both arteriolar and venous vessels. Fludrocortisone, a mineralocorticoid agonist that promotes retention of Na^+ and water, also can be used but can cause supine hypertension.

Structural heart disease: Anatomic causes include depressed EF (causing VT/VF), AS, HCM, atrial myxoma, PE, pulmonary HTN, and ischemia.

Medications: Check the patient's history for new medications. Common medications causing syncope include cardiovascular, neurologic, antiparkinsonian, and antidepressant medications. Medications for BPH (prazosin, terazosin, and tamsulosin) are a classic cause of syncope. For this reason, these meds are usually given at bedtime.

A thorough history, physical exam, supine and upright blood pressure, and ECG are essential parts of the initial evaluation, followed by additional testing in selected subgroups (e.g., carotid sinus massage, echocardiogram). If the diagnosis remains uncertain, stratify the patient to determine whether the patient is at increased risk of death (typically patients with severe structural heart disease or clinical or ECG features suggesting arrhythmic syncope).

Admit high-risk patients for further workup, which can include coronary angiogram and EP study. Low-risk patients, particularly with only 1 episode of syncope, usually do not require further evaluation.

If the history is typical for vasovagal syncope, and this is the first episode in a young patient with no suspected heart disease, the patient can be reassured and sent home.

Initial measures aimed at reducing events include avoidance of both precipitating factors and volume depletion. Patients should also be taught to sit or lie down at the onset of symptoms and to initiate physical isometric maneuvers (leg-crossing and handgrip). Value of pharmacologic agents (e.g., beta-blockers, fludrocortisone, midodrine) is less certain. Frequent episodes, despite initial management, require evaluation with continuous ambulatory electrocardiography. Patients with severe cardioinhibitory response (i.e., bradycardia, prolonged PR interval, AV block) during syncope could benefit from pacemaker placement. Patients in high-risk occupations should be worked up after the 1st episode of syncope.

CARDIOMYOPATHIES

PREVIEW | REVIEW

- What are the risk factors for sudden death in patients with HCM?
- What are the 3 main medications used in the treatment of HCM?
- Which auscultatory finding is pathognomonic for constrictive pericarditis?
- What are some causes of restrictive cardiomyopathy?
- List some of the etiologies of DCM.

NOTE

There are 4 main types of cardiomyopathy: dilated, hypertrophic, restrictive, and arrythmogenic right ventricular. There is also an "unclassified" category that includes certain acquired cardiomyopathies. Always rule out ischemic cardiomyopathy with stress testing or coronary angiography.

We cover hypertensive heart disease (e.g., see Pulmonary Hypertension on page 13-68 and Right Ventricular Failure on page 13-64 and), valvular heart disease (see Valvular Heart Disease on page 13-37), and ischemic heart disease (see Angina on page 13-12) elsewhere in this section. Some guidelines consider these cardiomyopathies, but most don't.

DILATED CARDIOMYOPATHY

Patients with **dilated cardiomyopathy** (DCM) have ventricular dilation and depressed myocardial contractility in the absence of abnormal loading conditions such as hypertension or valvular disease. African Americans have nearly a 3-fold risk for developing DCM when compared to Caucasians.

The prognosis of patients with symptomatic HF and DCM is poor, with 50% mortality at 5 years. Heart failure due to dilated cardiomyopathy is treated similarly to other causes of HF (see Heart Failure, next).

Etiologies of DCM:

- Familial (e.g., noncompaction cardiomyopathy—excessively prominent trabeculae)
- Idiopathic (viral = most common)
- Obesity
- Diabetes mellitus
- Hyperthyroidism
- Acromegaly
- Tachycardia-induced
- Late hemochromatosis
- Drugs and toxins, including:
  - Alcohol
  - Cocaine
  - Cancer chemotherapy (especially anthracyclines like doxorubicin and daunorubicin)
  - Ephedra
  - Cobalt
  - Anabolic steroids
  - Chloroquine
  - Clozapine
  - Amphetamines
  - Methylphenidate
  - Catecholamines
  - Organic solvents (glue sniffer's heart)

Think Chagas disease in patients from Central and South American countries.

HYPERTROPHIC CARDIOMYOPATHY

Hypertrophic cardiomyopathy (HCM) is the most common genetic cardiovascular disease. It has an autosomal dominant pattern of inheritance and is characterized by a thickened but not dilated left ventricle (Figure 13-20) in the absence of other cardiac or systemic conditions (e.g., HTN, aortic valve stenosis). HCM is the most common cause of sudden cardiac death in young age (< 35 years of age), including competitive athletes.

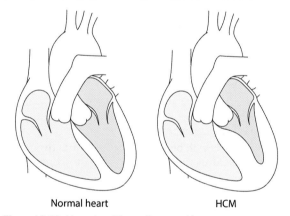

Normal heart   HCM

Figure 13-20: Hypertrophic cardiomyopathy

Patients with HCM usually present with heart failure, chest pain (typical or atypical), or syncope. They can be asymptomatic and recognized because of abnormal physical exam (e.g., murmur).

Physical exam in HCM: The patient usually has a harsh, crescendo-decrescendo systolic murmur, typically in the left 3rd space, which increases with Valsalva and decreases with sustained handgrip, squatting, and passive leg raise. There is a carotid pulse that has a brisk upstroke, but, because outflow obstruction occurs late in systole, it is bifid in 2/3 of HCM patients. The briskness of the upstroke further distinguishes it from aortic stenosis. Palpation at the apex can surprise you with a double- or triple-tap impulse. A mitral regurgitation murmur can also be heard from systolic anterior motion of the mitral valve due to a suction-like effect of the outflow obstruction.

The ECG with HCM is abnormal in > 90% of patients. Most common abnormalities include LVH, ST-T changes with sometimes-marked T wave inversion in the lateral precordial leads, and Q waves in inferior and lateral leads.

Diagnosis is with echocardiogram. Cardiac MRI can be considered if the diagnosis is uncertain or for better assessment of cardiac anatomy prior to septal ablation or surgical myectomy (see below). There is no single classic morphologic form, and virtually all possible patterns of hypertrophy have been described. Some patients have dynamic obstruction related to systolic anterior motion of the mitral valve. Left ventricular outflow tract (**LVOT**) obstruction can occur: This is called obstructive HCM. Approximately 25% of patients with HCM have a resting LV outflow gradient (> 30 mmHg).

A majority of patients with HCM have normal life expectancy with little or no disability; however, subgroups of patients are at risk for complications including sudden death, progressive heart failure, and atrial fibrillation.

Risk factors for sudden death in HCM (and potential indications for ICD):

- Septal thickness > 30 mm
- Personal history of syncope
- Family history of sudden death in 1st degree family member
- NSVT on Holter monitor
- Failure to augment systolic BP on exercise tolerance testing (< 10 mmHg increase at peak exercise)

Treatment for HCM:

- **Beta-blockers** (obstructive and nonobstructive HCM) and verapamil (obstructive HCM) improve diastolic filling by slowing heart rate.
- **Disopyramide** with beta-blockers for obstructive HCM when other drugs fail to achieve symptom control
- **IV phenylephrine** (or other pure vasoconstrictor) is recommended for treating acute hypotension in HCM patients who do not respond to IV fluids.
- **ICD placement** is recommended for HCM patients with prior documented cardiac arrest, ventricular fibrillation, or hemodynamically significant VT. ICD is also reasonable to place if there is a history of sudden cardiac death in ≥ 1 first-degree relative(s), LV wall thickness ≥ 30 mm, or ≥ 1 recent unexplained syncopal episode(s).
- **Septal reduction therapy** via open-heart surgery (septal myectomy) or percutaneous, transcatheter injection of ethanol. This reduces the obstruction in patients with severe drug-refractory symptoms and LVOT obstruction.
- **Septal myectomy** is preferred for patients with severe drug refractory heart failure symptoms (NYHA III and IV).

RESTRICTIVE CARDIOMYOPATHY

Restrictive cardiomyopathy must be differentiated from constrictive pericarditis (more under Constrictive Pericarditis on page 13-65) because the signs and symptoms can be similar (dyspnea, fatigue, and right-sided heart failure). Although constrictive pericarditis is often quickly treated with good results, restrictive cardiomyopathy is not reversible.

Arrhythmias, such as atrial fibrillation, occur early in the course of these diseases. Constrictive pericarditis is a pericardial problem; restrictive cardiomyopathy is a myocardial problem.

Causes of restrictive cardiomyopathy include amyloidosis, sarcoidosis, hemochromatosis, and lipid storage diseases.

Physical exam findings with restrictive cardiomyopathy include S_3 or S_4, mitral and/or tricuspid regurgitation, and inspiratory increase in venous pressure—i.e., Kussmaul sign. (Constrictive pericarditis will also have these findings, but in addition, a paradoxical pulse may be present [1/3 of cases]; a pericardial knock during early diastole is pathognomonic for constrictive pericarditis.) Look for pericardial calcification on chest or cardiac CT scan.

On echocardiogram, the myocardium may be thickened with a granularity that suggests an infiltrative process. Despite hypertrophy on the echocardiogram, the ECG may show normal or low voltage. Cardiac catheterization with pressure recordings can also help distinguish the 2 entities. For example, elevated filling pressure is common in restrictive cardiomyopathy but rare in constrictive pericarditis.

Thoracotomy is occasionally done to ensure that you do not miss a treatable constrictive pericarditis (which is treated with pericardiectomy).

Treat restrictive cardiomyopathy with diuretics and management of underlying etiology.

ARRHYTHMOGENIC RIGHT VENTRICULAR CARDIOMYOPATHY

ARVC is a genetic disease where heart muscle is progressively replaced by fibrous and fatty tissues, causing ventricular arrhythmias and RV wall deterioration and dysfunction.

UNCLASSIFIED CARDIOMYOPATHIES

The following are a few of the acquired cardiomyopathies that do not fall within the preceding categories.

Stress cardiomyopathy (a.k.a. takotsubo cardiomyopathy) often presents with sudden onset of chest pain that is suggestive of acute coronary syndrome. ECG typically reveals anterior ST elevations of acute myocardial infarction. However, angiography reveals normal coronaries. Left ventriculogram or echocardiogram most commonly shows apical ballooning with akinesis of the apical and distal anterior wall. There is a spade-shaped presentation

CARDIOLOGY

as well with basal akinesis and normal apical kinesis. An emotional or stressful life event may precipitate the presentation. The expression of beta receptors on the ventricular myocardium is more vulnerable to surges of epinephrine that precipitate these cases.

1/3 of these patients will recover from their LV dysfunction. 1/3 will remain the same, but the last 1/3 may have deterioration of their LV function. Patients should be treated supportively for HF (see next topic).

Peripartum cardiomyopathy in pregnant women can occur anytime from the beginning of the last trimester through the first 6 months postpartum.

Severe myocarditis can cause cardiomyopathy. Myocarditis is an inflammatory disease of the myocardium typified by infiltration of mononuclear cells in the myocardium. This inflammation is typically attributed to viral causes but may have other causes, including bacteria (e.g., *Rickettsia*, *Chlamydia*), fungi, or toxins. Myocarditis may present acutely, subacutely, or chronically with HF and depressed ejection fraction. Myocarditis should be considered in patients without risk factors for other causes of cardiomyopathy.

Troponin levels may be elevated in myocarditis, but they do not follow the typical pattern of ischemia; rather, levels are stable over time. Echocardiogram may demonstrate poor LV function but cannot differentiate myocarditis from other causes of cardiomyopathy.

Definitive diagnosis is by endomyocardial biopsy. For cases of viral myocarditis detected early, antiviral therapy can be considered. Immunosuppression and antiinflammatory therapy have had mixed results in trials and are not routinely recommended. Patients with viral myocarditis presenting with symptoms of HF should be treated with the usual guidelines-directed medical therapy.

HEART FAILURE

OVERVIEW

PREVIEW | REVIEW

- In the 2013 ACC/AHA classification, what are the 2 major types of heart failure?

Heart failure (HF) is a complex clinical syndrome resulting from any structural or functional cardiac disorder that impairs the ability of the ventricle to fill or to eject blood. Left ventricular ejection fraction (LVEF) is considered important in classification of patients with HF.

The lifetime risk of developing HF is 20% for Americans ≥ 40 years of age. African American males have the highest risk for HF and the highest 5-year mortality rate (Atherosclerosis Risk in Communities [ARIC] Study—ongoing).

The 2013 ACC/AHA definitions:

- Heart failure with reduced ejection fraction (HFrEF): EF ≤ 40%, systolic HF
- Heart failure with preserved ejection fraction (HFpEF): EF > 50%, including diastolic HF

CO is well maintained in mild HF, usually at the expense of increased left ventricular end-diastolic volume (LVEDV) and increased heart rate.

Numerous adaptations occur in response to heart failure in the peripheral circulation, kidney, skeletal muscle, and other organs. The changes contribute to the overall clinical manifestations and ultimately become maladaptive.

In response to exercise, LVEDV and plasma norepinephrine rise in patients with HF more than in controls, but the resulting CO increase does not rise in proportion to O_2 consumption—so the patient has dyspnea on exertion and is easily fatigued. The adrenergic system and the renin-angiotensin-aldosterone system play a major role in progression of heart failure and maladaptive mechanisms.

LOW-OUTPUT HF

PREVIEW | REVIEW

- Define Stage A through Stage D heart failure (ACC/AHA classification). What are the goals of therapy for each of these stages?
- What is the sequence of drugs used to treat HF based on ACC/AHA stages?
- What are the most common causes of low-output HF?
- Which factors result in a poor prognosis in HF?
- What is the sequence of events that worsens HF?
- When are beta-blockers started in the treatment of HF?
- With which type of HF do aldosterone antagonists prolong survival?
- True or false? Digoxin can be beneficial in HFrEF patients to decrease hospitalizations for HF.
- In which population is hydralazine + isosorbide dinitrate beneficial?
- True or false? Ivabradine can be beneficial in stable HF patients to decrease hospitalizations for HF.
- Which patients with chronic HF should receive anticoagulation?
- CRT is indicated for which HF patients?
- Know all drugs used for emergency treatment of severe HF!
- What does dopamine do at low doses (< 2 µg/kg/min)? At doses of 2–5 µg/kg/min?

- True or false? MCS is beneficial in selected patients with Stage D HFrEF in whom definitive management (cardiac transplantation) or cardiac recovery is anticipated or planned.

NYHA Classification

New York Heart Association (NYHA) classification of heart failure (classes and definitions) is a functional classification based on how much the patient is limited during physical activity. In clinical use, it is being superseded by the ACC/AHA classification (next). NYHA classification:

Class I: Cardiac disease but no limitation in physical activity

Class II: Slight limitation of normal physical activity (fatigue, palpitations, dyspnea, and/or angina)

Class III: Marked limitation of physical activity. Slight activity causes symptoms.

Class IV: Symptoms may be present at rest. Unable to carry on any physical activity without discomfort.

ACC / AHA Staging and Management

The 2013 ACC/AHA staging system for HF acknowledges heart failure as a progressive disorder and has goals of therapy for each stage (A through D). Know the definition, goal of therapy, and medications for each stage of HF.

Stage A HF patients are at high risk for heart failure but have no structural heart disease or symptoms of HF. This stage includes patients with any of the following:

- Hypertension (HTN)
- Atherosclerotic disease
- Diabetes
- Obesity
- Metabolic syndrome
- Use of cardiotoxins (such as anthracycline)
- Family history of cardiomyopathy.

So yes, you read this right: Just having HTN means you have Stage A heart failure!

Goals for Stage A therapy are to treat the disorder (e.g., HTN, atherosclerotic disease) and control/avoid other risk factors that can lead to or contribute to HF, such as hyperlipidemia, obesity, diabetes mellitus, tobacco use, and known cardiotoxic agents (e.g., excess alcohol/illicit drug use). Regular physical activity is recommended in all HF patients.

Stage A drugs include ACEIs/ARBs/statins in appropriate patients.

Stage B HF patients have structural heart disease but without signs or symptoms of heart failure. This stage includes patients who have a history of a previous MI, those with LV remodeling from left ventricular hypertrophy (LVH) or low LVEF, and those with asymptomatic valvular heart disease.

Goals of Stage B therapy are to prevent HF symptoms and prevent further cardiac remodeling.

Stage B drugs are ACEIs/ARBs, beta-blockers, and statins if there is a history of MI/ACS. Use ICD if indicated and revascularization or vascular surgery as appropriate.

Stage C HF patients have structural heart disease with prior or current symptoms of HF. These are patients with structural heart disease as described above in Stage B, and who additionally have signs and symptoms of HF (e.g., dyspnea, fatigue, and decreased exercise tolerance).

Goals for Stage C therapy are symptom control, patient education, improved health-related quality of life, and prevention of hospitalization and mortality.

Stage C drugs are:

- Loop diuretics for all volume-overloaded NYHA II–IV patients
- RAAS inhibitors (ACEI or ARB or combination ARB + neprilysin inhibitor) for all patients with chronic HFrEF to reduce morbidity and mortality
- Combination ARB + neprilysin inhibitor to replace ACEI or ARB monotherapy in patients with chronic symptomatic HFrEF, to further reduce morbidity and mortality
- Hydralazine/isosorbide dinitrate for symptomatic African American NYHA III–IV patients after optimal treatment with ACEI/ARB and beta-blockers
- Aldosterone antagonist for NYHA II–IV patients (estimated GFR > 30 mL/min and K^+ < 5 mEq/L [5.00 mmol/L])
- Statins and beta-blockers as used in Stage B (i.e., if MI/ACS) and ACEIs/ARBs as used in Stage A

Use ICD and/or cardiac resynchronization therapy (CRT) if indicated and revascularization or vascular surgery as appropriate.

Stage D HF patients have marked symptoms at rest and frequent hospitalizations despite maximal medical therapy.

Goals for Stage D therapy are to control symptoms, improve health-related quality of life, reduce hospital readmissions, and establish the patient's end-of-life goals.

Stage D drugs are the same as those for Stage C.

Options for Stage D patients include consideration of "extraordinary measures"—including heart transplant, chronic inotropes, temporary or permanent mechanical circulatory support (ventricular assist devices), experimental surgery or experimental drugs—and include consideration of palliative care, hospice, and ICD deactivation.

Until definitive therapy (coronary revascularization, mechanical circulatory support, or heart transplantation) is performed or the acute precipitating problem resolves, patients with cardiogenic shock should receive temporary IV inotropic support to maintain systemic perfusion and preserve end-organ performance.

CARDIOLOGY

The most common causes of HF with reduced EF (HFrEF) are:

- Coronary artery disease (40–60%)
- Dilated cardiomyopathy (30%)
- Valvular disease (15%)
- Hypertension (10%)

HF is the most common diagnosis in hospitalized elderly patients. Only 50% of patients with HF die from actual pump failure; ~ 40% die from arrhythmias!

Determining Prognosis in HF

Factors corresponding to a worse prognosis in severe HF include:

- Lower ejection fraction
- Hyponatremia
- CKD
- Anemia
- Elevated troponin
- High brain natriuretic peptide (BNP)
- Increased width of QRS
- Persistent sinus tachycardia
- Poor functional capacity (NYHA III and IV)
- High norepinephrine and catecholamine levels

Mechanism of HF

Heart failure with reduced ejection fraction (HFrEF) results in decreased CO. This in turn causes an increased A-a O_2 difference and decreased renal perfusion. The decreased CO can be due to systolic dysfunction, diastolic dysfunction, or both. Note that diastolic dysfunction can occur with normal CO (see below). After a certain point, decreased CO from any type of HF causes decreased renal perfusion. This stimulates the release of renin, which allows the conversion of angiotensinogen to angiotensin I. Angiotensin I is converted to angiotensin II in the lungs. Angiotensin II then stimulates the secretion of aldosterone, which then causes retention of Na^+ and water, causing a greatly increased filling pressure (moving the Starling curve to the right).

Let's see if we have all of that: Low CO → low renal perfusion → high renin → high angiotensin I → high angiotensin II → high aldosterone → retention of Na^+ and water → high filling pressure → exacerbation of HF (Figure 13-21). The increased heart rate in HF is due to both an increased sympathetic tone and an increased level of catecholamines in an attempt to compensate for reduced stroke volume. The higher the catecholamine pool, the worse the prognosis.

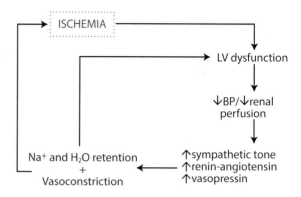

Adapted from Califf RM, Bengtson JR. NEJM. 1994 Jun 16;330(24): 1724-1730.

Figure 13-21: Spiral of worsening HF

ADH is normally released from the hypothalamus in response to increased osmotic states. In HF, inappropriate release of ADH can be seen. The high ADH state in heart failure causes hyponatremia, which is associated with poor prognosis.

Atrial (or A-type) natriuretic peptide (ANP) and brain natriuretic peptide ([BNP]; a.k.a. B-type natriuretic peptide) are released from the heart myocytes; the release is stimulated by stretching of the atrium (for ANP and BNP) and the ventricle (for BNP). ANP and BNP increase excretion of Na^+ and water, cause vasodilation, and inhibit the effects of aldosterone. These peptides offset the effects of renin, angiotensin, and ADH but cannot antagonize them adequately.

In severe heart failure, the BNP increases 20–100-fold. High levels of these peptides (especially BNP) correlate directly with a poor prognosis in HF. BNP is also elevated in restrictive cardiomyopathy but not constrictive pericarditis and is used to differentiate between these disorders.

In ~ 50% of patients with HF, the ejection fraction (HFpEF; formerly known as diastolic dysfunction) is preserved. Myocardial ischemia, severe concentric LVH, HCM, and diabetic cardiomyopathy cause diastolic dysfunction, at least initially. With diastolic dysfunction, the CO is often normal; HF develops from increased filling pressure (from decreased relaxation due to increased stiffness). So the problem is not that the ventricle is not squeezing enough, but rather that it is not relaxing enough. This is reflected in elevated left and right end-diastolic pressure (LVEDP and RVEDP), tachycardia, and an S_4.

Treatment for HF

General Measures

See ACC / AHA Staging and Management on page 13-59 for treatment according to ACC/AHA stage. Exercise training in patients with stable chronic HF can result in an 11% reduction in combined all-cause death or hospitalization (2009 HF-ACTION trial). We will now discuss the individual drugs and how they affect/improve survival in heart failure.

(Note: In our discussion, the term class refers to NYHA classification; the term stage refers to the ACC/AHA classification.)

Pharmacologic management of low-output heart failure is aimed at reducing ventricular preload and afterload and diminishing, inhibiting, and/or antagonizing neuro-hormonal vasoconstrictor activation. This contrasts with historical treatment strategies, which aimed to directly increase cardiac contractility.

The optimal treatment of HF aggressively addresses the major risk factors, including hypertension, diabetes, obesity, metabolic syndrome, hyperlipidemia, and coronary artery disease (CAD). Use therapies that promote regression of LVH or reverse remodeling of the dilated heart; these include inhibitors of catecholamines and the renin-angiotensin-aldosterone pathway.

ACE Inhibitors and ARBs

Angiotensin-converting enzyme inhibitors (ACEIs; e.g., captopril, enalapril, lisinopril, benazepril, fosinopril, quinapril, ramipril) are 1st line therapy. ACEIs block formation of angiotensin II. They decrease systemic vascular resistance, pulmonary capillary wedge pressure, right atrial pressure, and end-diastolic and end-systolic dimensions; and they improve cardiac performance, as evidenced by increased CO and stroke volume and by improved fractional shortening, as determined by echocardiography. Hence, they decrease tachycardia due to HF. They also decrease the incidence of ventricular arrhythmia and prolong survival. In addition, they reverse the remodeling in the myocytes that causes progression of heart failure.

Angiotensin II receptor blockers (ARBs) block the effect of angiotensin II. ARBs may be used in place of ACEIs (if ACEI-intolerant) and are equally effective (the 2 are commonly grouped in discussion as ACEIs/ARBs). ARBs are often given when patients develop refractory cough on ACEIs. Do not use ACEIs and ARBs together!

Per the 2017 AHA/ACC Focused Update on the 2013 Guidelines for the Management of Heart Failure, inhibition of the RAAS system with ACEIs or ARBs or ARB + neprilysin inhibitor (e.g., sacubitril/valsartan) is recommended for all patients with chronic heart failure with reduced ejection fraction to reduce morbidity and mortality. This newer class of drugs, angiotensin receptor-neprilysin inhibitors (ARNIs), inhibits neprilysin, an enzyme that degrades natriuretic peptides and other vasoactive peptides.

Monitor patients on ACEIs/ARBs for renal impairment and hyperkalemia. Important side effects include angioedema and acute renal insufficiency in patients with bilateral renal artery stenosis. ACEIs/ARBs are contraindicated in pregnancy.

Commonly used ARBs:

- Candesartan (Atacand)
- Valsartan (Diovan)
- Irbesartan (Avapro)
- Olmesartan (Benicar)
- Eprosartan (Teveten)
- Losartan (Cozaar)
- Telmisartan (Micardis)

Candesartan and valsartan are preferred agents in ACE-intolerant patients since they have the strongest trial data supporting their use.

Beta-Blockers

Beta-blockers are standard heart failure treatment. In HF, the sympathetic nervous system is overstimulated. This raises norepinephrine levels, which can cause cardiac remodeling, lead to arrhythmias, and increase mortality risk. Mortality is clearly improved by carvedilol (~ 65% relative risk reduction), metoprolol succinate (~ 66%), and bisoprolol (~ 35%). They are indicated to reduce morbidity and mortality in patients with HFrEF and current or prior symptoms.

Previously, it was taught that starting these drugs while patients are decompensated is contraindicated. The 2013 ACCF/AHA Guidelines for the Management of Heart Failure recommend initiation of beta-blockade at any stage of heart failure, after an ACEI has been initiated. 3 beta-blockers are recommended for the treatment of systolic heart failure: carvedilol, metoprolol succinate, and bisoprolol. Carvedilol is a nonselective beta-blocker that also has some alpha-blocker effect. Extended-release metoprolol succinate and bisoprolol are beta-one selective beta-blockers and are dosed once daily. Use beta-blockers in conjunction with ACE inhibitors in Class I–IV heart failure.

Diuretics

Give loop diuretics if needed for volume control (i.e., to decrease edema and pulmonary congestion) during Stage C therapy. Remember: Therapy with ACEIs/ARBs and beta-blockers should begin before patients even have symptoms.

Diuretics are effective in treating volume overload in both HF with reduced EF and HF with preserved EF. Loop diuretics have no mortality benefit, unlike ACEIs/ARBs, beta-blockers, and aldosterone antagonists.

Promptly treat HF patients admitted with significant fluid overload with IV loop diuretics. In those already receiving outpatient loop diuretics, the initial IV dose should be more than their chronic oral daily dose and be given as either intermittent boluses or continuous infusion. Adjust diuretic dose for symptom relief, to reduce volume, and to avoid hypotension.

If a loop diuretic given 2× daily in doses equivalent to furosemide 200 mg/day is inadequate, a thiazide or thiazide-like diuretic (e.g., metolazone) can be added, which results in a synergistic effect. This combination can result in severe hypokalemia, so close monitoring is necessary.

CARDIOLOGY

Aldosterone antagonists (a.k.a. mineralocorticoid antagonists) reduce morbidity and prolong survival in NYHA II–IV and with reduced EF < 35%:

- **Spironolactone** decreased mortality by 30% at 24 months in patients with Class IV HF or Class III with a history of Class IV in the previous 6 months (1999 RALES trial).
- **Eplerenone** is similar to spironolactone but with greater specificity for the mineralocorticoid receptor—thus fewer side effects (e.g., gynecomastia). Eplerenone decreased mortality by 15% at 16 months in patients with recent MI, EF < 40%, and evidence of HF or diabetes mellitus (2003 EPHESUS trial). Monitor patients closely for hyperkalemia.
- NYHA Class II patients benefit from aldosterone antagonists only if they have prior HF hospitalizations and elevated plasma natriuretic peptides.

More notes on diuretics:

- **Thiazides** block Na^+ and Cl^- resorption in the distal convoluted tubule. Examples are hydrochlorothiazide and metolazone.
- **Furosemide, bumetanide, torsemide,** and **ethacrynic acid** are loop diuretics. They block Na^+ resorption in the ascending limb of the loop of Henle. Bumetanide can also have some action on the proximal tubule.
- **Triamterene** and **amiloride** act by blocking Na^+ reabsorption in the cortical collecting tubule. Like the aldosterone antagonists, they are potassium-sparing diuretics: they cause hyperkalemia, not hypokalemia.

With azotemia, use spironolactone or triamterene with caution because these can cause hyperkalemia; thiazides are effective for blood pressure but not edema. For edema, furosemide works best. Much more information on diuretics is in Nephrology & Urology, Book 2.

Digoxin

Digoxin decreases hospitalizations for HF in patients with HFrEF. It is started after the above therapies are established if the patient is still symptomatic. In HF, digoxin appears to reset the baroreceptors and dampen the renin-angiotensin effects; it has very little inotropic effect. It also is used to control the ventricular rate in patients with HF and atrial fibrillation. Digoxin has no mortality benefit. Many drugs affect digoxin metabolism; see Table 13-12 for drugs that increase digoxin levels.

Table 13-12: Drugs That Increase Digoxin Levels
Alprazolam
Amiodarone
Macrolides and tetracycline antibiotics
Cyclosporine
Diphenoxylate or propantheline (decrease bowel motility)
Indomethacin
Itraconazole (antifungal)
Omeprazole
Propafenone (Class Ic antiarrhythmic)
Quinine
Spironolactone

Nitrates

Nitrates are occasionally used next (good venodilator, moderate arterial dilator). Remember the nightly 6-hour nitrate-free window to prevent tolerance (discussed under Antianginal Drugs on page 13-13).

With ventricular failure, patients can have increased systemic (peripheral) vascular resistance (SVR) with a normal or low BP, and they still benefit from an arteriolar vasodilator.

Hydralazine and Isosorbide Dinitrate

Hydralazine is an afterload reducer (arterial vasodilator); it also increases heart rate. Hydralazine is frequently used with nitrates to get the added benefit of decreased preload.

The combination of hydralazine and isosorbide dinitrate is recommended to reduce morbidity and mortality in African Americans with NYHA III–IV HFrEF, as adjunctive therapy to ACEIs (or ARBs) and beta-blockers (2004 A-HeFT). The combination can also be helpful in patients with current or prior symptomatic HFrEF who cannot be given ACEIs/ARBs (e.g., drug intolerance, hypotension, renal insufficiency).

Ivabradine

Ivabradine, approved by the FDA in 2015, reduces hospitalizations from worsening HF.

The 2017 ACC/AHA Heart Failure Focused Update recommends consideration of ivabradine in patients who:

- have stable, chronic HF (EF ≤ 35%) with symptoms (NYHA Class II–III),
- are in sinus rhythm at a rate of ≥ 70 bpm, and
- are taking maximally tolerated doses of beta-blockers.

Valsartan / Sacubitril

The 2017 ACC/AHA Guidelines have added this combination pill to the armamentarium for HF. In patients with HFrEF who were treated with ACEIs and subsequently changed to valsartan/sacubitril, the risk of death and rehospitalization decreased.

Anticoagulation

For patients with chronic HF and permanent, persistent, or paroxysmal atrial fibrillation plus an additional risk factor for cardioembolic stroke (Hx HTN, DM, previous stroke/TIA, or ≥ 75 years of age), give individualized anticoagulation (warfarin, dabigatran, apixaban, or rivaroxaban).

Clinical practice guidelines—the 2013 ACCF/AHA Guidelines for the Management of Heart Failure and the 2017 ESC Guidelines for the Management of Acute Myocardial Infarction—also recommend anticoagulation in HF patients with a cardioembolic source (history of systemic or pulmonary embolism, or a mobile left ventricular thrombus). In the absence of above-mentioned indications, anticoagulation is not recommended in patients with HFrEF.

Decompensated HF patients admitted to hospital should receive VTE prophylaxis.

Other Therapy

The 2013 ACCF/AHA Guidelines for the Management of Heart Failure recommend implantable cardioverter-defibrillator (ICD) for primary prevention of sudden cardiac death, and to reduce total mortality, in patients with nonischemic dilated cardiomyopathy or ischemic heart disease who are ≥ 40 days post-MI and either

- EF ≤ 35% and NYHA II/III symptoms on optimal medical therapy or
- EF ≤ 30% and NYHA I symptoms on optimal medical therapy.

ICD candidates must also have an expected survival > 1 year. See Implantable Cardioverter-Defibrillators on page 13-24 for Class I indications for ICD therapy.

Ventricular dyssynchrony is caused by electrical disturbances that cause the heart to pump blood in an inefficient way. It is suggested by severe HF (NYHA III/IV), severely decreased ejection fraction (LVEF ≤ 35%), and QRS exhibiting LBBB configuration with QRS duration ≥ 120 msec.

Cardiac resynchronization therapy (CRT) involves pacing the right and left ventricles and is recommended for patients with EF ≤ 35%, sinus rhythm, LBBB with a QRS duration of ≥ 150 msec, and NYHA II, III, or ambulatory with NYHA IV symptoms despite optimal medical therapy. This is per the 2013 ACCF/AHA Guidelines for the Management of Heart Failure.

Emergency Treatment for Severe HF

Know: With severe ventricular failure, patients may require short-term treatment with inotropes (dopamine, dobutamine, and milrinone).

Dobutamine is an inotropic agent that does not have the vasoconstrictor activity of dopamine and actually has some vasodilatory effects.

Milrinone is an inotropic/vasodilator agent with phosphodiesterase inhibitor activity (peak III cAMP—an isoenzyme of cAMP). It is indicated for short-term IV treatment of HF. It does not cause thrombocytopenia (unlike amrinone) or tachycardia.

Dopamine:

- At < 2 µg/kg/min dopamine stimulates the dopaminergic receptors and causes mesenteric dilation.
- At 2–5 µg/kg/min, it has a predominantly beta-agonist effect (positive inotropy) and increases renal perfusion.
- At > 10 µg/kg/min, it mainly has an alpha-agonist effect and causes vasoconstriction. Generally, never use > 10 µg/kg/min!

Mechanical circulatory support (MCS) is beneficial in selected patients with Stage D HFrEF in whom definitive management (e.g., cardiac transplantation) or cardiac recovery is anticipated or planned. Nondurable MCS (percutaneous and extracorporeal ventricular assist devices) are reasonable as a bridge to recovery/decision in carefully selected HFrEF patients who have acute, profound hemodynamic compromise. Durable MCS can be used to prolong survival for carefully selected HFrEF patients.

Revascularization (CABG or PCI) is indicated for patients on optimal medical therapy with angina and suitable anatomy, especially left main stenosis (> 50%) or left main–equivalent disease. For end-stage HF, cardiac transplant is the best option. There is a 65% 5-year survival and a 55% 10-year survival!

Harmful for HFrEF patients:

- Definitely avoid or withdraw most antiarrhythmics, calcium blockers (except amlodipine), NSAIDs, and thiazolidinediones (e.g., rosiglitazone, pioglitazone).
- Long-term use of positive inotropic drugs is potentially harmful, except as palliation for patients with end-stage (Stage D) disease who cannot be stabilized with optimal medical therapy.

HIGH-OUTPUT HF

PREVIEW | REVIEW

- With which diseases does high-output heart failure occur?

High-output ventricular failure is seen with peripheral shunting (large AV fistulas, severe hepatic hemangiomatosis, and Paget disease!) and low systemic vascular resistance, as seen in sepsis. You can also see it in patients with hyperthyroidism, beriberi, carcinoid, or anemia. Remember, though, these patients often have a normal, rather than high, CO measurement by the time of diagnosis—because of the worsening ventricular failure!

RIGHT VENTRICULAR FAILURE

"The most common cause of right heart failure is left heart failure!" is what you heard on rounds. And, indeed, right ventricular failure (RVF) is mainly caused by pulmonary hypertension (1° or 2°)—typically secondary to left ventricular failure (LVF). RVF is also seen with large RV infarctions and cor pulmonale. Remember: If the patient has signs of RVF (JVD and liver congestion) but pressures are equal in all chambers in diastole, think external compression (constriction or effusion).

As LVF progresses, orthopnea usually worsens, but it may then actually improve temporarily as RV function worsens due to the pulmonary hypertension.

Paroxysmal nocturnal dyspnea does not improve with sitting up, as orthopnea does.

PULMONARY EDEMA

PREVIEW | REVIEW

- What is the treatment for acute pulmonary edema?

Immediate treatment for acute pulmonary edema:

- Patient should be sitting with legs dangling, if possible, to decrease venous return.
- Give supplemental O_2 if hypoxemic (pulse ox < 90%).
- Give IV furosemide (causes venodilation even before the diuresis).
- IV nitroglycerin or nitroprusside can be used if systolic BP is > 100 mmHg.
- Strongly consider the use of dobutamine if systolic BP < 90 mmHg.

PERICARDIAL DISEASES

PREVIEW | REVIEW

- What are some causes of nonconstrictive pericarditis? What ECG changes can you see?
- What are the 2 clinical hallmarks of constrictive pericarditis?
- How is BNP used to differentiate constrictive pericarditis from restrictive cardiomyopathy?
- In which conditions are the measured diastolic pressure of all 4 chambers equal?
- What treatments can be helpful in recurrent pericarditis?
- Name the 3 hallmarks of cardiac tamponade.

NONCONSTRICTIVE PERICARDITIS

90% of nonconstrictive pericarditis is idiopathic and probably viral in origin; often, there is a preceding URI or gastroenteritis.

Causes of nonconstrictive pericarditis:

- Idiopathic (90%); probably viral
- Tuberculosis (TB)
- Connective tissue diseases
- Sepsis
- Renal failure (uremic)
- Cancer
- Postradiation
- Hypothyroidism
- MI (Dressler syndrome)
- Open heart surgery (postpericardiotomy syndrome)
- Certain drugs, especially procainamide and hydralazine

Suspect TB as the cause if the patient is at high risk or if the symptoms of pericarditis do not resolve after 2 weeks of treatment.

Dressler syndrome can really be considered a form of postpericardiotomy syndrome, as both Dressler syndrome and postpericardiotomy are autoimmune processes that occur several weeks after the precipitating event. Even if the history is very suggestive, you must consider the following entities and exclude them to make the diagnosis: MI, pulmonary embolus, and endocarditis. Other causes include uremia and connective tissue disease.

Patients with pericarditis commonly present with very severe chest pain, sometimes pleuritic, which (classically) improves when leaning forward. The pain is retro-sternal and left precordial and referred to the neck, arms, or left shoulder. Typically, the patient has some fever and tachycardia. A pericardial friction rub (which does not always occur and can be evanescent) is diagnostic for pericarditis.

The ECG may show diffuse concave-up ST elevation (vs. localized, concave-down ST elevation in an acute MI) and, occasionally, depressed PR segments, especially in lead II. ECG changes occur in 4 stages:

- Stage 1: diffuse ST-elevation segments with upward concavity with PR depression
- Stage 2: normalization of ST segments after several days
- Stage 3: inverted T waves
- Stage 4: Weeks or months after onset of acute pericarditis, ECG returns to normal.

Pericarditis can cause transient increases in troponin (secondary to associated myocarditis). Treat pericarditis by stopping any possible causative drugs and giving NSAIDs. Do not treat idiopathic pericarditis with steroids because there can be a relapse when they are stopped. Treatment with colchicine has been shown to reduce recurrence.

CONSTRICTIVE PERICARDITIS

Constrictive pericarditis occurs when resorption of pericardial effusion is followed by obliteration of the pericardial cavity with scarring. Constrictive pericarditis must be differentiated from restrictive cardiomyopathy (see Restrictive Cardiomyopathy on page 13-57) because the signs and symptoms can be similar.

(Again: Although constrictive pericarditis is often quickly treated with good results, restrictive cardiomyopathy is not reversible.)

Constrictive pericarditis may follow:

- Viral or idiopathic pericarditis
- Traumatic hemopericardium
- TB
- Cardiac surgery
- Mediastinal irradiation
- Purulent infection
- Histoplasmosis
- Rheumatoid arthritis
- SLE
- Neoplastic disease (especially breast cancer, lung cancer, and lymphoma)
- Chronic renal failure with uremia treated by chronic dialysis

In constrictive pericarditis, ventricular filling is normal during early diastole but falls abruptly when the elastic limit of the pericardium is reached.

Constrictive pericarditis is characterized by rapid, early diastolic filling of the LV, causing a loud presystolic knock just after S_2. Pulsus paradoxus can occur but is usually mild.

There are 2 clinical hallmarks of constrictive pericarditis on neck vein examination:

1) Kussmaul sign: Because the heart is encased in a "shell," the negative pressure during inspiration is transferred to the venous inflow tract, resulting in a lack of the normal decrease in jugular venous distention (JVD) during inspiration. When severe, JVD can even increase during inspiration.

2) Large, right-sided x and y descents. This is seen as a brisk collapse of the jugular veins during diastole.

Constrictive pericarditis can cause calcification of the pericardium (~ 50%). You can see this best on the lateral chest x-ray because it is typically found over the right ventricle, but you also can see it on the posteroanterior view and on CT. A lateral chest x-ray that shows calcification over the right ventricle is pathognomic for constrictive pericarditis.

CT and MRI are best for measuring pericardial thickness, but echo is also used. A pericardial thickness of > 5 mm is suggestive of, but not sufficient for, diagnosis. The pericardium can be of normal thickness in ~ 20–25% of cases of constrictive pericarditis.

Brain natriuretic peptide (BNP) plasma levels can help differentiate between constrictive pericarditis and restrictive cardiomyopathy. BNP increases with HF. With restrictive cardiomyopathy, there is a component of HF, and BNP levels are markedly elevated (e.g., 8× max normal). With constrictive pericarditis, there is little or no actual HF, and BNP levels are typically just above normal.

In both tamponade and constrictive pericarditis, cardiac cath shows the same pressure during diastole in all 4 chambers. You can often make the differentiation between tamponade and constrictive pericarditis at the bedside using several hallmark signs (Table 13-13).

Table 13-13: Distinguishing Tamponade and Constrictive Pericarditis		
Findings	**Tamponade**	**Constrictive Pericarditis**
Duration of symptoms	Hours to days	Months to years
Chest pain, friction rub	Often present	Absent
Pulsus paradoxus	Present	Usually absent
Kussmaul sign	Absent	Usually present
Diastolic knock	Absent	Often present
Pericardial calcification	Absent	Often present
Thickened pericardium on CT/MRI	Absent	Present
Pericardial effusion	Present	Absent
Jugular venous waveforms	Prominent x descent	Prominent x and y descents
Diastolic pressures	Equal	Equal
Echo findings	Pericardial effusion, collapse of RV/RA	Marked respiratory variation in transmitral flow
Systemic disease	Cancer, uremia, recent cardiothoracic surgery, chest trauma	TB, previous XRT, remote cardiothoracic surgery

Constrictive pericarditis must be treated with an open thoracotomy and pericardiectomy. Unfortunately, this resolves the problem only 50% of the time!

Think of constrictive pericarditis in the cancer survivor who has undergone prior radiation therapy to the chest and now presents with progressive dyspnea, typically occurring over several months to years.

RECURRENT PERICARDITIS

Recurrent pericarditis is a condition in which the only disabling problem is the associated chest pain. It does not progress to constrictive pericarditis. It rarely results in arrhythmias. Treat with colchicine and/or NSAIDs. Do not use glucocorticoids for treatment of pericarditis, as they increase morbidity and recurrence rates. Pericardiectomy often does not have good results and is tried only after medical treatment options have been exhausted.

PERICARDIAL EFFUSION

Pericardial effusion is generally diagnosed with an echocardiogram, but CT and MRI are the most accurate, especially if the resultant tamponade is due to localized pockets of effusion. Chest x-ray may show an enlarged cardiac silhouette, although in rapidly developing effusions, patients can present before sufficient volume accumulates to alter the heart's appearance on x-ray. Electrical alternans on ECG is noted with alternating amplitude of the QRS complex and is evidence of the heart swinging in the pericardium. Check blood work to exclude liver dysfunction, hypothyroidism, or coagulopathy, potential causes for the effusion.

Pericardial biopsy can help diagnose TB. Sometimes, you need an endomyocardial biopsy to differentiate constrictive vs. restrictive etiology.

Surgical drainage is preferable in traumatic hemopericardium and postsurgical effusion and when bacteria or TB is suspected as the cause of tamponade. Pericardiocentesis is often used to treat viral, idiopathic, neoplastic, hypothyroid, and renal failure–related tamponade. Pericardiocentesis is usually only helpful diagnostically if there is a malignancy.

TAMPONADE

Know! Tamponade occurs when a pericardial effusion leads to critical cardiovascular compromise. There is obstruction to the inflow of blood to the ventricles and equalization of pressures in all 4 cardiac chambers. The most common causes are trauma, cancer, uremia, and acute pericarditis. When there is rupture of the free wall of the heart, as in trauma or post-MI, tamponade develops quickly; otherwise, it generally develops slowly.

The 3 hallmarks of acute tamponade:

1) Hypotension and muffled heart sounds
2) Pulsus paradoxus (systolic BP drops > 10 mmHg during inspiration)

3) Jugular venous distention with no collapse during diastole (i.e., an attenuated y descent)

Tamponade causes soft, distant heart sounds. Compare and know the difference between this and constrictive pericarditis (see Constrictive Pericarditis on page 13-65).

Treatment of tamponade is surgery and pericardiocentesis.

CONGENITAL HEART DISEASES

PREVIEW | REVIEW

- What is the most common congenital heart abnormality found initially in adults?
- True or false? Ostium secundum ASD often has right axis deviation and/or RBBB on ECG.
- When should surgery be performed for a secundum ASD?
- Which type of cyanosis would you expect to see in someone with a PDA?
- What is the most common congenital heart defect in children?
- What are the 2 most common causes of sudden cardiac death in an exercising young person? What 3rd cause do you consider in young women?

NOTE

Most adult patients with congenital heart disease are asymptomatic! Know that the magnitude of any shunt does not depend on the total blood flow rate but is commonly a constant ratio of pulmonic to systemic flow (Qp:Qs).

ASD

Ostium Secundum ASD

Secundum atrial septal defect comprises 70% of all atrial septal defects (ASDs). It is the most common form of congenital heart disease diagnosed in adulthood (F > M), except for bicuspid aortic valve. With a large secundum ASD, there is a systolic ejection murmur at the left sternal border (2° to increased flow across the pulmonic valve), occasionally a diastolic murmur (from increased flow across the tricuspid valve), and a fixed split S_2. The left-to-right shunt causes diastolic overloading of the right ventricle and increased pulmonary blood flow with inspiration and expiration.

ECG shows right axis deviation and/or right bundle branch block (RBBB). Chest x-ray shows an enlarged RV with shunt vasculature. Notice all of the right-sided stuff with ASD—makes sense because ASD causes a volume load on the right side of the heart. Patients can develop 2° atrial fibrillation.

Standard treatment had been open surgical closure, but now most secundum ASDs are closed percutaneously. If there is a > 2:1 left-to-right shunt, closure is done, even if the patient is asymptomatic. In this case, the ASD would eventually cause an increase in pulmonary vascular resistance and associated complications.

Generally, severe fixed pulmonary hypertension is considered a contraindication to surgical repair of the ASD.

Ostium Primum ASD

Ostium primum ASD is seen most commonly in Down syndrome. Patients may have a loud pansystolic murmur 2° to mitral and/or tricuspid regurgitation. The regurgitation occurs because the ostium is low on the septum, interfering with the function of the AV valves or left mitral valve. ECG may show 1st degree AV block, left axis deviation, and RBBB.

Surgery for any type of ASD essentially cures the problem. Functional Class III/IV patients can revert to functional Class I with excellent survival! Eisenmenger syndrome (left-to-right cardiac shunt, pulmonary arterial disease, and cyanosis) is a contraindication to ASD surgery.

Sinus Venosus ASD

Sinus venosus ASD is seen with anomalous pulmonary venous return because it occurs high on the septum. It is a cause of 10% of ASDs.

PDA

Adult patients with patent ductus arteriosus (PDA) are usually asymptomatic, although heart failure and infectious endocarditis can occur. Females are affected more than males. PDAs are typically discovered early by detection of the distinct murmur.

PDA causes a continuous, machinery-like murmur at the LUSB. As pulmonary pressures rise, the murmur becomes less continuous. Differential cyanosis (e.g., clubbed toes, normal fingers) with pulmonary hypertension is possible.

Chest x-ray shows calcification of the ductus arteriosus in adults.

If the patient develops pulmonary hypertension, consider Eisenmenger syndrome (more under Eisenmenger Syndrome on page 13-68).

Surgical or percutaneous closure has excellent results in patients with heart failure or pulmonary hypertension symptoms and in asymptomatic patients with moderate-to-large PDAs. Surgery is not advised in the case of severe, irreversible pulmonary hypertension.

PULMONARY STENOSIS

Balloon valvuloplasty is the procedure of choice for treating pulmonary stenosis. It has favorable long-term clinical and hemodynamic results.

VSD

Ventricular septal defects (VSDs) are the most common congenital defect in children. They are uncommon in adults because most have either closed spontaneously or have been surgically closed in childhood. 80% of small VSDs close spontaneously in the first 10 years of life. Large VSDs typically require surgery (although even 10% of these eventually close spontaneously). Expect to hear a holosystolic murmur at the left lower sternal border. Larger VSDs cause softer murmurs; smaller VSDs cause louder murmurs. Any adult with a residual VSD should have a Qp:Qs (right-to-left shunt) measurement (usually by right heart catheterization). Those with Qp:Qs of ≥ 2:1 should be referred for closure to avoid the possibility of progression to Eisenmenger syndrome (more information is in Eisenmenger Syndrome on page 13-68).

COARCTATION OF THE AORTA

Know that a bicuspid aortic valve occurs in ~ 50% of patients with coarctation of the aorta (COA)! Other associated anomalies include mitral valve problems, left ventricular myocardium problems, and membranes in the left atrium. Notice that all of the heart problems seen with coarctation of the aorta are left-sided! The classic physical findings are either a delayed femoral/brachial pulse (a distinct delay between the branchial pulse and the femoral pulse) or an absent femoral pulse. Patients can have upper-body hypertension and can get hypertensive aneurysmal dilatation and rupture of the circle of Willis. Look for rib notching on chest x-ray due to the collateral vessels getting very large and eroding the ribs. Many patients with Turner syndrome have coarctation of the aorta and a bicuspid aortic valve.

ANOMALOUS CORONARY ARTERY

Coronary anomalies are the 2nd most common cause of sudden death associated with strenuous exercise in competitive athletes (1st is HCM).

Premortem detection is extremely difficult and requires a high index of suspicion. This can present as exertional chest pain or exertional syncope in a young, otherwise healthy individual. Syncope after exercise can occur in healthy people, but syncope during exercise is never normal.

In many cases of anomalous coronary artery there is a benign retroaortic course. However, there can be an abnormal course of 1 of the 2 coronary arteries between the 2 great vessels, the pulmonary artery and aorta. At rest, there is plenty of room for the vessel to pass without compromise; however, in extreme exercise, the CO can increase 4- to 8-fold. This expands the elastic pulmonary artery and aorta, resulting in compression of the coronary artery as it courses between the great vessels. This compression creates coronary ischemia and arrhythmias.

While invasive coronary catheterization is the diagnostic gold standard, coronary CTA or MRA are excellent and highly accurate noninvasive imaging methods to identify anomalous coronary arteries.

TETRALOGY OF FALLOT

Tetralogy of Fallot (TOF) is the most common cyanotic congenital heart disease. A minority of cases have a known genetic defect—usually 22q11.2 deletion syndrome (10–16%), then trisomy 21 (3–8%). TOF comprises the following 4 defects:

1) Large VSD

2) Right ventricular outflow tract obstruction

3) Overriding aorta

4) RVH

A helpful mnemonic to remember the 4 components of tetralogy of Fallot is V-ROAR-V, where **V** stands for **V**SD, **R** stands for **r**ight ventricular outflow obstruction, **OA** for **o**verriding **a**orta, and **RV** for **RV**H. Virtually all those born with TOF undergo repair and have a normal life expectancy.

SUDDEN DEATH IN EXERCISING YOUNG PEOPLE

Etiologies of sudden death in exercising young people:

- HCM (36%)
- Coronary anomalies (17%)—especially in the 30–40-year-old age group
- Possible HCM (8.2%)
- Myocarditis (5.9%)
- Arrhythmogenic RV cardiomyopathy (4.3%)
- Ion channelopathies including long QT syndrome (LQTS; 3.6%)
- Also consider primary pulmonary hypertension as the cause in young women.

OTHER

Marfan syndrome causes decreased strength of the aorta (with aortic regurgitation and dissection) and mitral regurgitation. Cystic fibrosis can eventually cause pulmonary hypertension. Rubella (eradicated from the Americas) causes congenital pulmonic stenosis, PDA, and multiple pulmonary artery stenoses. Bicuspid aortic valve is discussed in Aortic Stenosis on page 13-39.

PULMONARY HEART DISEASE

PREVIEW | REVIEW

- What is the only effective treatment for Eisenmenger syndrome?

COPD AND SLEEP APNEA

The most common causes of pulmonary heart disease are COPD and sleep apnea syndrome. These 2 are covered extensively in Pulmonary Medicine, Book 2, so we will cover the other causes here.

EISENMENGER SYNDROME

Eisenmenger syndrome occurs in patients with a large, intracardiac shunt when the pulmonary vascular resistance becomes greater than systemic vascular resistance—so, the shunt becomes right-to-left instead of the usual left-to-right. It is a result of severe pulmonary hypertension, which can develop early (or late) in patients with large, cardiac, left-to-right shunts of virtually any type: VSDs, PDAs, and ASDs. Cyanosis is common, and Eisenmenger's is an absolute contraindication to pregnancy (more under Pregnancy and the Heart on page 13-69). Heart-lung transplant is the only effective treatment for Eisenmenger syndrome.

CHRONIC THROMBOEMBOLIC OBSTRUCTION

Chronic thromboembolic obstruction mainly occurs as a result of impaired fibrinolytic resolution of acute thromboembolism, leading to organization, incomplete recanalization, and chronic obstruction of the pulmonary vascular bed. Most patients treated for acute pulmonary thromboembolism do not develop chronic pulmonary hypertension. Chronic thromboembolic obstruction can also result from other causes of secondary pulmonary hypertension such as large left-to-right shunts and chronic LVF.

Progression of this disease probably results from pulmonary arteriolar changes (rather than more PEs); these are similar to the changes that develop with large septal defects. The resultant increased pulmonary vascular resistance causes RVF. Surgical removal of the thromboembolic material results in significant improvement. In patients who have failed or are unable to take anticoagulants, vena cava filters may be used in patients with deep vein thrombosis (DVT).

PULMONARY HYPERTENSION

Pulmonary hypertension (PH) is divided into 5 different groups, based on etiology (Table 13-14).

The initial tests in suspected PH are ECG and echocardiogram. Pulmonary artery pressures can be estimated by echocardiography. Echo is also necessary to exclude less obvious cardiac causes of secondary pulmonary hypertension. Pulmonary arterial hypertension (PAH) includes the sporadic idiopathic pulmonary hypertension that commonly occurs in young women (though men can be affected as well), is refractory, and results in death within 5–10 years.

Treatment: Calcium channel blockers (in patients who are reactive to vasodilator testing) and sildenafil may be helpful. Endothelin antagonists and prostacyclin can also be of use. Heart-lung transplant is occasionally used.

It is important to differentiate between the different causes of PH because treatments may be beneficial to only certain types. For example, chronic thromboembolic pulmonary hypertension (CTEPH) may respond to surgical removal of the thromboembolic material. A heart catheterization rules out secondary causes such as right-to-left shunt, PH due to lung disease, or chronic LVF. A perfusion lung scan rules out pulmonary embolism (PE). Pulmonary capillary wedge pressure (PCWP) is, of course, increased only in the pulmonary hypertension caused by, or concurrent with, LVF. A discussion of PAH can be found in Pulmonary Medicine, Book 2; more on hypertension in pregnancy is located in Women's and Men's Health, Book 4.

PREGNANCY AND THE HEART

PREVIEW | REVIEW

- What are the 2 cardiac-related absolute contraindications to pregnancy?

Absolute contraindications to pregnancy include PAH and Eisenmenger syndrome (particularly deadly if cyanosis is present); these are discussed in Pulmonary Hypertension on page 13-68 and Eisenmenger Syndrome on page 13-68. More information on cardiology disorders in pregnancy is in Women's and Men's Health, Book 4.

CARDIOLOGY

Table 13-14: WHO Classification of PH				
Pulmonary Arterial Hypertension	**Pulmonary Hypertension with Left Heart Disease**	**Pulmonary Hypertension Associated with Lung Diseases and/or Hypoxemia**	**Pulmonary Hypertension Due to Chronic Thrombotic and/ or Embolic Disease (CTEPH)**	**Miscellaneous**
• Idiopathic (IPAH) • Familial (FPAH) • Associated with (APAH): • Connective tissue disorder • Congenital systemic-to-pulmonary shunts • Portal hypertension • HIV infection • Drugs and toxins • Other (thyroid disorders, glycogen storage disease, Gaucher's disease, hereditary hemorrhagic telangiectasia, hemoglobinopathies, chronic myeloproliferative disorders, splenectomy) • Associated with significant venous or capillary involvement: • Pulmonary veno-occlusive disease (PVOD) • Pulmonary capillary hemangiomatosis (PCH) • Persistent pulmonary hypertension of the newborn	• Left-sided atrial or ventricular heart disease • Left-sided valvular heart disease	• Chronic obstructive pulmonary disease • Interstitial lung disease • Sleep disordered breathing • Alveolar hypoventilation disorders • Chronic exposure to high altitude • Developmental abnormalities	• Thromboembolic obstruction of proximal pulmonary arteries • Thromboembolic obstruction of distal pulmonary arteries • Nonthrombotic pulmonary embolism (tumor, parasites, foreign material)	• Sarcoidosis • Histiocytosis X • Lymphangio-matosis • Compression of pulmonary vessels (adenopathy, tumor, fibrosing mediastinitis)

THE ELECTROCARDIOGRAM

THE 12-LEAD ECG

PREVIEW | REVIEW

- Does a positive deflection on ECG tracing indicate the depolarization wave is moving toward or away from the lead?

First, we will briefly go over the basics of electrocardiograms (ECGs). Refer to Figure 13-22 as we go through this.

A lead tracing is positive if the wave of depolarization spreads toward the positive pole of that lead, and it is negative if it spreads away from the positive pole. The tracing is zero if the wave is maximal at a 90° angle to it. For instance, if II is zero, look for the maximum projection to be at aVL (either + or –).

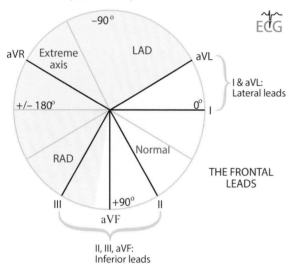

Figure 13-22: Axis determination diagram

With the 12-lead ECG, the wave of depolarization is recorded on both the frontal and horizontal planes and gives a 3-dimensional representation of the heart. The projection of the electrical activity of the heart onto the frontal plane is recorded by the frontal leads I, II, III, aVR, aVL, and aVF. On the horizontal plane, it is recorded via electrodes placed in the V1-6 position. These are referred to as the precordial leads. Occasionally, a V3R and V4R (placed same as V3 and V4, except on the right side of the chest) are used to better monitor the right side of the heart (e.g., to detect right-sided ischemia). Depolarization moving toward the lead causes a positive deflection (P wave and QRS), as does repolarization moving away from the lead (T wave).

The frontal leads give inferior-superior-left-right information. For example, II, III, and aVF cover the inferior area. ST variations/Q waves occur in these leads with inferior ischemia and infarction.

The horizontal leads relay anterior-posterior-lateral information. Think of V1 as looking at the right side of the heart while V6 looks at the left side. The QRS in V1 is positive when the right ventricle (RV) is depolarizing (and negative when the LV is depolarizing), whereas the QRS in V6 is positive when the LV is depolarizing.

AXIS DEVIATIONS

PREVIEW | REVIEW

- Know how to very quickly determine the axis of an ECG. Brand Figure 13-22 into your brain!
- What are the causes of left axis deviation?
- What are the causes of right axis deviation?
- Does RAD always warrant additional workup in an adult?

The normal mean QRS axis is between –30° and +100°. > +100° is right axis deviation (RAD), whereas < –30° is left axis deviation (LAD, not to be confused in this context with "left anterior descending," also abbreviated LAD). A quick, fairly accurate method to determine axis is to look at I and aVF. If both are prominent, you can quickly tell in which quadrant the mean vector lies. Visualize the following:

- Both (+) = normal
- I (+) and aVF (–) suggests LAD
- Both (–) = extreme right or left axis
- I (–) and aVF (+) suggests RAD

LAD is usually due to left anterior hemiblock and, therefore, is a marker for CAD—as are all fascicular blocks.

RAD is often a normal finding in children and young adults. Other causes include left posterior hemiblock (LPHB), RVH, and acute or chronic RV overload syndromes, such as pulmonary hypertension/embolism and pulmonic stenosis. If an adult is incidentally found to have RAD, do further workup.

RATES AND INTERVALS

PREVIEW | REVIEW

- Describe one way to determine heart rate from a 12-lead ECG.

The ECG is recorded on paper with a 1 mm^2 graph, with a thicker line every 5 mm. See Figure 13-23. Because the paper moves at 25 mm/second, each thicker line is 1/5 of a second—or 0.2 seconds (200 msec), and each thin line (mm) represents 0.04 seconds (40 msec). The interval covering 5 thicker lines (or "big squares") is 1 second.

There are a couple of quick ways to determine the heart rate. The RR interval is one way, although any prominent wave of the standard QRS can be used to determine the interval. Using a calculator, a quick and accurate method for determining heart rate is 1,500/RR interval in mm. So, if the beat interval is 28 mm, the rate is 1,500/28 = 54 bpm. A less accurate, but easier, method is to divide 300 by the number of big squares in the RR interval. If the beat interval is 28 mm, this is not quite 6 big squares. You divide 300 by 6 and get 50, but you know the heart rate is actually a little faster because the interval is not quite 6 big squares. A derivative of this is the method taught in Dale Dubin's book *Rapid Interpretation of EKG's*, in which you memorize 2 sets of triplicates: 300–150–100 and 75–60–50. These match to the heart rates corresponding to RR intervals of 1, 2, 3, 4, 5, and 6 big squares.

Normal rate is 60–100 bpm. Sinus tachycardia is defined as a sinus rhythm of > 100 bpm; sinus bradycardia is < 60 bpm. So, an RR interval < 3 big squares indicates tachycardia; > 5 big squares indicates bradycardia.

INTERVALS

PREVIEW | REVIEW

- Name the causes of prolonged QT intervals.

PR INTERVAL

The PR interval indicates the time between atrial and ventricular depolarization. Normal duration is 3–5 small squares (120–200 msec). Longer than 200 msec (1 big square) is the definition of 1st degree AV block. Shorter than 120 msec (3 small squares) may indicate WPW (delta wave), junctional rhythm (with retrograde P wave), or left

atrial overload (widened P wave); more information is located in the P Wave topic.

QRS DURATION

QRS duration is normally < 100 msec (i.e., 1/2 a big square). QRS > 120 msec can be caused by bundle branch block, ventricular beat/rhythm/ventricular pacemaker, drugs such as tricyclics, and WPW. 100–120 msec is often due to an incomplete bundle branch block (BBB).

QT INTERVAL

The QT interval corrected for rate is normally 340–470 msec, depending on gender and age. $QT_c = QT/(RR)^{0.5}$; that is, the QT interval (in msec or seconds) divided by the square root of the beat interval in seconds. Again: The RR interval in this calculation must be in seconds. (Consider the difference in dividing by the square root of 0.7 vs. the square root of 700!) When scanning ECGs, a rule of thumb is: The QT interval normally is ~ 40% of the RR interval—do the calculation for QT_c if it appears shorter or longer.

With prolonged QT_c, there is a tendency to develop *torsades de pointes*.

Prolonged QT_c has many causes:

- Congential long QT syndromes
- Tricyclic overdose
- Hypocalcemia
- Hypomagnesemia
- Hypokalemia
- Starvation
- CNS insult
- Hypothermia

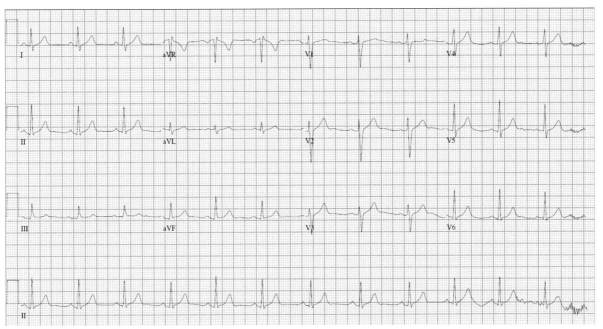

Figure 13-23: Normal ECG on ECG paper

- Type Ia and III antiarrhythmics (e.g., quinidine, procainamide = Ia; e.g., amiodarone, sotalol = III)
- Opioids, such as hydrocodone and methadone
- Antipsychotics, including chlorpromazine, haloperidol, and thioridazine
- Liquid protein diet

Short QTc can be caused by hypercalcemia and digoxin.

Patients with congenital long QT syndrome should be instructed to avoid strenuous exercise (which can precipitate arrhythmias) and avoid drugs that prolong the QT interval (see above). Congenital prolonged QT syndrome is usually treated with a beta-blocker.

WAVEFORMS AND SEGMENTS

PREVIEW | REVIEW

- What are the P wave findings for right atrial hypertrophy? For left atrial hypertrophy?
- What are the 5 causes of an R wave in lead V1?
- What does failure of R waves to progress across the precordial leads indicate?
- When are peaked T waves seen?
- What do focal, flipped T waves signify?
- U waves indicate a predisposition to which serious condition?
- What are the common causes of U waves?
- What is the significance of an inverted U wave?
- Name the 3 main causes of ST-segment elevation.
- What are the causes of ST-segment depression?

P WAVE

The P wave results from the depolarization of the atrium. The normal P wave is < 2 mm in height and < 120 msec (3 small squares) in duration, and the normal axis is –50 to +60 degrees. (Where else have you seen 120 msec? The normal PR interval is 120–200 msec.) See Figure 13-24.

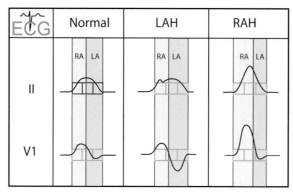

Figure 13-24: P wave in atrial enlargement

Most information from the P wave can be derived from II, aVR, and V1. As the wave of depolarization spreads from the SA node high in the right atrium and through the right and then left atrial myocardium, the mean vector is downward and to the patient's left—so the normal P wave is positive in II and negative in aVR.

A retrograde P wave is negative in II and positive in aVR—indicating an ectopic focus originating in the inferior part of the atrium or at the AV junction, resulting in a wave of depolarization traveling toward aVR (picture this!). A retrograde P wave from the AV junction often causes a tracing with a short PR interval.

Because atrial depolarization traverses from the patient's right to left, the left/initial side of the P wave represents the right atrium, while the right/terminal side of the P wave represents the left atrium (mid-P wave is both).

The normal P wave is positive in lead II and positive or biphasic in V1; when biphasic, the P wave is positive on the left side and a little negative on the right side (Figure 13-24). This is because the wave of depolarization through the atrium is toward V1 in the right atrium (left side of P wave) and somewhat away from V1 in the left atrium (right side of P wave).

With right atrial enlargement (a.k.a. right atrial hypertrophy; RAH), the right atrial (initial) portion of the P wave is widened and therefore overlaps onto the left atrial portion of the P wave. The P wave width stays normal (< 120 msec), but look for an increased P wave amplitude in II and V1 (the positive portion). Actually, the P wave being peaked in II is more important than its being tall.

Decreased P wave amplitude is seen in severe hyperkalemia.

With left atrial enlargement (a.k.a. left atrial hypertrophy), the right side of the P wave is enlarged, resulting in a wide P wave with a shortened or absent PR interval (i.e., < 120 msec). Other typical findings are a widened, notched P wave in II and an enlargement of the negative portion of the P wave in V1. The most sensitive ECG finding for left atrial enlargement is a negative P wave in V1, with a duration of > 40 msec (1 small square). On the other hand, the most specific ECG finding is a notched P wave (usually in II) with an interpeak distance of > 40 msec.

COPD: Because of the hyperexpanded lungs, the heart assumes a more vertical position, and there is resultant RAD of the P wave. A +90° P wave axis is highly suggestive of COPD. The pulmonary hypertension can result in right atrial enlargement with associated P wave changes.

R WAVE

The R wave should be negligible (or very small) in lead V1. The presence of a noticeable R wave in V1 should alert you to one of the following:

- RBBB
- RVH
- WPW pattern

- Prior RV infarction
- Duchenne muscular dystrophy (rare in adults)

Also look for normal progression of R waves across the precordial leads, with the R waves gradually becoming taller from V1 to V3/V4. Poor R wave progression can indicate prior anterior MI.

T WAVE

The T wave is ordinarily in the same direction as the QRS.

Causes of peaked T waves:

- Hyperkalemia
- Acute MI (early stage)
- Intracerebral hemorrhage
- In septal leads (V1–2): evolving post-MI

Focal, flipped (i.e., inverted) T waves may accompany:

- Ischemia
- RBBB, RVH, and elevated RV pressure (in V1–2)
- LVH (in V1–2)
- LBBB (in lateral leads—I, aVL, V6)
- LVH with strain (in precordial leads)

Diffuse, flipped T waves may accompany:

- Pericarditis
- Diffuse ischemia; postresuscitation
- Metabolic abnormalities
- Intracerebral hemorrhage

U WAVE

The U wave occurs just after the T wave. It is commonly small and is best seen in V2–3. If seen, it is usually a < 1-mm, rounded deflection in the same direction as the T wave. If the U wave is prominent, there is an increased tendency for *torsades de pointes*. Prominent U waves are present with hypokalemia, bradycardia, digoxin, and amiodarone.

Inverted U waves are significant—even if the rest of the ECG is normal! Causes are ischemia, HTN, AV valve disease, and RVH. Inverted U waves occur in up to 60% of patients with an anterior MI, up to 30% of patients with an inferior MI, and up to 30% of angina patients.

ST SEGMENT

There are 3 main causes of ST-segment elevation: acute MI, vasospastic (i.e., Prinzmetal) angina, and pericarditis. It can also be present with early repolarization variant, intracerebral hemorrhage, stress (i.e., takotsubo) cardiomyopathy, hypertrophic cardiomyopathy, LVH,

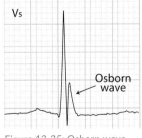

Figure 13-25: Osborn wave
Source: Jason E. Roediger, CCT, CRAT

LBBB, cocaine abuse, myocarditis, and hypothermia (J, a.k.a. Osborn, waves; see Figure 13-25).

ST-segment depression occurs with:

- Subendocardial ischemia (especially if downsloping or flat), such as seen in classic angina
- Acute posterior MI (in V1–2)
- Reciprocal depression in V1–2 with some inferior wall MIs—especially those with lateral or posterior extension. There may also be reciprocal ST depression in inferior leads with some anterior/septal MIs.
- LVH with LV strain (ST depression with flipped T waves in precordial leads)
- Isolated RV infarction, when there is ST elevation in V1 and ST depression in V2
- RVH that may cause RAD and ST-segment depression preceding a flipped T wave in V1
- Digoxin toxicity
- Hypokalemia

QRS COMPLEX

In the QRS complex, both ventricles depolarize simultaneously after depolarization of the interventricular septum. The normal mean vector of depolarization of the interventricular septum points from the patient's left to the right across the septum. You see this as a small initial deflection that is positive in V1 (r wave) and negative in V6 (q wave). See Figure 13-26 on page 13-74.

Note 1: By convention, a smaller wave in the QRS complex is written in lowercase, whereas a larger wave is written in uppercase.

Note 2: The terms "axis" and "vector" both describe the direction of voltage from the atria to the ventricles. "Axis" is generally used when discussing the ECG specifically, and "vector on the frontal plane" is used when discussing clinical findings or physiologic changes.

The left ventricle is normally much more massive than the right ventricle; therefore, the mean QRS vector (reflecting depolarization of the ventricles) is strongly to the patient's left. You see a large negative deflection in V1 and positive deflection in V6. So, in the frontal plane, the mean vector is between –30° and +100°.

The normal duration of the QRS is < 100 msec.

QRS changes seen with ventricular hypertrophy and conduction disturbances are discussed next.

VENTRICULAR HYPERTROPHY

PREVIEW | REVIEW

- What are the ECG criteria for LVH? RVH?
- What ECG changes would you expect to see in the presence of a large pulmonary embolism causing acute cor pulmonale?

LVH

Left ventricular hypertrophy (LVH) causes prolonged activation of the myocardium.

This prolonged activation results in a reversal of repolarization that proceeds from the endocardium to epicardium and is reflected by a flipped T wave in the septal leads (V1–2).

LVH causes an exaggeration of the negative deflection in V1 and the positive deflection in V6. Other ECG criteria for LVH include S in V1 + (R in V5 or R in V6) > 35 mm or (R in V5 or R in V6) > 25–35 mm. This is read "the S in V1 + the R in V5 is > 35 mm," and so on (Figure 13-26).

The diagnosis of LVH is strengthened by an intrinsicoid deflection (i.e., R peak time) of > 50 msec (1.25 small squares). This is the time from the beginning of the QRS complex to the peak of the R wave. Note: When you notice an obvious intrinsicoid deflection, make sure to check the PR interval—you might be looking at a delta wave in WPW!

When there is left axis deviation, the ECG criteria for LVH change! Use: S in III > 15 mm.

A left ventricular strain pattern may be present with LVH. LV strain is precordial ST-segment depression and flipped T waves seen in a patient with ECG criteria for LVH.

RVH

ECG criteria for right ventricular hypertrophy (RVH) are right axis deviation > 100°, ST-segment depression in the right precordial leads (i.e., V1, V2) due to repolarization (possibly with inverted T waves in same leads), R wave in V1 > 6 mm (or R:S ratio in V1 > 1), and R:S ratio in V5 and V6 < 1. Remember to look for that R wave in lead V1! The ST-segment depression and flipped T wave in V1 +/− V2 generally indicate RV stress/hypertension that hypertrophy causes (Figure 13-26).

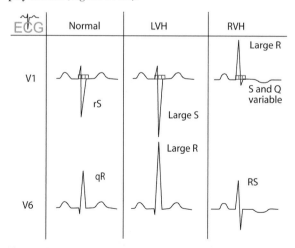

Figure 13-26: Ventricular hypertrophy

Because RVH is such an abnormal condition, with the mass of the right ventricle increasing to the point of shifting the mean QRS vector to a right axis, the specificity for

RVH is very high when ECG criteria are met—although, as with LVH criteria, the sensitivity is low.

Pulmonary embolism (PE): Note that with acute, severe pulmonary embolism causing acute cor pulmonale, the ECG shows acute RV strain with RV and RA dilation +/− ischemia. There is often an RBBB, sometimes RAD, and usually clockwise rotation. A prior ECG for comparison, and serial ECGs to demonstrate S1Q3T3 pattern (S wave in lead I, Q wave in lead III, and an inverted T wave in lead III) are an indication of RV strain and are a specific, but not sensitive, indication for acute PE.

CONDUCTION DISTURBANCES

PREVIEW | REVIEW

- What do you see on an ECG in LBBB? RBBB?
- What is so serious about a recent MI and the development of a bifascicular block?

AV BLOCKS

Atrioventricular (AV) blocks are due to conduction disturbances at the AV node. Know the 3 degrees and their patterns.

1st degree AV block prolongs the PR interval to > 200 msec (1 big square).

2nd degree AV block has 2 patterns:

- Mobitz 1 (i.e., Wenckebach): progressive prolongation of the PR interval until there is a dropped QRS (ventricular beat)
- Mobitz 2: Normal PR intervals, but periodically there is a dropped QRS. 2:1 AV block is 2 P waves for each QRS; 3:1 is 3 P waves for each QRS, and so on. Mobitz 2 almost always has a wide QRS complex (if narrow, it's probably Mobitz 1).

3rd degree AV block: No depolarizations are conducted through the AV node. The P wave and QRS have independent regular rhythms (AV dissociation). If the QRS complex has a normal width (< 100 msec), there is a junctional ectopic pacemaker. Junctional pacing rate is 40–60 bpm, whereas ventricular pacing is 20–40 bpm.

BUNDLE BRANCH BLOCK

Overview

Just a little after the AV node, the fast conduction pathway, known as the bundle of His, splits in 2. These 2 fast conduction pathways travel down the interventricular septum, and 1 then goes to the right ventricle, while the other splits again and proceeds to the anterior and posterior sections of the left ventricle. If conduction in 1 of these pathways is blocked, the depolarization downstream to that pathway is delayed because the myocardial tissue in that area can then be depolarized only via the depolarization wave from much more slowly conducting adjacent myocardial tissue. Refer to Figure 13-27.

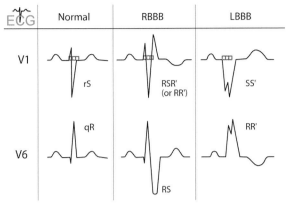

Figure 13-27: Bundle branch block

LBBB

Left bundle branch block (LBBB): The QRS is prolonged with a duration of 120–180 msec (3–4.5 small squares). Because the left ventricle depolarization is now transmyocardial, it is depolarized over a longer period, resulting in a notched or slurred R wave (RR′) in the lateral leads (I, aVL, and V6), and there is a corresponding SS′ (a.k.a. QS) in V1. 50% of patients have a normal axis; 50% have LAD (–30° to –90°).

The T wave vector and sometimes the ST segment are opposite in direction to the mean QRS vector in LBBB. Therefore, as illustrated in Figure 13-27, you see negative T waves following the positive RR′ in I, aVL, and V6—and positive T waves following the negative QRS in V1–3.

Right-to-left depolarization of the septum overcomes the expression of any septal Q waves with an MI—including the inferior leads. So, just as new septal Q waves do not appear in a patient with LBBB and an acute MI, MI-related septal Q waves disappear if LBBB develops because of the MI. Therefore, LBBB makes it impossible to use the ECG as an evaluation tool in a patient you suspect of having an MI.

Criteria for LBBB:

- QRS = 120–180 msec (3–4.5 small squares)
- Broad R wave (or RR′) in I and V6
- rS or QS in leads I, V5, and V6
- The T wave is often opposite the mean QRS vector in anteroseptal and lateral leads.

Incomplete LBBB fulfills the above criteria, except there is a QRS between 110 and 120 msec, an LVH pattern, and as R peak time > 60 msec in lateral precordial leads.

RBBB

Right bundle branch block (RBBB): The direction of septal depolarization is normal—left to right—but the right ventricle is depolarized over a longer period, resulting in an RR′ or RSR′ ("rabbit ears") in V1 and an S wave in V6.

Visualize how the RSR′ in V1 is formed: The initial R wave is due to normal left-to-right septal depolarization, the S wave is due to depolarization of the left ventricle, and the final R′ is due to the delayed depolarization of the right ventricle. In the lateral leads, the S wave is wide or slurred (40 msec) and is due to delayed depolarization of the right ventricle.

The T wave is usually negative in V1; sometimes it is negative in V2.

Criteria for RBBB:

- QRS > 120 msec (3 small squares)
- RSR′ ("rabbit ears") or RR′ in V1
- Prolonged S wave > 40 msec in leads I, V5, and V6

Incomplete RBBB fulfills the above criteria, except QRS = 110–120 msec.

IVCD

A nonspecific intraventricular conduction delay (IVCD) is the term used to describe a wide QRS (> 120 msec) that does not meet criteria for either right or left bundle branch block.

LAFB

With left anterior fascicular block (LAFB), a.k.a. left anterior hemiblock (LAHB), QRS duration is 100–120 msec. Septal activation is in a left-to-right (normal) and inferior direction. This inferior septal depolarization is sometimes reflected by a Q wave in the lateral leads (I and aVL). Because the last part of the heart to depolarize is the left posterobasal to anterolateral wall, the mean frontal QRS vector has a left-facing axis (–45° to –90°). Left axis deviation (LAD) more negative than –45° with a normal QRS duration is nearly always due to LAFB. Actually, LAFB is the component that causes the LAD in 50% of patients with LBBB.

Criteria for LAFB:

- LAD –45° to –90°
- qR pattern in lead aVL
- QRS < 120 msec
- R peak time in aVL ≥ 45°

LPFB

Left posterior fascicular block (LPFB; a.k.a. left posterior hemiblock [LPHB]): This problem is rare, and the ECG pattern is rather nonspecific because you can also see it in patients with RVH, lateral infarction, and emphysema. You can be sure that it is a LPFB only if it is a recent change—all else being the same. The septal depolarization is left to right but directed superiorly, causing a small Q wave in the inferior leads. Because final depolarization in the heart is in the inferior and posterior walls with the vector pointing inferior and to the right, there are large R waves in the inferior leads (II, III, aVF) and large abnormal S waves in the lateral limb leads (I, aVL). (Here, think "down, up, up" for the first 3 limb leads—the complete opposite of LAFB.) This also results in a mean QRS axis of +80° to +140°. The T wave is normal.

Criteria for LPFB:

- Small Q and large R (qR) waves in III and aVF
- Small R wave and large S (rS) in leads I and aVL
- Rightward axis (+90° to +/–180°)
- QRS < 120 msec

Bifascicular Block

Conduction abnormalities sometimes result in a combination of RBBB and either left anterior fascicular block, left posterior fascicular block, or complete LBBB. This condition is sometimes called bifascicular block, a term that has fallen out of favor but is still widely used.

Anterior MI and calcific aortic stenosis can cause bifascicular block. Remember that acute MI + a new bifascicular block indicates a high risk for progression to complete heart block.

WIDE QRS

Wide-complex QRS can be caused by BBB, ventricular origin of the complex, and/or aberrant conduction.

ARRHYTHMIAS

PREVIEW | REVIEW

- What is the difference between an ectopic beat and an escape beat?
- What are the ECG findings with A-fib?
- What are the ECG findings with MAT?
- What are the ECG findings with PVC?

ECTOPIC VS. ESCAPE

An ectopic beat occurs from an ectopic (abnormal) focus earlier than the expected next beat. It can originate in the atria, AV junction, or ventricle.

Throughout the heart are foci of cells with pacemaker capability, which can take over if there is a delay in depolarization, such as when the sinoatrial (SA) node ceases to function normally or there is a severe conduction disturbance. These are called escape beats. Atrial, non-SA node pacemaker activity has an inherent rate of 60–80 bpm. AV junction (not AV node!) pacemaker rate is 40–60 bpm. Ventricular pacemaker rate is 20–40 bpm (idioventricular rhythm).

Note that ectopic beats are different from escape/pacemaker beats. Ectopic beats are early. Escape beats are at the rate of inherent pacemaker activity.

ATRIAL ARRHYTHMIAS

ECG criteria for atrial fibrillation (A-fib):

- No P waves
- Irregularly irregular rhythm (intervals between QRS complexes follow no repetitive pattern)

A-fib is the result of multiple ectopic foci firing continuously or disorganized atrial activity. It is thought to be due to a micro-reentry mechanism. No P waves are seen, although there is loud, chaotic atrial noise throughout the tracing.

Atrial flutter (frequently described as Type I, or typical, but more accurately described as counterclockwise, or isthmus dependent):

- High atrial rate: characteristic rate ~ 300 bpm (range 240–340 bpm), typically with a 2:1 AV block
- Sawtooth-like flutter waves
- Whole number ratio of flutter waves to QRS complexes

Atrial flutter is due to a wave of depolarization repeatedly going around and around the atrium—usually with an anatomic obstacle, such as an AV valve, in the pathway. This results in the sawtooth-appearing P wave with an atrial rate of ~ 300 bpm (but it varies between 240 and 340 bpm). There is commonly a 2:1 or 3:1 AV block with a resulting ventricular rate of 150 or 100 QRS complexes/minute, respectively.

There is also a second form of atrial flutter that has been referred to as Type II, or atypical, but is best termed clockwise, left atrial, or non-isthmus dependent. It has a much higher atrial rate: 340–440 bpm.

Wandering pacemaker is exactly what the name implies. The pacing impulse migrates from one atrial pacemaker focus to another. It is a benign condition seen mostly in young people—especially athletes. The varying focus is reflected by varying shapes of the P wave.

Multifocal atrial tachycardia (MAT) is similar to wandering pacemaker, except that MAT occurs at a higher rate with more chaotic switching between pacemakers. MAT is often seen in patients with COPD, hypoxia, severe hypokalemia, and hypomagnesemia or in those taking digoxin or theophylline. Atrial rate is 100–130 bpm. The rhythm is irregularly irregular.

Sinus pauses result in a long TP interval. An ectopic escape beat (different P wave) may precede the resumption of the rhythm. If an atrial pacemaker takes over the rhythm, the rate is usually 60–80 bpm. If a junctional pacemaker focus takes over the rhythm, this is termed a junctional (a.k.a. escape) rhythm. With a junctional rhythm, there is a change in the P wave—it may not be visible, or it may be a retrograde P wave very close to the QRS (short PR interval). Junctional rate is normally 40–60 bpm.

VENTRICULAR ECTOPIC BEATS AND HEART BLOCK

Premature ventricular contraction (PVC):

- The QRS complex occurs earlier than expected (premature), is wider than normal, and has a higher amplitude than normal.
- P wave is obscured in the QRS complex.
- T wave is inverted.
- The next RR interval is longer than normal. This is called a full compensatory pause. The SA node is not reset by the ventricular depolarization—hence, the P waves march out normally.

A ventricular escape beat can occur if the sinus pause is long enough and no atrial or junctional pacemakers kick in. The PVC comes early; the escape beat comes late.

Remember: junctional escape = narrow (40–60 bpm), and ventricular escape = wide (20–40 bpm). Medication and certain illnesses can affect these rates.

MYOCARDIAL INFARCTION

PREVIEW | REVIEW

- Describe the sequence of ECG changes with the different phases of an MI.
- What ECG changes occur with a septal MI? Anterior? Lateral? Know all these!

COMMON FINDINGS

Know this topic! Common findings in myocardial infarction: Within the first minute or so of acute ischemia, the T waves flip. After 1–2 minutes, they become positive and peaked (hyperacute). Then injury to the cells occurs, causing ST-segment elevation. Q waves correlate with cell death. These associations of ECG changes with the actual pathophysiologic processes are somewhat artificial but clinically useful.

Again:

1) T-wave changes (ischemia), then
2) ST-segment changes (injury), and then
3) Q waves (cell death)

LOCATION OF MI VS. ECG CHANGES

Left ventricle:

- Septal MI = changes in V1–2
- Anterior MI = V2 or V3–4
- Anteroseptal MI = V1–4
- Lateral MI = I, aVL
- Anterolateral = I, aVL, V3 or V4–6 (if V1–6 = extensive anterolateral MI)
- Inferior MI = II, III, aVF
- Apical MI = II, III, aVL and any of V1–4
- Posterior MI = tall R in V1–2; ST depression in V1–2
- High lateral MI = I, aVL

Right ventricle:

- RV infarction is best determined by changes in the right precordial leads. ST elevation in V4R to V6R is fairly sensitive and specific for RV infarction (~ 90% each). It is diagnostic of RV infarction if the ST elevation is greater in V4R than in V1–3.
- With the standard ECG, suspect an RV infarction if, with an inferior infarction, there is also ST-segment elevation in V1–2. Also, be suspicious if you see ST-segment elevation in V1 along with ST-segment depression in V2!

NOTES

With acute inferior MI, there may be reciprocal ST depression in the septal leads (V1–2). With an anterior/septal MI, there may be reciprocal ST depression in the inferior leads.

The trick for reading the ECG with a suspected acute posterior MI is to hold the ECG upside-down and backwards, while holding it up to a light to see the tracing. Study V1–2. A posterior MI assumes the morphology of other MIs with this trick. (R waves look like Q waves and ST depression appears to be ST elevation.)

Posterior MI is often seen in conjunction with inferior- and lateral-wall MIs. So, if you see either of these, look closely for signs of a posterior MI.

Signs of acute infarct and ischemia may be obscured by LBBB, WPW, HCM, and ventricular pacemakers.

REMEMBER

PREVIEW | REVIEW

- Which conditions can cause diffuse, inverted T waves?
- Which conditions can cause a prolonged QT?
- AV node dysfunction is seen in which type of MI? What about bifascicular block?
- Which conditions cause resting ST elevation?

Know these ECG changes thoroughly:

- Diffuse, inverted T waves: ischemia, pericarditis, bundle branch block (when there is a large R), drugs (e.g., digoxin, antiarrhythmic drugs), metabolic abnormality (e.g., hypocalcemia), and CNS insult (intracerebral hemorrhage)
- Prolonged QT: drug effect (e.g., quinidine, sotalol, dofetilide; see more under *Torsades de Pointes* on page 13-52), hypocalcemia, hypomagnesemia, and CNS insult. This is a precursor to *torsades de pointes*.

CARDIOLOGY

ECG

- Peaked T waves: hyperkalemia (If severe, ECG looks like a sine wave.)
- Large U waves are seen with hypokalemia, bradycardia, and digoxin toxicity.
- A low-voltage ECG tracing suggests pericardial effusion, hypothyroidism, obesity, restrictive cardiomyopathy (think amyloid), and COPD.
- AV node dysfunction can result from an inferior MI and with digitalis and verapamil toxicity.
- Bifascicular block is seen with anteroseptal MI and calcific aortic stenosis.
- What causes ST-segment elevation during a stress test? Stress-induced coronary artery spasms.
- What causes resting ST elevation?
  - Acute MI
  - Post-MI wall motion abnormalities in the infarcted areas
  - Spontaneous spasm of the coronary artery
  - Pericarditis

ANALYSIS SUMMARY

OVERVIEW

Here is a simplified approach to analyzing the ECG:

First, check the rate and rhythm. Next, check the intervals—especially the PR, QRS, and QT. Then, check waveforms.

The ECG case studies on the following pages give you a little practice. Figure 13-28 provides a memory aid for ECG interpretation. This memory aid is copied below each ECG on the following pages.

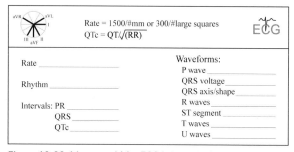

Figure 13-28: Memory aid for ECG interpretation

Study tip: To the top left of each ECG is the presenting information. After you have done your reading of the ECGs, check the Findings from ECG Case Studies on page 13-90. Do not look at that information until you have read the ECGs!

ECG CASE STUDIES

Case 1: A 57-year-old man with previous myocardial infarction and chronic hypertension on digoxin, beta-blockers, and ACEI

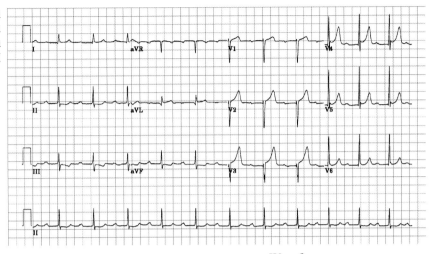

Waveforms:

Rate _____

Rhythm _____

Intervals: PR _____

QRS _____

QTc _____

P wave _____

QRS voltage _____

QRS axis/shape _____

R waves _____

ST segment _____

T waves _____

U waves _____

Case 2: A 36-year-old man with history of cocaine abuse and "slow heart rate" since his teens

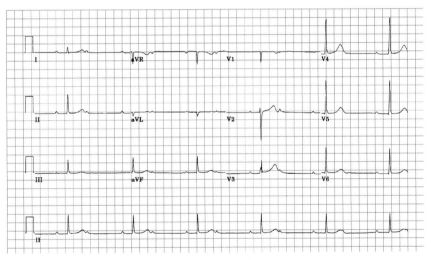

Waveforms:

Rate _____

Rhythm _____

Intervals: PR _____

QRS _____

QTc _____

P wave _____

QRS voltage _____

QRS axis/shape _____

R waves _____

ST segment _____

T waves _____

U waves _____

Case 3: A 76-year-old man with chronic heart failure

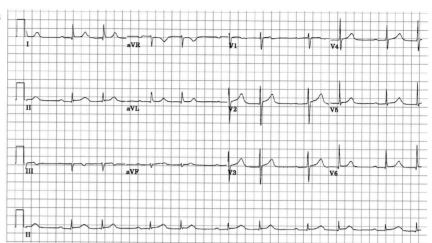

Rate _____

Rhythm _____

Intervals: PR _____
             QRS _____
             QTc _____

Waveforms:

P wave _____

QRS voltage_____

QRS axis/shape_____

R waves _____

ST segment _____

T waves _____

U waves _____

Case 4: A 36-year-old man with history of drug abuse and "slow heart rate" since he was young

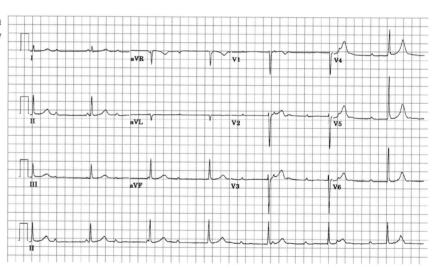

Rate _____

Rhythm _____

Intervals: PR _____
             QRS _____
             QTc _____

Waveforms:

P wave _____

QRS voltage_____

QRS axis/shape_____

R waves _____

ST segment _____

T waves _____

U waves _____

Case 5: A 54-year-old woman with history of chronic smoking

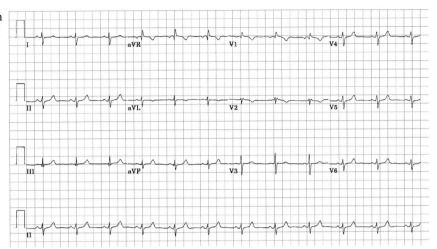

Rate _____

Rhythm _____

Intervals: PR _____
    QRS _____
    QTc _____

Waveforms:

P wave _____
QRS voltage _____
QRS axis/shape _____
R waves _____
ST segment _____
T waves _____
U waves _____

Case 6: A 77-year-old man with a history of chronic heart failure

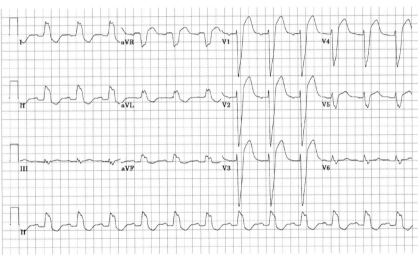

Rate _____

Rhythm _____

Intervals: PR _____
    QRS _____
    QTc _____

Waveforms:

P wave _____
QRS voltage _____
QRS axis/shape _____
R waves _____
ST segment _____
T waves _____
U waves _____

Case 7: A 67-year-old man with a history of a cardiac murmur and prior repair of a congenital heart defect

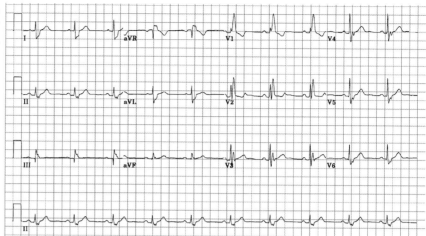

Rate _____

Rhythm _____

Intervals: PR _____
            QRS _____
            QTc _____

Waveforms:

P wave _____
QRS voltage _____
QRS axis/shape _____
R waves _____
ST segment _____
T waves _____
U waves _____

Case 8: A 77-year-old man with a history of myocardial infarction and recurrent syncope

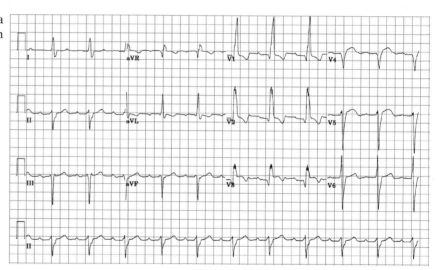

Rate _____

Rhythm _____

Intervals: PR _____
            QRS _____
            QTc _____

Waveforms:

P wave _____
QRS voltage _____
QRS axis/shape _____
R waves _____
ST segment _____
T waves _____
U waves _____

Case 9: A 65-year-old man with recurrent palpitations

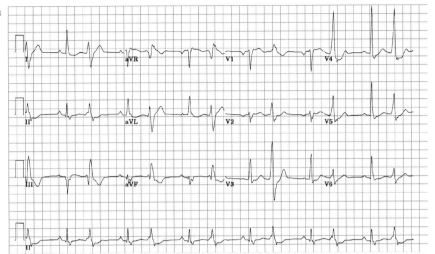

Waveforms:

Rate _____   P wave _____

                         QRS voltage _____

Rhythm _____   QRS axis/shape _____

                         R waves _____

Intervals: PR _____   ST segment _____

         QRS _____   T waves _____

         QTc _____   U waves _____

Case 10: A 45-year-old man with a history of rheumatic fever as a child and cardiac murmurs

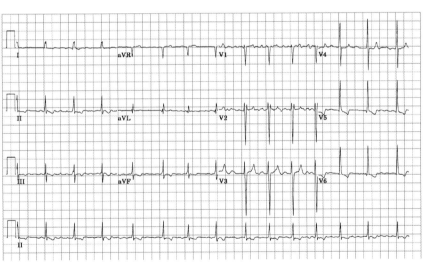

Waveforms:

Rate _____   P wave _____

                         QRS voltage _____

Rhythm _____   QRS axis/shape _____

                         R waves _____

Intervals: PR _____   ST segment _____

         QRS _____   T waves _____

         QTc _____   U waves _____

Case 11: A 44-year-old man with a history of 2-pack-per-day smoking for 15 years

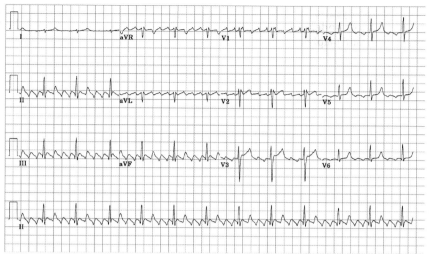

Rate _____

Rhythm _____

Intervals: PR _____
         QRS _____
         QTc _____

Waveforms:

P wave _____

QRS voltage_____

QRS axis/shape _____

R waves _____

ST segment _____

T waves _____

U waves _____

Case 12: A 34-year-old man with history of palpitations since childhood

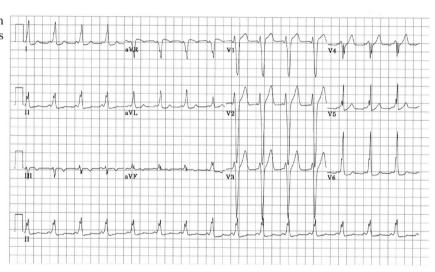

Rate _____

Rhythm _____

Intervals: PR _____
         QRS _____
         QTc _____

Waveforms:

P wave _____

QRS voltage_____

QRS axis/shape_____

R waves _____

ST segment _____

T waves _____

U waves _____

Case 13: A 74-year-old woman with recent episodes of light-headedness and palpitations

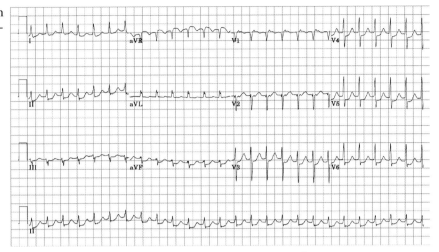

Rate _____

Rhythm _____

Intervals: PR _____

QRS _____

QTc _____

Waveforms:

P wave _____

QRS voltage_____

QRS axis/shape_____

R waves_____

ST segment _____

T waves _____

U waves _____

Case 14: A 71-year-old man with history of previous myocardial infarction and coronary artery bypass surgery admitted for chest pains and syncope

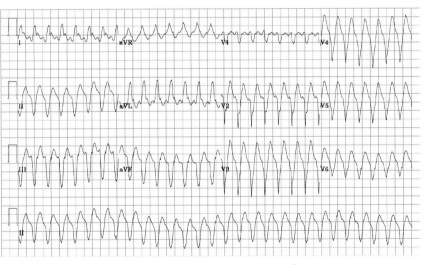

Rate _____

Rhythm _____

Intervals: PR _____

QRS _____

QTc _____

Waveforms:

P wave _____

QRS voltage_____

QRS axis/shape_____

R waves_____

ST segment _____

T waves _____

U waves _____

CARDIOLOGY

ECG

Case 15: A 47-year-old man with Type 1 diabetes and chronic renal insufficiency admitted with diabetic ketoacidosis and serum potassium of 7 mEq/L

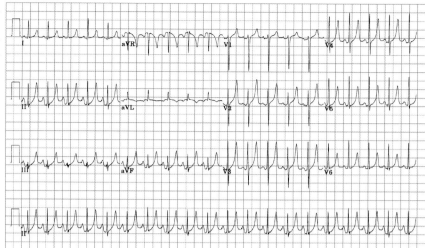

Rate _____

Rhythm _____

Intervals: PR _____

QRS _____

QTc _____

Waveforms:

P wave _____

QRS voltage _____

QRS axis/shape _____

R waves _____

ST segment _____

T waves _____

U waves _____

Case 16: A 39-year-old woman successfully resuscitated from ventricular fibrillation with no evidence of acute myocardial infarction

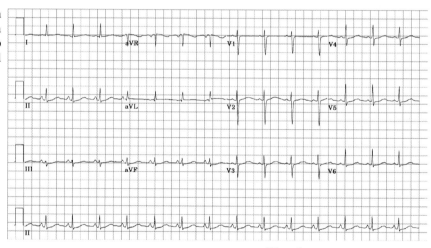

Rate _____

Rhythm _____

Intervals: PR _____

QRS _____

QTc _____

Waveforms:

P wave _____

QRS voltage _____

QRS axis/shape _____

R waves _____

ST segment _____

T waves _____

U waves _____

Case 17: A 65-year-old man admitted for pleuritic chest pains 1 week following a bout of flu-like symptoms

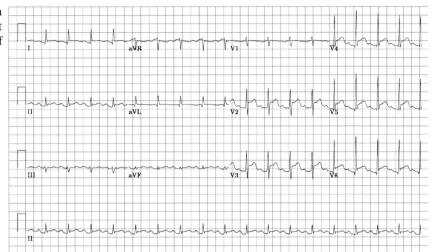

Rate _____

Rhythm _____

Intervals: PR _____

QRS _____

QTc _____

Waveforms:

P wave _____

QRS voltage _____

QRS axis/shape _____

R waves _____

ST segment _____

T waves _____

U waves _____

Case 18: A 65-year-old man admitted with a 2-hour episode of severe retrosternal chest pains and shortness of breath

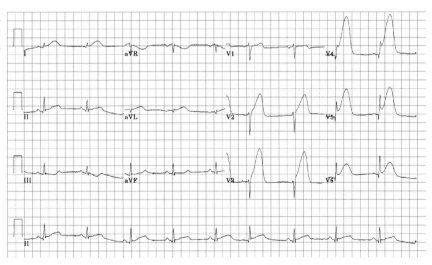

Rate _____

Rhythm _____

Intervals: PR _____

QRS _____

QTc _____

Waveforms:

P wave _____

QRS voltage _____

QRS axis/shape _____

R waves _____

ST segment _____

T waves _____

U waves _____

Case 19a: An 80-year-old woman is seen in the emergency department 3 hours after waking up with severe retrosternal pressure and lightheadedness.

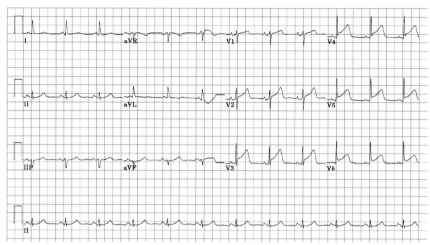

Rate _____

Rhythm _____

Intervals: PR _____

QRS _____

QTc _____

Waveforms:

P wave _____

QRS voltage _____

QRS axis/shape _____

R waves _____

ST segment _____

T waves _____

U waves _____

Case 19b: 20 minutes following infusion of a thrombolytic, a repeat ECG is performed.

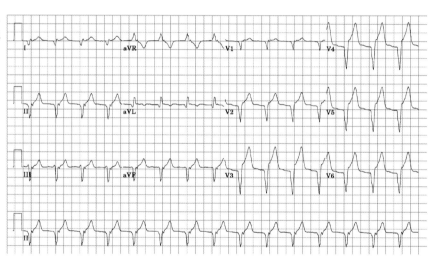

Rate _____

Rhythm _____

Intervals: PR _____

QRS _____

QTc _____

Waveforms:

P wave _____

QRS voltage _____

QRS axis/shape _____

R waves _____

ST segment _____

T waves _____

U waves _____

Case 19c: 90 minutes after thrombolysis, the patient is pain free.

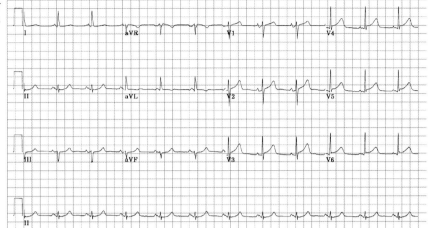

Rate _____

Rhythm _____

Intervals: PR _____

          QRS _____

          QTc _____

Waveforms:

P wave _____

QRS voltage _____

QRS axis/shape _____

R waves _____

ST segment _____

T waves _____

U waves _____

Case 20: A 65-year-old man with severe epigastric pains, nausea, and vomiting of 2-hour duration

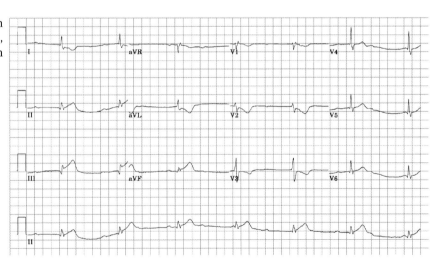

Rate _____

Rhythm _____

Intervals: PR _____

          QRS _____

          QTc _____

Waveforms:

P wave _____

QRS voltage _____

QRS axis/shape _____

R waves _____

ST segment _____

T waves _____

U waves _____

CARDIOLOGY

ECG

FINDINGS FROM ECG CASE STUDIES

Case 1: Note the 1st degree AV block with PR of 340 ms. Left ventricular hypertrophy. Probable early repolarization—the sharp S wave in V4–5 enhances the likelihood of the ST segment being due to repolarization. Possible inferior ischemia.

Case 2: Note the sinus rhythm with Mobitz Type 2 second-degree 2:1 AV block. This initially looks like Mobitz 2, but there is a subtle increase in the PR interval, and this also has a narrow QRS complex (Mobitz 2 usually has a wide complex).

Case 3: Note the 2nd degree Mobitz Type 1 (Wenckebach) 3:2 AV block. The 1st P wave is visible, the 2nd is just peeking out of the previous T wave, and the 3rd is fused with the previous T wave. Possible COPD.

Case 4: Note the sinus rhythm with complete, 3rd degree AV block.

Case 5: Note the sinus rhythm with right-axis deviation and incomplete RBBB consistent with pulmonary disease pattern.

Case 6: Note the sinus rhythm with complete LBBB and left atrial enlargement. This LBBB is a little atypical, but notice the large slurred S in the anteroseptal leads and the T wave opposite the mean QRS in the anterolateral leads. Also notice the terminal portion of the QRS in V1–3 is slurred, which is consistent with LBBB.

Case 7: Note the sinus rhythm with RBBB.

Case 8: Note the sinus rhythm, 1st degree AV block, RBBB and left anterior fascicular block (bifascicular block). Note also Q waves from V1 to V4 are consistent with anteroseptal infarct.

Case 9: Note the sinus rhythm with frequent ventricular premature beats in bigeminy. Note the full compensatory pause after the PVC.

Case 10: Note the atrial fibrillation and flipped Ts in the inferiolateral leads.

Case 11: Note the atrial flutter with 4:1 block, vertical axis, and incomplete RBBB.

Case 12: Note the sinus rhythm, short PR interval, and delta wave, consistent with Wolff-Parkinson-White syndrome. This is one of those ECGs on which you may mistake the delta wave for prolonged intrinsicoid deflection (as seen with LBBB and LVH) until you check the PR interval and find it is short!

Case 13: Note the narrow QRS tachycardia with retrograde P waves evident in precordial leads V1 and V2 consistent with AV node reentrant tachycardia at a rate of approximately 150 bpm. Also note the pronounced ST-segment depression in the inferiolateral leads—it is likely that the rapid rate is a factor in the ischemia.

Case 14: Note the wide QRS tachycardia with negative concordance in the precordial leads, which is consistent with ventricular tachycardia. Negative concordance is the QS pattern throughout the precordial leads; there is no hint of R wave progression.

Case 15: Note the tall and peaked T waves consistent with hyperkalemia. This tracing also shows LVH by the voltage criteria.

Case 16: Note the prolonged QT of 530 ms and a QTc of 640 ms. When measuring the QT interval, you must look at all the leads and choose the longest QT interval—in this case, use lead V2.

Case 17: Note the diffuse ST-segment elevations that are consistent with pericarditis. There is PR segment depression, best seen in II; this is also often seen with pericarditis. Also note the concave-up ST segment elevation more consistent with pericarditis than MI.

Case 18: Note the marked ST-segment elevation in precordial leads is consistent with acute extensive anterolateral infarction. Associated T waves are hyperacute.

Case 19a: Note the ST-segment elevations in the precordial leads is consistent with acute anterolateral STEMI. Even though the ST segment is mildly concave up, the lack of an S wave in V4–5 makes early repolarization unlikely—as does the presenting complaint!

Case 19b: Tracing with a wide QRS is seen with either accelerated idioventricular rhythm (reperfusion arrhythmia) or "slow" ventricular tachycardia at 90 bpm. Note the change in QRS duration and axis shift and the retrograde P waves showing a V-A association (i.e., the ventricle is resetting the atrium!).

Case 19c: A repeat ECG shows significant resolution of the precordial ST-segment elevations.

Case 20: Note the acute inferior infarction with reciprocal ST segment changes in the right precordial leads and the complete AV block shown by AV dissociation with an atrial rate of 75 bpm and a ventricular rate of 40 bpm.

AMBULATORY ECG MONITORING

CONTINUOUS AMBULATORY ECG (HOLTER) MONITORS

Intermittent arrhythmias may not be captured during a 12-second ECG. A Holter monitor continuously records the ECG over 24–48 hours or longer. The monitor is returned and analyzed to detect arrhythmias. Holter monitors are useful in patients with episodic lightheadedness, dizziness, palpitations, syncope, or chest discomfort. Holters are not typically useful for ischemia.

EVENT MONITORS

Similar to Holter monitors, event monitors are worn by patients at home to record their ECG over 2–4 weeks. These are used in patients whose symptoms occur infrequently, once or twice a month. A Holter monitor for 2 days is likely to miss such events; on the other hand, an event monitor is likely to capture it.

For symptoms that are even less frequent but significant enough, an implantable loop recorder may be advised. It is generally placed under the skin of the left upper chest and can be interrogated with a standard pacemaker programmer.

THE MEDSTUDY HUB: YOUR GUIDELINES AND REVIEW ARTICLES RESOURCE

For both the review articles and current internal medicine practice guidelines, visit the MedStudy Hub at

medstudy.com/hub

The Hub contains the only online consolidated list of all current guidelines focused on internal medicine. Guidelines on the Hub are easy to find, continually updated, and linked to the published source. MedStudy maintains the Hub as a service to the medical community and makes it available to anyone and everyone at no cost to users.

CARDIOLOGY

ECG